SAFETY

A Personal Focus

SAFETY
A Personal Focus

DAVID L. BEVER, Ph.D.

Coordinator of Health Education
Department of Human Services
George Mason University
Fairfax, Virginia

THIRD EDITION
with 215 *illustrations*

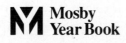

Mosby
Year Book

St. Louis Baltimore Boston Chicago London Philadelphia Sydney Toronto

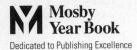
Mosby
Year Book
Dedicated to Publishing Excellence

Publisher: Ed Murphy
Editor: Vicki Van Ry-Malinee
Editorial Assistant: Cathy Waller
Project Manager: Barbara Merritt
Editing and Production: York Production Services
Book and Cover Design: Gail Morey Hudson

THIRD EDITION

Previous editions copyrighted 1984, 1988

Printed in the United States of America

Mosby–Year Book, Inc.
11830 Westline Industrial Drive, St. Louis, Missouri 63146

Library of Congress Cataloging-in-Publication Data

Bever, David L.
    Safety, a personal focus / David L. Bever.—3rd.
      p.   cm.
    ISBN 0-8016-6376-8

    1. Accidents—Prevention.   2. Safety education.   I. Title.
HV675.B48 1992
363.1'07—dc20
                            91-35830
                            CIP

92 93 94 95 96 CA/DC 9 8 7 6 5 4 3 2 1

To my parents
Jean and Keith Bever
on their 50th Wedding Anniversary
Love, Dave

Preface

Have you or a member of your family or one of your friends ever been injured seriously in an accident? Have you ever known someone who was assaulted or had his or her home burglarized? Do you live near a landfill, a nuclear plant, or a roadway with heavy traffic? Have you lived in an area of the country that has suffered earthquake, hurricane, or tornado damage? At one time or another all of us have dealt with a situation that has forced us to focus personally on some issue of safety.

When we speak of one's safety, we are referring to a dynamic condition in which a person attempts to minimize the risks from hazards that he or she may face. Whether one is riding an all-terrain vehicle, scuba diving, working in a steel mill, or walking to a parked car late at night, there are certain inherent risks that must be reduced if one is to have a happy, productive life. However, before this can be done, one must understand the wide variety of hazards that produce those risks.

As we advance into the 1990s and the era of high technology, the concept of safety takes on a new and more comprehensive meaning. No longer can we think of safety in terms of accident causation and prevention; we must define it in a much broader context. Issues that have come to national attention in recent years, such as violent crime, occupational illnesses, and toxic wastes, certainly affect the safety of millions of people. At the same time there has been a need to illustrate the close interrelationship between one's health and safety. A health-related topic such as alcohol abuse plays a prominent role in any discussion of motor vehicle and recreational safety. On the other hand, any discussion of occupational safety must address health-related issues, such as cancer and reproductive disorders, which may occur in workers exposed to hazardous chemicals.

In writing the third edition of this book, I have intended to present a new and stimulating approach to safety: one that is broadly based in terms of topical coverage, yet offers sufficient depth to provide significant information to the reader. Designed as a text for an introductory course in safety, this book offers both majors and nonmajors a solid instructional foundation.

SPECIAL FEATURES

There are seven features in this text that will enhance student learning in your safety course.

1. A personal approach

Many of the safety issues in this text touch everyone's lives. For this reason I have attempted to write in a style that personalizes the information and allows students to relate to the people described in each chapter. Another means of personalizing the book has been to use a conversational writing style that sets up a form of dialogue between myself and the reader. If a book is going to make an impact on people's lives, they must be able to relate to its content. In keeping with this personal approach, page perforations have been added to the third edition so that faculty and students can utilize the text materials to their fullest advantage.

2. Distinctive coverage

This book covers subject matter never before offered in a safety text. The topics of personal violence and crime are surveyed in depth in Chapter 6. Coverage includes crime prevention, self-defense techniques, firearm safety, and victim assistance information. In Chapter 8 (Occupational Safety) new sections are devoted to the recently implemented hazard communication standard, computer video display terminals, and the special hazards to which women in the workplace are exposed. A significant portion of Chapter 9 (Natural and Man-Made Disasters) involves discussions of hazardous material transport, toxic waste disposal, and the status of nuclear energy production since Three Mile Island and Chernobyl.

3. Timely and up-to-date presentation of topics

In a fast-paced and rapidly changing society, presentation of the most current information is essential in a text. By working closely with personnel from the National Safety Council, the National Institute for Occupational Safety and Health, the Centers for Disease Control, the National Highway Traffic Safety Administration, the Federal Emergency Management Agency, the Environmental Protection Agency, and the Consumer Product Safety Commission, I have received the latest statistical data generated by these organizations. Utilization of this information has resulted in up-to-date coverage of such topics as the Loma Prieta Earthquake, Hurricane Hugo, hotel and motel fire safety, mandatory safety belt laws, passive restraints, hazardous waste management, the operation of all-terrain vehicles (ATVs), and the use of jet skis, hot tubs, and tanning booths.

4. Comprehensive treatment of subject matter

A student's first experience in safety education should be one that provides the subject matter in its breadth. In its 12 chapters this book covers both traditional topics, such as home, fire, and motor vehicle safety, and a wide array of popular new topics, such as crime prevention and self-defense. In keeping with a comprehensive approach, I have subdivided the major chapters into detailed subtopics, thus providing depth to the presentation of the issues.

5. Systematic approach

Safety involves a multitude of topics and issues. There is a need to present this abundant material within a systematic framework so that the student can progress in an orderly fashion.

In the first three chapters the foundation for this systematic approach is developed. The cornerstone of the foundation is Chapter 1; in this chapter the concept of safety with its four interrelated factors is defined. Detailed examples illustrate how the safe individual must first understand the difficulties of a particular activity and second, develop skills for performance. The immediate state of the performer (both physiological and psychological components) is another personal factor that significantly affects one's safety. The fourth factor, condition of the environment, defines those external components that must be controlled if one is to minimize negative outcomes while maximizing positive experiences.

Chapter 2 and its detailed investigation of data interpretation prepares the reader to use information provided in succeeding chapters. The chapter discusses descriptive and inferential statistics, methods of data presentation, valid and reliable sources of safety statistics, and a variety of modern approaches to accident investigation. The third and final chapter in this foundation addresses the issue of what must be done if an emergency does occur. Although the major emphasis of the text is prevention, it is essential that a framework for action be provided in case one's safety is placed in jeopardy.

In the succeeding nine chapters (4-12) the factors of safe performance are utilized consistently, as are statistical data from the most recent and updated sources. And, as mentioned earlier, if safe performance cannot be maintained, alternatives must be examined.

An Emergency Care appendix has been added to the third edition. In Appendix A the reader will find first aid information for the following emergencies: Airway Obstruction, Respiratory Arrest, Cardiac Arrest, and Soft Tissue Injuries. This information supplements the action principles that are introduced in Chapter 3.

6. Pedagogical aids

To facilitate its use by instructors and students, this text employs the latest pedagogical aids.

Chapter Introductions. Introductions at the beginning of each chapter describe the major issues that will be examined.

Figures and Tables. Strong visual materials are used throughout each chapter to illustrate important points.

Case Studies. Short descriptive sketches are utilized throughout the text to stimulate reader interest.

Boxed Information. Material of special interest has been set off from the narrative of the text in boxes.

Chapter Summaries. Each chapter ends with a detailed summary that is particularly valuable for examination preparation.

Key Terms. At the end of each chapter is a list of key terms that have been discussed in the narrative. They are used to reiterate the importance of this material and provide the student with an additional method for review.

Applying What You Have Learned. New in the third edition, these hands-on projects allow students to take an active role in their own safety. The practical nature of the assignments will help to stimulate discussion of important concepts in each chapter. Perforation of pages allows students to remove these sections in the book so that assignments can be completed in a timely and efficient manner. This also provides faculty additional opportunities for measuring student progress.

Key Resource Organizations. For the individual seeking additional material concerning a particular topic, a comprehensive listing of resource organizations and their addresses is included at the end of each chapter.

7. Supplements

Instructor's Manual. For instructors, a manual is available that provides recommendations on how to use the text and manual most effectively and successfully. Each chapter contains teaching suggestions, including practical, hands-on experiences for students; discussion questions; major behavioral objectives that can be used as guidelines for preparing unit and lesson plans; and essay and objective test questions.

To enhance the ''hands-on'' approach of SAFETY: A PERSONAL FOCUS and to assist faculty in utilizing the text, detailed instructions have been given for the preparation of the suggested student activities and experiences. These teaching tips inform instructors as to what materials are needed and which agencies or individuals can provide specific safety expertise.

Acknowledgments

Shortly after I became involved in the development of SAFETY: A PERSONAL FOCUS, I realized the magnitude of such a project. Without the help, suggestions, and support of literally hundreds of people it would have been an impossible task.

First and foremost I want to thank all of the U. S. government agencies and their employees for the expertise, reference materials, and pictures they provided. Drucilla Besley of the Consumer Product Safety Commission, Mark Goodman of the Federal Bureau of Investigation, Ralph Hitchcock of the National Highway Traffic Safety Administration, Jim Gallahan of the Federal Emergency Management Agency, Gary Traub of the U. S. Coast Guard, and Christine Branche of the Division of Injury Control of the Centers for Disease Control are but a few of the individuals and organizations contributing invaluable assistance.

I would also like to express my appreciation to the publisher's reviewers for their contributions to the completion of the book:

Ronald Budig   Paul Wiley
Illinois State University   Southeastern Oklahoma State University

Ronald Puhl   Roy Yarbrough
Bloomsburg University   Liberty University

For her outstanding work in the preparation of the manuscript, Ann Derhammer of Hammer Associates, Burke, Virginia, receives my heartfelt thanks. I would like to thank Mr. Dwaine McCollum of the City of Fairfax Fire and Rescue Service, Mr. Paul Torpey of the Fairfax County Fire and Rescue Department, and Ms. Sandy Schnetzka of York Production Services for their technical assistance. At the same time I would like to express my gratitude to those students and staff at George Mason University who continually provided input, ideas, and support. They were there when I needed a helping hand. My thanks to Harold, Rodney, Rod, Craig, Tim, Peter, Amy, Chris, Coach, Sean, Scott, and Denise.

Finally, I want to thank Cathy Waller, my editorial assistant at Mosby–Year Book. During the past year she has kept me going, through both the good times and the bad. Her encouragement, suggestions, and expertise kept me on the right track.

David L. Bever

Contents

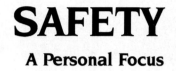

SAFETY
A Personal Focus

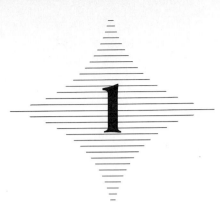

What Is Safety?

Injury is probably the most underrecognized major public health problem facing the nation today.

National Academy of Sciences: Injury Control

SAFETY DEFINED

"Is it safe to go there at night?" "I'm worried about her safety." "He's not a very safe driver." "Does that gun have a safety?" The word **safety** is widely used, yet few people seem to agree on its actual meaning. Numerous researchers have attempted to define or describe it. Mroz uses the following definition: "Safety is the prevention of accidents and the mitigation of personal injury or property damage which may result from accidents."[11] Strasser, Aaron, and Bohn use a more elaborate approach and state that "safety is a condition or state of being resulting from the modification of human behavior, and/or designing of the physical environment to reduce the possibility of hazards, thereby reducing accidents."[20]

Although these definitions vary in length and complexity, a common bond that ties them together is the notion that safety involves accident prevention and mitigation. As defined by the National Safety Council, an accident is "that occurrence in a sequence of events which usually produces unintended injury, death, or property damage."[14] Another definition often used describes an accident as "a sudden, unplanned event which has the potential for producing injury or damage."[14] Classic examples of accidents include motor vehicle collisions, falls in the home, fires, and the unintentional discharge of weapons. Most of the time these occurrences are sudden and unplanned, and have the potential for causing injury or damage.

Traditionally safety personnel have concentrated their efforts in two areas: (1) accident prevention—developing ways to eliminate the occurrence of these unplanned and potentially damaging events, and (2) accident mitigation—developing methodologies that reduce the damage caused by these unplanned events. An example of accident prevention would be the control of fire hazards in the home. Ensuring that electrical sockets are not overloaded, storing flammable materials outside the house

1

in a shed, and carefully following manufacturer's instructions when using a wood-burning stove or kerosene heater are methods of fire prevention. In terms of fire safety in the home, mitigation would entail such things as installing smoke detectors and fire extinguishers as well as developing plans of escape. Mitigative efforts would not prevent the occurrence of an accident, but could lessen the effects.

Wait a minute! There seems to be a problem with our definition of safety. What about situations that have the potential for producing injury, death, or property damage, but occur over a long period or are planned? Although they do not elicit their devastating results as quickly as a motor vehicle crash, environmental hazards such as air pollutants, toxic chemical wastes, noise, and radiation also have the potential for producing injury, death, or property damage. It may take a number of years of exposure to coal dust before a miner develops black lung disease or an asbestos worker suffers from the debilitating condition known as asbestosis. A report by the U.S. Environmental Protection Agency estimated that as many as 16 million workers may be exposed to potentially hazardous noise levels in their workplace.[25] No longer is the industrial safety specialist concerned only with worker accidents; this individual must now be aware of a broad range of hazardous materials and the occupational diseases with which they are related.

A second area that comprises a variety of hazards and risks is that of personal security. We would be remiss if a definition of safety did not reflect a legitimate concern for the injury, death, and property damage caused by criminal activity. In the past 10 years the violent crime rate per 100,000 people has increased approximately 20%; at least 6% of all U.S. households are affected by violent crime annually.[22] Violent crimes include murder, forcible rape, aggravated assault, and robbery. A similar increase in property crimes (burglary, vandalism, and larceny-theft) has also occurred in the last decade. Unlike the accident, with its unplanned and unintended personal injury and property damage, criminal activity is generally planned and deliberate.

How do we categorize people injured by toxic chemical wastes, radiation, or coal dust? What about victims injured during an attempted rape or robbery—aren't we concerned with their safety? Perhaps it is necessary to define the concept of safety in a broader sense than that of accident prevention or mitigation.

An individual is frequently faced with an assortment of hazards and risks. Depending on how these are handled, there is a wide variation in consequences. In one situation the results may be enjoyable; however, in other circumstances they may include severe injury or serious property damage.

For this text, the following definition of safety is used: **Safety is an ever-changing condition in which one attempts to minimize the risk of injury, illness, or property damage from the hazards to which one may be exposed.**

To better use the definition of *safety,* one must have an understanding of the terms **injury, hazard,** and **risk.** The word *injury* (hurt, damage, or loss sustained) comes from the Latin words *in* and *jus,* meaning ''not right.'' For the purposes of this text, **injury** will be defined as any kind of damage to the body resulting from a single exposure to some type of energy or force. For example, motor vehicle injuries are manifest almost immediately after victim impact with another object (that is, the victim's face and the windshield, dashboard, or steering wheel).

On the other hand, **illness,** from the standpoint of our definition of *safety,* can be defined as damage to the body resulting from repeated exposures to some type of energy or force. Illness generally occurs after a number of weeks or months. Children who suffer lead poisoning from chewing paint from window sills may not exhibit problems for several months. The same is true for workers in the poultry industry who suffer from an occupational illness known as carpal tunnel syndrome, a nerve disorder affecting the hands. This condition is the result of repeated stresses placed on the wrists of workers who use scissorlike devices to cut the poultry into pieces. It may take several years for this condition to appear.

Two of the terms in our definition of safety, **hazard** and **risk,** are interrelated. **Hazard** is defined as a condition or set of conditions that have the potential to produce injury and/or property damage.[10] A hazard by itself will not produce injury; it needs an outside stimulus to activate it and thus cause harm. An open container of gasoline may be categorized as a hazard; however, it won't cause harm until it is activated by a heat source such as a cigarette.

Risk refers to the probability that a hazard will be activated and produce injury or property damage. Risk involves two components: (1) the likelihood that a negative situation will occur, and (2) the severity of injury or damage if the hazard is activated.

A safe individual is one who can enjoy the greatest benefits at the lowest possible risk and cost (both physical and psychological). The concept of minimizing risks and controlling hazards to maximize the quality and quantity of people's lives will be emphasized throughout the text.

INJURY TODAY: SCOPE OF THE PROBLEM

More progress was made during the decade of the 1980s than in any prior decade in terms of the reduction in the total number of accidental deaths. Accidental deaths were reduced by over 10% from 105,312 in 1979 to 94,500 in 1989. Additionally, the death rate per 100,000 population dropped 19% from 46.9 to 38.1, the lowest rate ever recorded.[14]

Even with the significant decreases in deaths and death rates in the past 10 years, accidents remain the fourth leading cause of death for all ages, and the leading cause of death for Americans under age 44. To obtain a better perspective of the accident problems that we are likely to face in the 1990s, let's examine Fig. 1-1.

Of the 94,500 accidental deaths in the United States in 1989, the age groups from under 1 year to 44 years accounted for 52,400 of the total deaths, or 55.4%. Although the younger age groups accounted for a large number of accidental deaths, they were not necessarily the most susceptible groups. The three groups that seemed to be at greatest risk for all accidents were persons 65 to 74, 75 years of age and older, and 15- to 24. The elderly are more likely to die in accidents because they cannot react

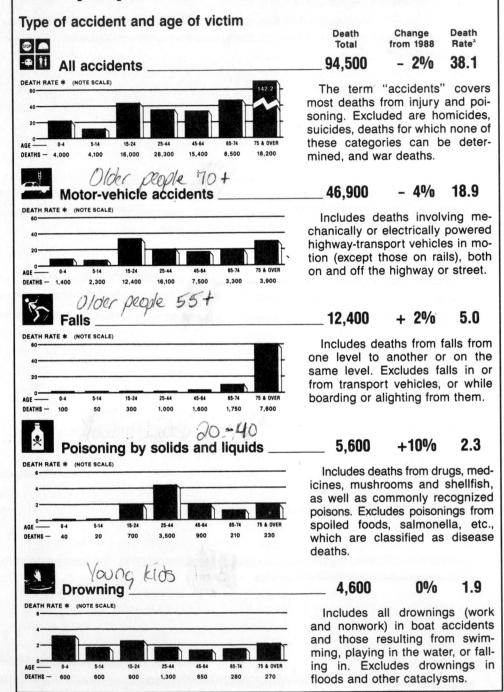

How people died accidentally in 1989

Type of accident and age of victim

	Death Total	Change from 1988	Death Rate[a]

All accidents _____ **94,500** **– 2%** **38.1**

DEATH RATE * (NOTE SCALE)

142.2

AGE	0-4	5-14	15-24	25-44	45-64	65-74	75 & OVER
DEATHS	4,000	4,100	16,000	28,300	15,400	8,500	18,200

The term "accidents" covers most deaths from injury and poisoning. Excluded are homicides, suicides, deaths for which none of these categories can be determined, and war deaths.

Older people 70+

Motor-vehicle accidents _____ **46,900** **– 4%** **18.9**

DEATH RATE * (NOTE SCALE)

AGE	0-4	5-14	15-24	25-44	45-64	65-74	75 & OVER
DEATHS	1,400	2,300	12,400	16,100	7,500	3,300	3,900

Includes deaths involving mechanically or electrically powered highway-transport vehicles in motion (except those on rails), both on and off the highway or street.

Older people 55+

Falls _____ **12,400** **+ 2%** **5.0**

DEATH RATE * (NOTE SCALE)

AGE	0-4	5-14	15-24	25-44	45-64	65-74	75 & OVER
DEATHS	100	50	300	1,000	1,600	1,750	7,600

Includes deaths from falls from one level to another or on the same level. Excludes falls in or from transport vehicles, or while boarding or alighting from them.

Young kids 20~40

Poisoning by solids and liquids _____ **5,600** **+10%** **2.3**

DEATH RATE * (NOTE SCALE)

AGE	0-4	5-14	15-24	25-44	45-64	65-74	75 & OVER
DEATHS	40	20	700	3,500	900	210	230

Includes deaths from drugs, medicines, mushrooms and shellfish, as well as commonly recognized poisons. Excludes poisonings from spoiled foods, salmonella, etc., which are classified as disease deaths.

Young kids 1-5

Drowning _____ **4,600** **0%** **1.9**

DEATH RATE * (NOTE SCALE)

AGE	0-4	5-14	15-24	25-44	45-64	65-74	75 & OVER
DEATHS	600	600	900	1,300	650	280	270

Includes all drownings (work and nonwork) in boat accidents and those resulting from swimming, playing in the water, or falling in. Excludes drownings in floods and other cataclysms.

FIG. 1-1   How people died accidentally in 1989.

(From National Safety Council: Accident facts, Chicago, 1990.)

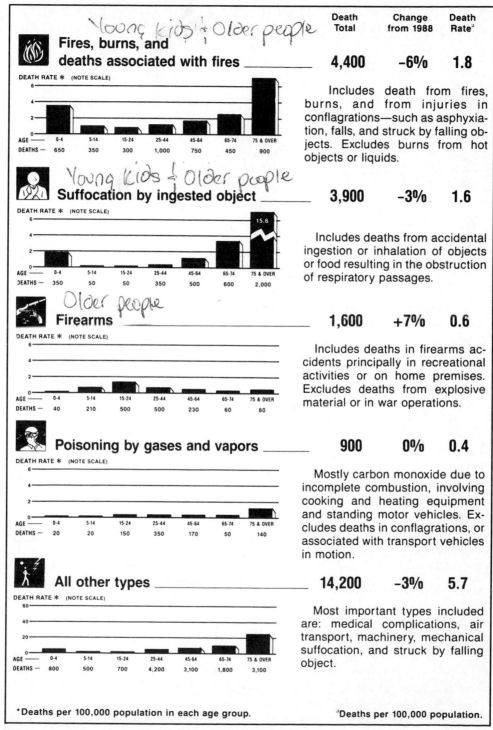

	Death Total	Change from 1988	Death Rate[a]

Young Kids + Older people (handwritten)

Fires, burns, and deaths associated with fires _____ 4,400 −6% 1.8

DEATH RATE * (NOTE SCALE)

AGE	0-4	5-14	15-24	25-44	45-64	65-74	75 & OVER
DEATHS	650	350	300	1,000	750	450	900

Includes death from fires, burns, and from injuries in conflagrations—such as asphyxiation, falls, and struck by falling objects. Excludes burns from hot objects or liquids.

Young Kids + Older people (handwritten)

Suffocation by ingested object _____ 3,900 −3% 1.6

DEATH RATE * (NOTE SCALE) — 15.6

AGE	0-4	5-14	15-24	25-44	45-64	65-74	75 & OVER
DEATHS	350	50	50	350	500	600	2,000

Includes deaths from accidental ingestion or inhalation of objects or food resulting in the obstruction of respiratory passages.

Older people (handwritten)

Firearms _____ 1,600 +7% 0.6

DEATH RATE * (NOTE SCALE)

AGE	0-4	5-14	15-24	25-44	45-64	65-74	75 & OVER
DEATHS	40	210	500	500	230	60	60

Includes deaths in firearms accidents principally in recreational activities or on home premises. Excludes deaths from explosive material or in war operations.

Poisoning by gases and vapors _____ 900 0% 0.4

DEATH RATE * (NOTE SCALE)

AGE	0-4	5-14	15-24	25-44	45-64	65-74	75 & OVER
DEATHS	20	20	150	350	170	50	140

Mostly carbon monoxide due to incomplete combustion, involving cooking and heating equipment and standing motor vehicles. Excludes deaths in conflagrations, or associated with transport vehicles in motion.

All other types _____ 14,200 −3% 5.7

DEATH RATE * (NOTE SCALE)

AGE	0-4	5-14	15-24	25-44	45-64	65-74	75 & OVER
DEATHS	800	500	700	4,200	3,100	1,800	3,100

Most important types included are: medical complications, air transport, machinery, mechanical suffocation, and struck by falling object.

*Deaths per 100,000 population in each age group.

[a]Deaths per 100,000 population.

FIG. 1-1 cont'd. How people died accidentally in 1989.

as quickly to dangerous situations or tolerate trauma as well as younger people. Persons 15 to 24 years old are more likely to die in accidents because they are prone to experimentation and tend to take more unnecessary risks.

Examining the various types of accidents in Fig. 1-1, we see that certain age groups are more susceptible to particular types of accidents than to others. The four age groups exhibiting these tendencies are children from birth to 4 years of age, young adults 15 to 24 years old, persons 65 to 74, and adults 75 and older.

Because they spend most of their time at home, the age groups birth to 4, 65 to 74, and 75 and older are more likely to die in fires, as indicated by their death rates. These three groups also have much higher death rates from choking than any other age groups, because both the very young and the old are susceptible to problems in chewing food.

Another common type of home accident contributing to the high death rate among the elderly are falls. Impairments of sight and mobility that increase with age make the elderly prime candidates for this type of accident. The very young have low death rates resulting from falls because their bodies are more flexible, thus allowing them to withstand the trauma of a fall.

The causes of death among the 15 to 24 age group are indicative of the risk-taking behavior of people in this group. Individuals 15 to 24 have the highest rates of death for accidents involving motor vehicles and firearms. This group also accounts for the second highest death rate for drowning. Those under four years of age have the highest drowning death rate.

Annually, 9 million persons suffer disabling injuries in accidents, and nearly $150 billion are spent as a result of these injuries. Costs to the nation include lost wages, medical expenses, insurance administration, and property damage. Fig. 1-2 gives a breakdown of the costs of accidents in 1989.

The Toll of Injury

A tremendous amount of suffering, grief, and stress for victims, their families, and friends must be included in the yearly toll of injury. It is hard to compute in dollars and cents—the real loss here is the loss of human potential. With a person's life expectancy now in the mid-70s, it seems even more tragic that a person should die at an early age, never to reach his or her full potential. Research has indicated that individuals reach their creative and productive peaks between 50 and 55 years of age.

In 1982, the Centers for Disease Control developed an additional measure of injury loss known as the YPLL Index.[17,18] This index reports the *years of potential life lost* before age 65 and draws attention to preventable mortality occurring early in life. It is not surprising to find that injuries are the leading cause of years of potential life lost. This observation is underscored by the fact that the average YPLL for death from heart disease is 12.1 years and for cancer 16 years, whereas the averages for accidental deaths and homicides are 35.1 and 30.6 years respectively. When expected lifetime earnings are applied to the YPLL Index, it has been shown that the average productivity loss per injury death is $335,000, while the cost per death for heart disease is $51,000, and the cost for each cancer death is $88,000.[17]

Costs of accidents in 1989

Accidents in which deaths or disabling injuries occurred, together with vehicle accidents and fires, cost the nation in 1989, at least

$148.5 billion

Motor-vehicle accidents . . . . $72.2 billion

This cost figure includes wage loss, medical expense, insurance administration cost, and insured property damage from moving motor-vehicle accidents. Not included are the cost of public agencies such as police and fire departments, courts, indirect losses to employers of off-the-job accidents to employees, the value of cargo losses in commercial vehicles, and damages awarded in excess of direct losses. Fire damage to parked motor-vehicles is not included here but is distributed to the other classes.

Work accidents . . . . $48.5 billion

This cost figure includes wage loss, medical expense, insurance administration cost, fire loss, and an estimate of indirect costs arising out of work accidents. Not included is the value of property damage other than fire loss, and indirect loss from fires.

Home accidents . . . . $18.2 billion

This cost figure includes wage loss, medical expense, health insurance administration cost, and fire loss. Not included are the costs of property damage other than fire loss, and the indirect cost to employers of off-the-job accidents to employees.

Public accidents . . . . $12.5 billion

This cost figure includes wage loss, medical expense, health insurance administration cost, and fire loss. Not included are the costs of property damage other than fire loss, and the indirect cost to employers of off-the-job accidents to employees.

Certain Costs of Accidents by Class, 1989 ($ billions)

Cost	TOTAL[a]	Motor-Vehicle	Work	Home	Public Nonmotor-Vehicle
Total	$148.5	$72.2	$48.5	$18.2	$12.5
Wage loss	37.7	19.5	8.3	6.1	5.5
Medical expense	23.7	5.2	8.1	6.6	5.0
Insurance administration[b]	28.4	20.7	6.1	0.9	0.7
Fire loss	9.4	(c)	3.5	4.6	1.3
Motor-vehicle property damage	26.8	26.8	(c)	(c)	(c)
Indirect work loss	22.5	(c)	22.5	(c)	(c)

Source: National Safety Council estimates. Cost estimates are not comparable with those of previous years. As additional or more precise data become available, they are used from that year forward, but previously estimated figures are not revised.

[a]Duplications between work and motor-vehicle and home and motor-vehicle are eliminated in the totals.

[b]Home and public insurance administration costs may include costs of administering medical treatment claims for some motor-vehicle injuries filed through health insurance plans.

[c]Not included, see comments by class of accident above.

FIG. 1-2 Costs of accidents in 1989.

(From National Safety Council: Accident facts, Chicago, 1990.)

INJURY EPIDEMIOLOGY

"It's not worth the risk." "That's a risky proposition." "There is little risk involved." No one is absolutely free from risk. The basic functions of everyday life require a person to take certain risks. Crossing the street, driving a car, and climbing stairs all involve a certain amount of risk taking. While most people repeatedly perform these activities with little effort, each year approximately 7,500 pedestrians are struck and killed by motor vehicles, 47,000 motor vehicle occupants die, and nearly 7,000 persons die as a result of falls in the home.[14]

In this world there are survivors and nonsurvivors—the outcomes of the survivors' endeavors are certainly more favorable. Questions arise such as: "Why is an activity relatively safe for one person, but not for another?" "Are there characteristic differences between persons who have numerous accidents and persons who seldom have accidents?" "How can an individual repeatedly perform the same activity without a problem and then suddenly receive a serious or fatal injury?" To answer these questions, it would seem appropriate that we first determine what affects the safe performance of an activity. As a starting point, let's take a look at a scientific field known as "injury epidemiology." Epidemiology is the fundamental science of studying the occurrence, causes, and prevention of disease. When we combine the terms *injury* and *epidemiology,* we have a discipline for studying the occurrence, causes, and prevention of injury.

Classically the epidemiologic model has been used in the investigation of a variety of communicable diseases (Fig. 1-3). The agent, perhaps a specific type of bacteria, is carried by either an animal (the vector) or an inanimate object (the vehicle) and transmitted to a host (a susceptible person) who develops the disease. Environmental conditions also determine whether effective transmission of the disease can occur; for

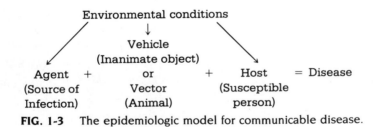

FIG. 1-3 The epidemiologic model for communicable disease.

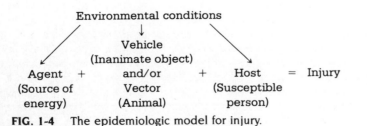

FIG. 1-4 The epidemiologic model for injury.

instance, weather and temperature conditions may prevent the growth of a bacterial agent, thus stopping the spread of the disease. On the other hand, conditions leading to a lack of hygiene may increase a person's chances of becoming infected.

In the case of injury production, basically the same model can be used (Fig. 1-4). Like infections, injuries have agents whose action is necessary to produce a specific type of damage. For injury or property damage to occur, an energy exchange is needed. This exchange may be chemical, electrical, mechanical, thermal, or radiant (from a radioactive source). A vehicle or vector transmits the energy. The vehicle of transmission for mechanical energy may be a car or truck; for radiation it may be steam leaking from a nuclear power plant; and in the case of a violent crime the vehicle of injury may be a knife carried by an attacker (the vector).

The host in our injury epidemiology model can either be a susceptible person who is injured or an object, such as a car or house, which is damaged by the energy source. Environmental conditions, either natural or man-made, also play a role in the transmission of energy and the resultant injury or property damage.

With the following examples we will demonstrate the practical application of the injury epidemiology model. Our first case is the investigation of the electrocution of a construction worker at her job site.

> Laurie A. had been working as a carpenter during the construction of a new supermarket, and at the time of her fatal injury she was cutting plywood panels for the building roof with a power saw.
>
> In this case the agent of injury was electrical energy; it was carried by a vehicle (power saw) and transmitted to a host (Laurie A.), who suffered cardiac arrest and subsequently died. Environmental factors that were found to have significantly increased Laurie's susceptibility to injury included the fact that she was working in the rain, her saw had defective insulation around its electric motor, and the construction site was not equipped with ground fault circuit interrupters (fast-acting circuit breakers that rapidly stop current flow to a power tool).

This model lends itself not only to injury investigation, but to other safety-related problems such as occupational diseases, chemical spills, nuclear accidents, and violent crime. For years to come, epidemiologists will be investigating the effects of ionizing radiation on persons involved in the Chernobyl nuclear accident. Investigators will be looking at individuals living within a wide radius of the accident site, since it is likely that high levels of radiation were carried on wind-blown smoke particles from the Chernobyl fires to neighboring cities in the Soviet Union.

> In December 1984 tragedy struck at the Union Carbide chemical plant in Bhopal, India in the form of a toxic chemical release. This event can also be examined from an epidemiologic perspective. After its accidental release from the plant, the agent (the chemical methyl isocyanate) vaporized, escaped into the air, and was carried on wind-blown particles (the vehicle) to densely populated villages (the hosts) surrounding the plant. Environmental factors such as wind conditions and a heavy population density near the plant increased the severity of the incident. Experts say that many of the survivors will suffer permanently disabling injuries or disorders. In the aftermath, over 2000 people were killed and the number of injured exceeded 80,000—and the effects linger on.

An area in which injury epidemiology is just beginning to be applied is that of violent crime. In a crime such as armed robbery, the agent would be the use of force (mechanical energy). The vector would be the assailant and the vehicle would be the weapon used. The victim would be considered the host; his or her injuries could include physical harm, psychological trauma, and loss of possessions. Environmental factors in such an epidemiologic investigation include characteristics of both attacker and victim, such as age, sex, size, location of the crime, and type of weapon used—just to name a few.

From the discussion above, one begins to get an understanding of the complexity of the concept of safety. Our epidemiologic model illustrates that a change in any of its components (agent, vehicle and/or vector, host, or environmental conditions) may alter the existing state of one's safety and either increase or decrease the possibility of injury or property damage.

In the next sections we will examine a variety of injury prevention and control strategies that will be used throughout this text.

The Haddon Matrix TEST

A forerunner in the study of injury epidemiology was Dr. William Haddon, Jr. In the late 1960s he developed the Haddon Matrix, a system for identifying motor vehicle hazards and developing countermeasures to reduce the likelihood of undesirable results.[6] The matrix has two dimensions. The first is based on the fact that injury or property damage from interactions with specific hazards involves processes that fall into three stages: (1) the pre-event phase, (2) the event phase, and (3) the post-event phase. The second dimension is divided into human factors, vehicle/vector factors, and environmental factors. Table 1-1 illustrates the basic Haddon Matrix.[8]

In the pre-event phase the various factors play a role in determining whether potentially damaging energy exchanges will actually take place. The event phase is the period in which an energy exchange takes place and damage or injury occurs. The post-event phase involves the period after energy damage has already occurred; numerous factors influence the severity of damage to people and property during this time.

Table 1-1 The Haddon Matrix

| Phases | Factors | | |
	Human	Vehicle/vector	Environment
Pre-event	1	2	3
Event	4	5	6
Post-event	7	8	9
Results	10	11	12

Adapted from W. Haddon, Jr.: A logical framework for categorizing highway safety phenomena and activity, The Journal of Trauma 12 (3):193-207. © by Williams & Wilkins, 1972.

Let's take a look at the Haddon Matrix in an investigation of motorcycle accidents. The cells in the matrix are numbered to show to which phase and factor hazards may apply.[8]

1. Pre-event, human: role of alcohol in crash initiation, motorcycle-riding experience
2. Pre-event, vehicle: mechanical failure (tires, brakes, driveshaft, gear box, chain)
3. Pre-event, environment: road surface conditions, inadequate signs or signals, obstructions to vision
4. Event, human: resistance of the properly or improperly protected motorcyclist's body against crash forces
5. Event, vehicle: the structural integrity of the motorcycle as it is exposed to crash forces
6. Event, environment: trees, poles, ditches, structures, and other vehicles that may impact with the motorcycle and the motorcyclist
7. Post-event, human: trauma to the protected or unprotected rider
8. Post-event, vehicle: amount of damage to the motorcycle
9. Post-event, environment: inadequacy of emergency response systems
10, 11, 12. These numbers represent the severity of damage to people, vehicles, and property, as well as the overall impact on society

The next step in using the matrix involves going back through these 12 steps and introducing countermeasures that could either prevent or reduce damage to people and property.

The Haddon Matrix is by no means limited to motor vehicle accident investigation. This model has many applications for a wide variety of safety-related issues. In the next example we will use the matrix to analyze loss-reduction countermeasures for residential fires.

1. Pre-event, human: improve family members' behaviors in terms of fire prevention.
*2. Pre-event, vehicle: placement of smoke alarms in the home
3. Pre-event, environment: location of nearest fire station, neighbor, or call box
4. Event, human: ability of family members to implement fire escape procedures
5. Event, vehicle: activation of an automatic residential sprinkler system
6. Event, environment: rapid response of fire department personnel
7. Post-event, human: sufficient insurance coverage to replace personal property and repair the structure
8. Post-event, vehicle: ease with which structural repairs can be made as a result of construction technology
9. Post-event, environment: operation of social response services; that is, Red Cross, local churches
10, 11, 12. These numbers represent the severity of damage to people and property.

One can see that the Haddon Matrix provides a basic set of guidelines for identifying potential problems as well as a strategy for selecting countermeasures.

---

*The term *vehicle* in this case refers to a residence/home.

FOUR FACTORS OF SAFETY

Another injury control model addressed in this text involves the four factors of safety that play a major role in the performance of any activity. These factors include:

1. **Understanding the difficulty of the activity**
2. **Ability level of the performer**
3. **Immediate state of the performer**
4. **Condition of the environment**

All four factors are closely related. If any of them cannot be adequately controlled, the performer's safety is put in jeopardy.

Understanding the Difficulty of the Activity

Before a person can safely complete an activity he or she must have a clear understanding of what is involved. In the case of riding a motorcycle, this entails a knowledge of motor vehicle laws, motorcycle operation, riding techniques, protective gear, and the inherent dangers of motorcycle riding. It is at this point that the risks must be considered. Who will be exposed to what risks, in what way, and for how long? What is the threat, and how serious is it? A thorough understanding of the activity will enable a person to weigh the potential risks of the activity against potential benefits; inadequate knowledge may, however, lead to a failure to recognize and properly evaluate hazards. Motorcycle riders not well informed of the dangers presented by motor vehicle operators who ignore or fail to see them are often unable to react promptly when a car or truck suddenly pulls out in front of them.

Ability Level of the Performer

Insufficient skill or attempting a skill beyond one's ability is often a contributing factor in accidents. The person involved in a motorcycle accident is generally someone who has been riding for less than 6 months. Also, about half of these victims are under 20 years of age. Common driving errors made by the novice motorcyclist include traveling at excessive speed, following too closely, and being unable to adjust to road conditions. Too often the beginning cyclist has failed to adequately develop the steering and braking skills essential for safe motorcycle operation.

Physical limitations may also affect performance. Factors such as size, strength, and coordination of the rider must be considered when purchasing a particular type of motorcycle. A beginning cyclist with a handicap such as hearing impairment, vision impairment, or an amputation would need special training to compensate for his or her condition.

As a person grows older, physiological functions such as hearing, vision, mobility, and reaction time are affected to varying degrees. These age-related impairments, in turn, affect the skill levels of elderly drivers. Motor vehicle operators over 75 years of age have the second highest death rate of all age groups.[14]

Immediate State of the Performer

The human organism at any point in time is significantly affected by temporary physiological and psychological factors.[7] The state of the performer is constantly changing; thus when the demands of the moment are greater than human capacity, adequate responses may not be forthcoming and an accident results. With this in mind, it is easy to understand how an accomplished cyclist who has been drinking after a fight with his or her spouse can have a serious or fatal accident.

Since the early 1900s researchers have attempted to identify those persons who tend to have more than their share of accidents; they are commonly referred to as "accident prone." Most investigations have indicated that there seem to be no physical differences between the accident prone and those who have few or no accidents. However, this did not seem to be the case when psychological factors such as attitude and emotional state were studied.

Attitudes and emotions play an important role in determining behavior. These psychological factors may act to favorably support activity performance, or they may serve to disrupt the normally safe individual and cause him or her to act in a reckless manner.

There is a strong relationship between the performance of an activity and a person's attitude toward that particular activity. An **attitude** is an enduring predisposition to react negatively or positively toward an object.[20] This object may be a person, group, activity, or belief. Attitudes are developed over a period of time and are not easily changed once formed. For example, when riding a motorcycle, the beginning cyclist may have a negative attitude about the use of protective gear. Consequently the rider fails to wear a helmet, gloves, boots, or other appropriate clothing and greatly increases his or her risk of serious injury should an accident occur.

Emotions also affect activity performance. Arnold defines **emotion** as "a felt tendency toward something intuitively assessed as good, favorable, beneficial, or away from something assessed as unfavorable, harmful, or bad."[7] Generally emotions are closely related to attitudes.

At times emotions may disrupt normal attitude-behavior patterns; for example, the cyclist who normally wears protective equipment may neglect to do so after a fight with his or her spouse. The emotion of anger results in a temporary loss of control and a change in behavior.

Temporary physiological factors may also influence the performance of an activity. After overexertion or at the end of the workday one's ability to perform is usually reduced. Reaction time increases and attentiveness decreases. The cyclist who has worked a physically exhausting shift may not be able to react quickly enough to avoid a motorist pulling into his path.

Drugs and alcohol may alter performance. Alcohol depresses the central nervous system and affects a person in a variety of other ways. Depending on the amount consumed, alcohol may slightly alter one's mood, or cause one to lose consciousness. Alcohol, even in small amounts, slows reflexes and impairs coordination. Drinking is a factor in at least half of the fatal motor vehicle accidents in the United States each year.[14]

Though limited data are available on the role of drugs other than alcohol, it has been estimated that as many as 13% of all traffic fatalities involve the use of some sort of drug other than alcohol. Most of these substances depress the central nervous system and thus affect perception, coordination, and level of consciousness.

A motorcycle rider who has consumed alcohol, drugs, or a combination of both is more likely to have difficulty controlling the vehicle, especially if a quick response becomes necessary. As mentioned earlier, if the demands of the moment are greater than human capacity, a potentially harmful situation may result.

Condition of the Environment

The environment includes both natural and man-made elements that surround an individual during the performance of an activity. The environment can affect the outcome favorably or negatively. On a clear day the cyclist may be able to exceed the speed limit repeatedly without being endangered; however, if the same maneuver is attempted on wet pavement and under conditions of poor visibility, the chances of a serious accident increase significantly. Environmental elements such as protective gear can have a profound effect on the motorcyclist's safety. Who will have a better chance of survival in an instance where a rider loses control and falls on loose gravel: (A) a rider wearing a helmet, a full set of leathers, boots, and gloves, or (B) a rider wearing shorts, a tee shirt, and flip flops? (Hint: Don't bet the ranch on rider B.)

The environment can be separated into two sets of factors, the natural environment and the man-made environment. Natural environmental factors that may directly or indirectly lead to an unsafe situation include rain, snow, dust, ice, wind, and temperature. For example, rain and snow may impair a motorcyclist's vision and directly cause an accident; high temperatures may cause the asphalt on the roadway to soften and thus indirectly lead to the same result.

The man-made environment includes homes, neighborhoods, the workplace, and machines and devices used in everyday living. As in the case of the natural environment, the man-made environment can enhance an individual's safety, or it may lead to serious trouble. Although most safety changes since the early 1900s have been positive, people continue to endanger themselves with new hazards. As the chemical industry has developed new products, there has been an increase in the number of jobs for chemical workers. The benefits brought to the economy by these new products often have been outweighed by the toxicity of these chemicals and their harmful effects on employees.

Using the example of the motorcyclist once again, the man-made environment can have a profound effect on safety—the most obvious problem being one of equipment failure. If the steering or braking system malfunctions while the cyclist is traveling at 55 miles per hour, his or her safety is in jeopardy. Roadway design is another man-made environmental factor that could present serious hazards for the motorcycle rider. An improperly banked exit ramp could cause a motorcycle to follow a straight path off the ramp because of inertia, rather than allowing it to follow the direction of the ramp.

The four factors of safety can be applied to any situation that involves a person's safety, whether it concerns nondeliberate acts such as accidents or deliberate acts such as criminal activity.

Since we have already illustrated how failure to control these factors may lead to an accident such as a motorcycle mishap, we will now examine how they may affect a person's ability to protect himself or herself against crime.

Let's consider a couple who goes into the city for an evening of dining and dancing. To safely perform this activity, they must have knowledge about the area to which they are traveling. Do they know how to get there? Is the area they are visiting relatively free from crime? People get into trouble when they get lost and venture into a high-crime neighborhood or park their cars in unfamiliar areas.

Regarding protection from criminal assault, the ability level of the performer mainly refers to physical characteristics that may deter an attacker. Factors such as height, weight, and strength of the potential victim have been shown to deter would-be muggers. The axiom "strength in numbers" also holds true. Visitors to the city who travel in groups of four or more are less likely to be attacked or robbed. On the other hand, physical limitations and age-related impairments increase the risk of becoming a victim of crime. The elderly and the physically handicapped are "easy targets" for the mugger because they are at a great disadvantage in terms of self-defense.

Closely related to the factor of physical ability to defend against attack is the immediate state of the performer. An individual who has been drinking may be unable to defend himself or herself, at least temporarily. Also, the person who has lost the ability to function well emotionally may be willing to take more chances in terms of personal security. The intoxicated individual who leaves a bar alone or with newfound friends may be asking for more than he or she bargained for.

The environment also plays a part in safety. A parking area where lighting and security are poor gives an attacker, especially one who is familiar with the neighborhood, a decided advantage. Other environmental factors affecting safety include time of day, population density of the area, and the local crime rate. A person who fails to consider any of these factors increases the risk of becoming a victim of crime.

Like the Haddon Matrix, the four factors of safety provide a model that can be used to identify hazards and develop strategies for both injury prevention and mitigation.

INJURY REDUCTION: MORE THAN BEHAVIORAL CHANGE

The tendency to attribute injuries to human error has nourished the hope that they can best be prevented through voluntary behavior change. **Safety education** classically has consisted of three elements:

1. Knowledge creates an awareness of accident potential and problem areas.
2. Attitudes enable a person to judge the potential value of making a behavior change.
3. Skill development allows the individual to consistently and safely perform an action.

Statistical information concerning types of injuries, persons involved, possible causes, costs, and damages is useful for creating an awareness of problem areas.

Though factual material is an important first step in the behavior-change process, this alone will not effect a change.

Studies in the industrial setting have shown that workers' attitudes strongly influence behavior on the job and their willingness to respond to new safety measures.[10] A person who sees no potential value in changing a particular behavior will probably not make a serious effort to change. Investigations by Walker and Cohen found that top-management support and participation in safety training programs was a key factor in reducing accident frequency on the job. A follow-up study correlated positive worker attitudes with their perception that management was sincerely concerned about their safety.[6,7]

The third element in the behavioral change triad is skill development. Many injuries result less from lack of knowledge than from failure to apply what is known.

The safe performance of an activity often involves **adjustive behavior:** the consistent successful performance of an action or skill in the face of possible unplanned interruptions. Adjustive behavior introduces the concepts of skill and judgment as they relate to maintaining a state of harmony between the individual and the environment. We must develop ways to teach people to perform adjustively (that is, use safety belts, wear helmets, use vehicle crash avoidance techniques) so that aggressive, risky behavior is undertaken only when necessary and only under the most appropriate conditions.

There is an increasing need for safety education to be realistic. It must give a true sense of the tensions and pressures that may occur when a person is put in an unsafe situation. Safety training must be pertinent to the individuals involved; they should be able to relate their new knowledge and skill to their current surroundings, including the home, workplace, school, and social or recreational settings.

Although it is not a radically new idea, the use of simulation training has significant potential for improving one's adjustive behavior. For years, flight simulators have been used to train pilots to handle a wide variety of in-flight emergencies. The railroad industry has used computerized mock-ups that simulate railway sights, sounds, and motion in the training of engineers, while the shipping industry has developed similar equipment for training personnel on ocean-going vessels.[21] Malfunctions and failures are programmed into the simulators, and students are introduced to problems of increasing complexity. Certain simulators can even reproduce the noise, heat, and humidity one would find in a ship's engine room. In this age of computerization, similar technologies could be used to improve instruction for such diverse groups as driver-education students, truck drivers, and industrial equipment operators.

Simulation training or experiential learning can be as simple or as complex as needed. In fire safety classes, rooms can be arranged to simulate hotel or motel hallways, so that students must actually practice fire escape procedures; likewise, controlled fires can be used to give them hands-on firefighting experience. Because of the realism built into this training, students react with the same sort of anxiety and sense of urgency that would occur in an actual situation.

A health promotion/injury prevention strategy developed by Green and associates in the late 1970s has refined the three elements of safety education. Known as the PRECEDE model, it looks at the determinants of behavior change from a slightly different perspective.[18] Predisposing factors provide the rationale or motivation for a behavior change—i.e., knowledge and attitudes about a particular safety-related problem. Enabling factors allow that motivation or behavior change to be realized—i.e., availability and accessibility of safety training, equipment, etc. Once a skill or behavior has been developed, reinforcing factors provide rewards or incentives for the behavior to continue.

Let's take a look at the PRECEDE model as it might apply to rape prevention and self-defense training on a university campus.

Predisposing factors: Through workshops in dormitories and sorority houses as well as in women's studies courses at the university, many of the myths and misconceptions about rape could be dispelled. At the same time, issues concerning self-reliance, self confidence, and empowerment would be addressed, as they apply to a woman's ability to physically defend herself against an attacker.

Enabling factors: To develop fighting skills, self-defense classes could be offered for credit through the university's physical education program. Seminars and training workshops also could be offered at a minimal cost by local community centers or by campus organizations.

Reinforcing factors: To ensure a continued level of skill in those who had been trained, workshops could be held throughout the academic year. Other incentives to maintain skill levels might include academic credit, discounts at local stores, and sportswear advertising the program.

Although education is an important part of any injury reduction program, it has rarely proved to be the complete answer. Behavior change to prevent or reduce injuries has been most successful when the behavior was easily observable and required by law. For example, in the absence of laws requiring the use of protective helmets, only about 50% of motorcyclists voluntarily wear them, but helmet-use laws result in almost 100% use.[26] Factors that influence the effectiveness of these laws include the probability of arrest for violation of the behavior, the extent to which enforcement is supported by members of the community, and the severity of punishment.

Even with intensive enforcement, many people violate speed limits, safety-belt use, and child-restraint laws. Research indicates that as the frequency and amount of individual effort increases, the number of persons adopting the required behavior decreases.

A third approach to injury prevention and reduction that will be covered in this text involves such changes in the environment as improved product design and built-in or automatic protection. High-mounted, midline brake lights, which became standard equipment on all passenger cars and trucks in 1986, have substantially reduced the incidence of rear-end crashes. Likewise, the use of child-resistant closures over the past 18 years has significantly reduced the number of poisoning fatalities in children. Double insulation of power tools, three-prong grounded plugs, and ground fault circuit interrupters are examples of built-in protection that we now take for granted.

Ultimately, a threefold approach including: (1) education/behavioral change, (2) laws and regulations, and (3) product design and automatic protection provides the greatest potential for a comprehensive injury-reduction program.

THE SAFETY MOVEMENT: HISTORICAL PERSPECTIVE

The nearly total dependence of the early colonies on Europe for goods led indirectly to the first safety innovation in America. The construction of the Boston Light (a lighthouse at the entrance of Boston Harbor) in 1716 was intended primarily to protect goods being shipped from Europe; however, it also provided increased safety for crews and passengers of these cargo vessels. Most of the early efforts to improve safety were implemented to protect property.[15]

Before the Revolutionary War, advances in safety were mainly concerned with fire protection. In 1736 Benjamin Franklin founded the first fire department in America in Philadelphia. That same year, the first fire insurance company was established in Charleston, South Carolina. By 1750 a number of fire insurance companies had been established throughout the colonies; the best known of these was the Contribution, which had Benjamin Franklin as one of its directors. A major competitor of the Franklin firm was the Green Tree Company, the first insurance company to offer varying rates to homeowners based on increased risk. This was the first attempt to encourage and reward preventive safety measures. The Green Tree Company offered lower premiums to homeowners who removed trees that were in close proximity to their residences. In case of a home fire, this allowed fire fighters and equipment better access to the fire, thus reducing damage.

During the Revolutionary War most of the country remained sparsely populated and relatively unsophisticated. Only about 5% of the population lived in towns and cities, while the remainder were on farms. Most Americans attributed accidents, injury, and death to "acts of God" or "luck." Their major concern was relatively simple—survival.

After the War of Independence the nation turned its attention toward industrialization and the manufacturing of goods. No longer would England be supplying the vast number of articles that it had before the revolution. With the advent of the industrial revolution, Americans began moving from the farms to the cities. The cottage industries of artisans and craftsmen gave way to mills and factories. Articles that were once handmade became mass produced through industrialization. With this increased sophistication in the production of goods came an increase in the number and complexity of hazards for the worker.

In 1794 a group of shoemakers in Philadelphia organized the first trade society in the United States, called the Federal Society of Journeymen Cordwainers.[9] It originated as a mutual aid society, which paid sickness and death benefits to members or their widows and children. The early trade societies were forerunners of today's unions, which continue to be concerned with worker safety.

As the populations of cities increased, it became apparent that some type of regulatory agency was needed to protect people from the new and increasing number of hazards. In 1799 the first board of health was established in Boston, with Paul Revere serving as its president. The board's duty was to inspect stores, vessels, factories, and houses where health hazards were expected to exist. Board members also had the power to levy fines and require the offender to remove the hazard at his own expense. In the past 180 years, similar approaches have been taken to protect the public at the local, state, and federal levels of government throughout the United States.

During the 1800s the United States came into its own as a world industrial leader. From 1800 to 1850 the process of industrialization was slow but steady. Progress in production of goods was often at the expense of worker safety. Generally the safety of workers was assumed to be their responsibility. Insurance carriers were strictly property oriented. This is evidenced by the establishment in 1835 by Zachariah Allen of the first factory mutual insurance company. To qualify for coverage by this company at reduced premiums, mills had to meet certain construction and fire safety standards; however, only the contents and structures could be insured—there were no clauses for the protection of workers.

With the introduction of three major industries in America during the mid-nineteenth century—railroading, mining, and steel production—hazards of a type and magnitude not previously known confronted the American worker. Amputations and crushing injuries were very common. Frequent hand and finger amputations among textile mill workers in Massachusetts led to the organization of the first state bureau of labor statistics in 1869. It was this nation's first attempt to collect data about accidents, and it was an indication that worker safety was becoming a public concern. During that same year the Pennsylvania legislature passed the first mine safety law, which required all mines to have at least two exits.[16] As in Massachusetts, the Pennsylvania law was passed after a number of mining disasters had occurred. Safety measures in the industrial setting were implemented only after extensive losses had been suffered by the work force. The influx of immigrants during the nineteenth century provided a major source of cheap, yet expendable, labor. If a worker was hurt on the job, there were plenty of other people waiting to take his or her place. For the remainder of the nineteenth century, little was done to improve safety conditions for the American worker.

In 1894 Underwriters Laboratories (UL) was founded in Chicago to investigate fire hazards related to the use of electricity.[16] Two years later the National Fire Protection Association was established to develop standards for fire-fighting equipment and methods of fire protection. Today both of these organizations continue to play a major role in the fire safety industry.

From 1900 to 1910, the nation's interest in safety remained unorganized. Most people accepted injury and death as the price of progress. Some of the major disasters that occurred during the early 1900s included: (1) the San Francisco earthquake and fire (1906, 452 deaths), (2) the burning of the steamship General Slocum in New York City's East River (1904, 1,021 deaths), (3) the Iroquois Theatre fire in Chicago (1903, 575 deaths), and (4) coal mine explosions in Monongha, West Virginia (1907, 361 deaths) and Jacobs Creek, Pennsylvania (1907, 239 deaths).[14] With few exceptions, government involvement in safety matters remained limited. A laissez-faire attitude was generally the rule of the day.

In 1911, two incidents had a dramatic impact on safety efforts in the United States. The first was the Triangle Shirtwaist Company fire in New York City, which claimed 145 lives; most of the victims were young girls. An inspection of the building after the fire indicated that exit doors had been locked, fire escapes were blocked by machinery, and fire-fighting equipment was inoperable. The public outcry after this tragedy was expressed by Rabbi Stephen Wise, who stated, "It is not the action of God but the inaction of man that is responsible. . . . This was no inevitable disaster which could not be foreseen."[19]

The second event that changed the direction of safety in the United States was the passage of the country's first workers' compensation law by the Wisconsin legislature. This law provided for hospital expenses and a percentage of wages for injured workers as well as benefits to their survivors in case of death. It was a powerful financial incentive for employers to prevent accidents rather than pay large premiums for compensation insurance.[15] Before this legislation employees were forced to sue their employers for damages if they were injured on the job. Because most employers used contributory negligence, assumption of risk, and negligence of a fellow worker as common defenses, few claimants were ever successful.

In 1912 the First Cooperative Safety Congress of the Association of Iron and Steel Electrical Engineers convened. The congress adopted a resolution to form a national organization for the promotion of safety: the National Safety Council, which was established in 1913. Another major development in 1913 was the founding of the U.S. Department of Labor. This was the beginning of federal influence in the field of safety.

During the next 25 years numerous groups, including the American Society of Safety Engineers, became associated with the National Safety Council in an effort to improve the safety of the American worker. The federal government continued to investigate and correct hazardous conditions across a broad spectrum of industries. The Walsh-Healy Act of 1936 was a forerunner of today's Occupational Safety and Health Act. The Walsh-Healy Act established standards, including health and safety requirements, for work done on federal contracts exceeding $10,000.[19]

Before World War II injury and death rates in the United States had been gradually declining. Wartime expansion of the work force led to increased injury and death rates because a large number of new workers had little or no on-the-job experience. An increase in the hours worked per week had a negative impact on home safety, where accident and death rates also increased. The only area in which there was a drop in injury and death rates was the motor vehicle category. This decrease was caused, in part, by fuel rationing and the limited availability of vehicle parts during the war. During the Korean War a similar fluctuation in death and injury rates occurred; however, with a return to peacetime and improved safety conditions, accident rates began another steady decline through the 1950s.

In the 1960s, statistics indicated that accidents and the resulting injuries, illnesses, and deaths were on the rise. This upward trend was exhibited in both industrial and motor vehicle accidents. In addition, attention was called to the significant number of injuries and deaths attributed annually to consumer products.[16] Four pieces of legislation promulgated between 1966 and 1974 to stem the increasing accident rates were the Highway Safety Act of 1966, the Occupational Safety and Health Act of 1970, the Consumer Product Safety Act of 1972, and the nationwide 55-mile-per-hour speed limit of 1974.

The Highway Safety Act requires states to have a highway safety program developed with uniform standards set by the U.S. Department of Transportation. The 18 program standards include such areas as motorcycle safety, emergency medical services, highway engineering, vehicle inspection, and accident investigation.[24] Legislation enacted as a result of the energy crisis in 1973 was the imposition of a 55-mile-per-hour nationwide speed limit. It has been estimated that since the early 1970s these laws have saved approximately 40,000 lives.

Between 1961 and 1969 the nation's all-industry accident frequency rate climbed from 5.99 to 8.87 per 100 full-time employees.[9] As early as 1964 the federal government was concerned with the increase in work-related accidents. President Lyndon B. Johnson convened a conference on occupational safety during that year. Six years later, in 1970, the Occupational Safety and Health Act became a reality. Under the act the Occupational Safety and Health Administration (OSHA) was created within the U.S. Department of Labor. Its major function is to provide safe and healthful conditions for every working man and woman by developing and enforcing job safety standards, monitoring job-related illnesses and injuries, and providing research to solve occupational safety and health problems.[23]

The Latin phrase *caveat emptor,* meaning ''let the buyer beware,'' has been a very practical suggestion for the American consumer. Until 1972 little had been done in the way of legislation to protect the public from unsafe products and the unreasonable risk of injury associated with them. With the passage of the Consumer Product Safety Act, Congress established the U.S. Consumer Product Safety Commission (CPSC). The CPSC monitors injuries associated with consumer products, sets and enforces safety standards for over 10,000 products, and in certain instances bans the sale and distribution of hazardous products.[12]

The effectiveness of groups such as OSHA and the CPSC can be gauged by looking at the decade of the 1980s. From 1979 to 1989 more progress was made than in any previous decade in reducing the total number of accidental deaths and the death rate. This trend has continued into the 1990s; death rates in the workplace have decreased 28% in the past 10 years, while the death rate for home accidents fell 9%.

In 1986, acting on a recommendation from the National Academy of Sciences, the

U.S. Congress established a Division of Injury Control within the Centers for Disease Control in Atlanta, Georgia. Activities of the Division of Injury Control involve the prevention, mitigation, treatment, and rehabilitation of both unintentional and intentional injuries. Ultimately its role will be to develop a coordinated national injury agenda for the 1990s and beyond.[18]

Although great strides have been made through a wide range of innovative safety measures, especially during the past 80 years, much remains to be done. Nearly 100,000 persons continue to die each year as a result of accidents and another 9 million suffer disabling injuries. Additionally, an estimated 6 million Americans are victims of violent crimes. President Theodore Roosevelt summed it up very succinctly more than 80 years ago when he said, "As modern civilization is constantly creating artificial dangers to life, limb, and health, it is imperative upon us to provide new safeguards against the perils."[20]

SUMMARY

In the past 265 years we have seen this nation change from one that was rather unsophisticated and rural to one that is quite complex and highly industrialized. Inevitably, as society has become more sophisticated, its problems and hazards have also become more sophisticated. Occupational illnesses that were unheard of at the turn of the century have become a major safety issue for today's industries. Many chemicals used in manufacturing processes have created a serious environmental problem with toxic wastes. As America continues to become more urbanized, a greater number of people are exposed to the criminal elements in society. Consequently, safety in the 1990s must include more than a study of the accident process. It must include a broad range of topics not included in traditional safety education. In this ever-changing society, the safe individual is one who can adjust appropriately to hazards and dangers and still enjoy life.

Key Terms

Adjustive behavior   The consistent, successful performance of an action or skill in the face of possible unplanned interruptions.

Attitude   An enduring predisposition to react negatively or positively toward an object.

Emotion   A felt tendency toward something intuitively assessed as favorable or away from something assessed as unfavorable.

Hazard   A condition or set of conditions that have the potential to produce injury and/or property damage.

Risk   The probability of a negative occurrence as well as its severity.

Safety   An ever-changing condition in which one attempts to minimize the risks of injury, illness, or property damage from the hazards to which one may be exposed.

Safety education   An attempt to develop the knowledge, attitudes, and skills that will allow an individual to enjoy maximum success with minimum risk.

References

1. American Society of Safety Engineers: The first 75 years: 1911-1986, Des Plaines, Ill., 1986.
2. Baker, S. P., and Teret, S. P.: Freedom and protection: a balancing of interests, American Journal of Public Health 71 (3): 295, 1981.
3. Centers for Disease Control: Premature mortality due to homicides—United States, Morbidity and Mortality Weekly Report 37 (36), 1988.
4. Centers for Disease Control: Premature mortality due to unintentional injuries—United States, Morbidity and Mortality Weekly Report 36 (49), 1987.
5. Centers for Disease Control: Public health surveillance of 1990 injury control objectives for the nation, Morbidity and Mortality Weekly Report 37 (55-61), Feb. 1988.
6. Denton, D. K.: The unsafe act: exploring the dark side of accident control, Professional Safety, July 1979, p. 34.
7. Ferry T. S., and Weaver, D. A., editors: Directions in safety, Springfield, Ill., 1976, Charles C. Thomas, Publisher.
8. Haddon, W., Jr.: A logical framework for categorizing highway safety phenomena and activity, The Journal of Trauma 12 (3):193, 1972
9. Jayroe, T.: 1776 thru 1976: 200 years of safety and the glass industry, Safety Newsletter, July 1976, p. 1.
10. Moriarty, B., and Roland, H. E.: System safety engineering and management, New York, 1983, John Wiley & Sons, Inc.
11. Mroz, J. H.: Safety in everyday living, Dubuque, Ia., 1978, Wm. C. Brown Group.
12. National Business Council for Consumer Affairs: Safety in the marketplace, Washington, D.C., 1973, U.S. Government Printing Office.
13. National Research Council and the Institute of Medicine: Injury in America, Washington, D.C., 1985, National Academy Press.
14. National Safety Council: Accident facts—1990 ed., Chicago, 1990.
15. Progress and problems in industrial safety, Monthly Labor Review, Dec. 1956, p. 1438.
16. Pyle, H. J., and Newman, E. L.: A bicentennial look at safety, Professional Safety, April 1976, p. 16.
17. Rice, D. P., MacKenzie, E. J., and associates: Cost of injury in the United States: a report to congress, San Francisco, Calif., 1989, Institute for Health and Aging, University of California and Injury Prevention Center, The Johns Hopkins University.
18. The National Committee for Injury Prevention and Control: Injury prevention: meeting the challenge, American Journal of Preventive Medicine 5 (3), 1989.
19. The safety revolution, National Safety News, May 1963, p. 37.
20. Strasser, M. K., Aaron, J. E., and John, R. C.: Fundamentals of safety education, ed. 3, New York, 1981, Macmillan Publishing Co.
21. Texaco, Inc.: Training by simulation, National Safety News, Jan. 1985, p. 40.
22. U.S. Department of Justice, Bureau of Justice Statistics: Report to the nation on crime and justice, ed. 2, Washington, D.C., NCJ-105506, 1988.
23. U.S. Department of Labor, Occupational Safety and Health Administration: All about OSHA, rev. ed., Washington, D.C., 1980, U.S. Government Printing Office.
24. U.S. Department of Transportation: Highway safety program manual no. 11: emergency medical services, Washington, D.C., 1974, U.S. Government Printing Office.
25. U.S. Public Health Service: 1987 conference on injury in America, Public Health Reports 102, (6), Nov.-Dec. 1987.
26. Watson, G. S., Zador, P. L., and Wilks, A.: The repeal of helmet use laws and increased motorcyclist mortality in the United States, 1975-1978, American Journal of Public Health 70:579, 1980.

Resource Organizations

American Academy of Safety Education
Executive Director
Missouri Safety Center
Humphreys Building
Central Missouri State University
Warrensburg, MO 64093

American Society of Safety Engineers
1800 East Oakton Street
Des Plaines, IL 60018-2187

Board of Certified Hazard Control
Management
8009 Carita Court
Bethesda, MD 20817

National Aeronautics and Space
Administration
Space Science and Applications
400 Maryland Avenue, S.W.
Washington, DC 20546

National Safety Council
444 North Michigan Avenue
Chicago, IL 60611

Public Risk Management Association
1117 N. 19th Street
Suite 900
Arlington, VA 22209

Safety Equipment Institute
1901 North Moore Street
Arlington, VA 22209

System Safety Society
14252 Culver Drive, Suite A–261
Irvine, CA 92714

Underwriters Laboratories
333 Pfingsten Road
Northbrook, IL 60062

Applying What You Have Learned

1. How would you apply the injury epidemiology model in an investigation of forcible rapes on your campus?

    a.) Agent: _____

    _____

    b.) Vehicle/vector: _____

    _____

    c.) Host: _____

    _____

    d.) Environmental conditions: _____

    _____

2. Discuss the four factors of safety in terms of teaching someone to water ski.

    a.) Understanding the difficulty of the activity:

    _____

    _____

    b.) Ability level of the performer:

    _____

    _____

    c.) Immediate state of the performer:

    _____

    _____

    d.) Condition of the environment:

    _____

    _____

Continued.

CHAPTER 1

Applying What You Have Learned—cont'd

3. Using the PRECEDE model, develop a strategy to get university students to wear bicycle helmets when riding.

    a.)   Predisposing factors:

_____

_____

_____

    b.)   Enabling factors:

_____

_____

_____

    c.)   Reinforcing factors:

_____

_____

_____

2 Safety Analysis: A Statistical Approach

A prerequisite for the scientific study of injury is the acquisition of data on which to base priorities and research.

National Research Council and the Institute of Medicine: Injury in America

ROLE OF STATISTICS IN SAFETY

Before an investigation of safety-related issues can be undertaken, it is essential that one understands some of the basic statistical concepts used in this field of study. In Chapter 2 we will attempt to allay some of the fears and misconceptions that people have about statistics. Many of us suffer from an age-old problem known as "math anxiety," a condition based on the assumption that statistics are so hard to understand that anyone who is not a mathematician has little chance for success.

The truth of the matter is that statistical data are relatively easy to understand if a person is familiar with simple arithmetic processes such as fractions, percentages, and proportions and has a basic understanding of the terminology involved. Often people become confused because they do not know the difference between "number of deaths" and "death rate." Although both types of data are important, comparing them would be like comparing apples and oranges—it just won't work. Some people have difficulty understanding graphic presentations of data, such as histograms and frequency polygons; however, once they understand the purpose of presenting data in this manner, they often prefer it because it allows rapid interpretation of large amounts of information.

Statistical data serve a number of functions in the field of safety. Data are frequently used to determine problem areas. Statistics concerning work-related injuries at a manufacturing plant may indicate that most accidents occur in a particular department. Statistics can be helpful in developing strategies in safety education. A recent study completed at the University of Chicago suggests that violent physical resistance by women may be a more appropriate method of defense against a rapist than nonviolent approaches that have been taught in the past.[22] Statistical information also has played an important role in the development of safer equipment. The eye-level, midline rear brake lights that have been standard equipment on all new motor vehicles since 1986 were developed in response to statistical studies that indicated that braking reaction times of drivers following vehicles with this lighting system were significantly reduced. Follow-up studies have since documented the efficacy of the midline, eye-level brake light system in reducing rear-end collisions.[12]

STATISTICS DEFINED

Statistics is an area of science concerned with the extraction of information from numerical data.[6] Anything dealing with the collection, presentation, analysis, and interpretation of numerical information belongs in the domain of statistics.[1]

Statistics are generally of two types, descriptive and inferential. **Descriptive statistics** give information about the characteristics of a particular group.[8] They give us a factual report of what has occurred. An example of a descriptive statistic is the 1989 death total for motor vehicle accidents, which was 46,900. Other descriptive statistics include the age, sex, and race of those killed in motor vehicle accidents.

Inferential statistics consist of estimations, generalizations, or predictions about a particular group. For example, before each major holiday the National Safety Council predicts how many people will be killed on the nation's highways during this period. These predictions are based on the number of motor vehicle deaths recorded during previous years for the same periods. Often the National Safety Council estimates for these holidays differ by as little as 1% from the actual number of fatalities.

A second example of inferential statistics is illustrated by the Law Enforcement Assistance Administration's National Crime Survey. Data from representative national samples of households and businesses provide the basis for making estimates of the extent and nature of crimes of theft and violence in the United States.[23] Approximately 60,000 households and 50,000 businesses compose the sample. The basic objective of inferential statistics, in this case, is to draw generalizations about a larger population from which a sample has been selected. Some experts on crime suggest that the National Crime Survey is more reliable than the Federal Bureau of Investigation's annual Uniform Crime Report, which is based on monthly reports from local and state law enforcement agencies throughout the United States.

Presentation of Data

Frequency distributions. It is difficult to work with large numbers of scores unless they are arranged in a more convenient form. An efficient way to present a significant amount of data is to group them in several classes. This statistical tool is known as a **frequency distribution.** Table 2-1 illustrates this form of data presentation.

Any set of measures or values is known as a distribution. An example of a distribution is a breakdown of the ages of the 94,500 people who died in accidents in 1989. One way to present these data would be to list the ages of every person who died; however, this would be impractical for two reasons: (1) a listing of all accidental death victims by age would take up an inordinate amount of space and be time consuming, and (2) listing the data in this manner would not give an overall impression of the victims' ages.

Table 2-1   U.S. accidental deaths by age, 1989

Age group	Number of deaths
0-4	4,000
5-14	4,100
15-24	16,000
25-44	28,300
45-64	15,400
65-74	8,500
75+	18,200
All ages	94,500

Source: National Safety Council: Accident facts, Chicago, 1990.

Table 2-2   Frequencies and percentages of accidental deaths by age, 1989

Age group	Number of deaths	% of deaths
0-4	4,000	4.2
5-14	4,100	4.3
15-24	16,000	16.9
25-44	28,300	30.0
45-64	15,400	16.3
65-74	8,200	9.0
75+	18,000	19.3
All ages	94,500	100

Source: National Safety Council: Accident facts, Chicago, 1990.

Percentages. Another form of data presentation is the use of percentages. A **percentage** is defined as "a given part of the whole expressed as a decimal."[10] It is derived by dividing the number of cases of interest by the total number of cases. Percentages can be used as a means of comparison or to demonstrate changes over time.

In Table 2-2 we have taken the age-group frequencies from Table 2-1 and converted them to percentages for ease of comparison. After examining the data, one can see that nearly 50% of those who die in accidents are between the ages of 15 and 44. The figures also indicate that age doesn't seem to protect people from accidents.

Between 1979 and 1989 accidental work-related deaths decreased from 13,000 to 10,400 while total employment increased from 98 million to 116 million workers.[13] Using percentages, these figures signify that between 1979 and 1989 accidental work-related deaths decreased 20% while total employment increased 18.4%. A major value of percentages is their ability to clarify the raw numbers.

Rates. Rates are percentages that are based on a particular population. Unlike percentages, rates control for population; that is, regardless of the total population of groups to be compared, rates will be based on the same figure, usually per 100,000 population.

The most widely used rate is the death or mortality rate. It is further divided into crude death rates and specific death rates. The crude death rate is the number of deaths that occur in a given year per 100,000 persons in the entire population. In 1989 the crude death rate for the United States was 872.3 per 100,000 population.[21] This figure gives us no information about the causes of death or descriptions of the victims, such as age, race, and sex. Crude death rates are used most often on an international level as a comparison between countries. These rates are also used by population specialists to determine growth rates. The formula for the crude death rate is:

$$\text{Crude death rate} = \frac{\text{Number of deaths} \times 100,000}{\text{Total population}}$$

The specific death rate provides more detailed information. Specific death rates provide information about the causes of death and types of accidents as well as the age, race, and sex of the victims. The formula for specific death rate is:

$$\text{Specific death rate} = \frac{\text{Number of deaths for a specific population} \times 100,000}{\text{Specific population}}$$

The **specific death rate** is the number of deaths that occur in a given year for every 100,000 persons in a particular population. For example, let us compare the specific death rates for workers in mining and transportation. In 1989 there were approximately 700,000 people in the mining industry, and 300 of them died in accidents. Using the formula above, we obtain a specific death rate of 43 per 100,000 persons. In transportation there were 5,900,000 workers in 1989; 1400 of them died. Using the formula, we obtain a specific death rate for transportation workers of 24 per 100,000 persons. Based on this information, we can see that mining is the more dangerous of the two occupations, even though more transportation workers died in 1989.[13]

The figures in Table 2-3 further illustrate the advantage of using rates to compare different groups. Looking at the age-specific death rates in Table 2-3, we can see that the death rate for persons 75 years of age and older is more than three times greater than the rate for persons 15 to 24.

Remember, all the rates are based on deaths per 100,000 persons in the popula-

Table 2-3 Frequencies, percentages, and specific rates of accidental deaths by age, 1989

Age group	Number of deaths	% of deaths	Death rate
0-4	4,000	4.2	21.3
5-14	4,100	4.3	11.7
15-24	16,000	16.9	43.8
25-44	28,300	30.0	35.2
45-64	15,400	16.3	33.1
65-74	8,500	9.0	46.8
75+	18,200	19.3	142.2
All ages	94,500	100	38.1

Source: National Safety Council: Accident facts, Chicago, 1990.

tion. In 1989 the population of persons 75 years of age and older in the United States was 12.8 million, while the population of 15-to-24-year-olds was 36.52 million.[13] By controlling for variations in population, we can get a more accurate picture of accidental deaths.

Another rate, discussed in a later chapter, is the injury/illness incidence rate. It is used widely in the field of industrial safety. The incidence rate is defined as the number of injuries and illnesses per 100 worker years or 200,000 hours of work.

Graphic presentations. Presentation of data in picture or graphic form enables the reader to view the results of a frequency distribution without reading all the raw data.[10] The histogram is probably the most widely used method for presenting data graphically. The various classes for which data have been collected are placed on the horizontal axis; the class frequencies are placed on the vertical axis. Fig. 2-1 is a histogram presenting data about the number of U.S. accidental deaths in 1989.*

Another graphic method of presenting frequency data is the frequency polygon. The polygon uses a series of interconnected points to represent the distribution of frequencies. Fig. 2-2 demonstrates the use of a frequency polygon in presenting a frequency distribution.

A third method of graphic data presentation is the pie chart. Generally, frequency data are converted to percentages before they are presented in a pie chart. Fig. 2-3 illustrates the use of a pie chart in presenting a percentage distribution.

The above methods for presenting data are generally employed when safety personnel wish to rearrange a large set of data into a more understandable and usable form. Throughout the remainder of this text frequency and percentage distributions,

---

*Source: National Safety Council: Accident facts, Chicago, 1990

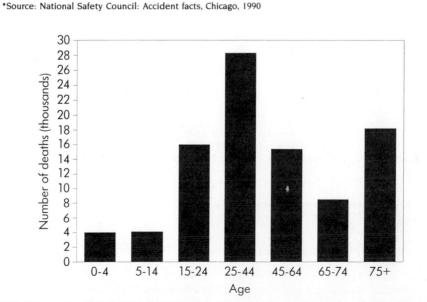

FIG. 2-1 Age distribution histogram for accidental deaths in the United States, 1989.
(From National Safety Council: Accident facts, Chicago, 1990.)

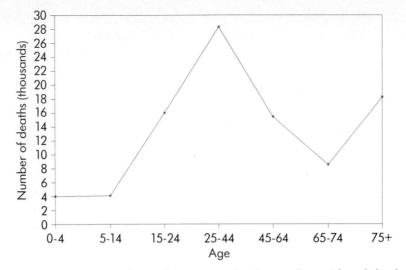

FIG. 2-2 Frequency polygon showing age distribution for accidental deaths, 1989. (From National Safety Council: Accident facts, Chicago, 1990.)

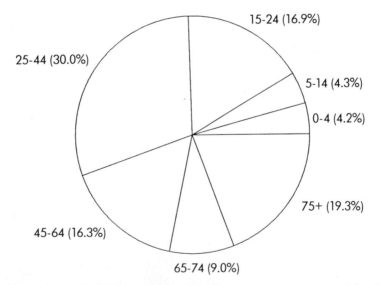

FIG. 2-3 Pie chart illustrating a percentage distribution for accidental deaths by age group, 1989.

rates, and graphic presentations will be used repeatedly to describe events in the field of safety.

Errors and Problems in Data Collection

A statement commonly heard among statisticians is ''If you put garbage into the computer, you will get garbage out of the computer.'' They are referring to a problem that arises when either incomplete or incorrect data are used to answer questions about a given population or situation. The collection of accurate data is vital in the field of safety.

Two important aspects of data collection are the validity and reliability of the observations or measurements that have been taken. **Validity** or accuracy is a measure of how closely data correspond to the actual state of affairs, while **reliability** or reproducibility is a measure of how closely a series of observations of the same thing match one another. Safety researchers have greatly improved the accuracy and reliability of accident and crime data through sophisticated techniques of sampling, instrument design, and computerization. However, when large amounts of data are collected by an equally large number of agencies and individuals, some degree of error can be expected.

Validity errors may be caused by incorrect sampling of a target population, failure to report information, or differences in reporting systems. Sampling errors often result when too few cases are selected to give an estimate of the population at risk; for example, one study of the rate of violent crime in the United States based its findings on data from cities with populations greater than 250,000. The study failed to take into account the lower crime rates found in more rural sections of the United States, and consequently the results exaggerated the actual violent crime picture.

At times administrators are under considerable pressure to show improvement in their safety record in the industrial setting or perhaps in the area of law enforcement. Not that we are condoning this type of behavior, but it is reasonable to believe that a certain amount of data are deliberately suppressed to protect people and organizations.

Certain types of accidents and crimes are reported with more accuracy than others. Accidents and crimes involving death or serious injury are usually well reported because emergency medical services or government agencies are often called on to help. Minor accidents may not be reported because treatment occurs in the home and property damage is minimal and not covered by insurance. A number of violent crimes are underreported because the victims believe that authorities can do nothing to correct the situation.

Differences in reporting systems also reduce the accuracy of safety statistics. Because not all jurisdictions have the same methods for classifying accidents and crimes, a certain amount of information will not be collected or appropriately identified. For example, national statistics concerning the number of annual injuries are collected by the National Safety Council and the U.S. Public Health Service; however, the injury totals presented by these organizations vary significantly because each group uses a different definition of injury.

The primary reason for the unreliability of certain statistics is the variation that occurs when different people make the same observations.[6] Depending on their definitions of occupational illnesses and injuries, industrial safety supervisors may not consider certain cases as recordable incidents. Consequently, whether or not an injury is recorded in the OSHA logbook may depend on which supervisor is working at the plant.

With the large amount of data that must be collected at an accident or crime scene, variation in observations of what occurred is not uncommon. Although variation in reporting will never be eliminated, it can be kept to a minimum by standardizing methods and procedures for collecting data and by continuing to update the training of personnel who must record this information.

Valid and Reliable Sources of Safety Statistics

Because of the potential for error in data collection, a person might wonder whether there are any valid and reliable sources of safety statistics. The answer is yes; a number of organizations gather statistical data on a wide range of safety-related topics. Data sources at local, state, and national levels provide us with a general idea of the extent and patterns of injury in the population.

National Safety Council. One of the most reliable sources of nationwide data pertaining to all types of accidents is the National Safety Council. Established in 1913 and chartered by Act of Congress, this nongovernmental, nonprofit organization has become a leader in safety services. Its annual publication, *Accident Facts,* provides detailed analyses of the different classes of accidents as well as information about accident trends.

National Center for Health Statistics A branch of the U.S. Public Health Service, the National Center for Health Statistics collects and publishes data about diseases and accidents. *The National Health Survey,* which is conducted and published by this agency, samples 45,000 households annually. Interviewers record health data, including injuries, that members of the households experienced 2 weeks before the interview. The accident information recorded covers motor vehicle, home, and work-related injuries.

National Injury Information Clearinghouse. This organization was established under guidelines set by the Consumer Product Safety Act of 1972. Its function is ''to collect, investigate, analyze, and disseminate injury data and information relating to the causes and prevention of death, injury, and illness associated with consumer products.''[20] Data are supplied to the clearinghouse by a number of sources including the National Electronic Injury Surveillance System (NEISS), copies of death certificates that indicate the involvement of consumer products, accident investigations conducted by the Consumer Product Safety Commission, and consumer complaints.

The primary source of statistical information for the clearinghouse is the National Electronic Injury Surveillance System. The NEISS consists of a network of hospitals located throughout the United States and its territories. The data from these hospitals provides national estimates of the number and severity of injuries associated with consumer products.

National Criminal Justice Reference Service (NCJRS). Established in 1972 by the U.S. Department of Justice, this agency serves as a clearinghouse of information about law enforcement and criminal justice. A major document published annually and available through the NCJRS is the *Sourcebook of Criminal Justice Statistics,* a compilation of national criminal justice and related statistics provided by law enforcement, governmental, and private agencies. Two other sources of nationwide information about criminal activity and victimization are the *National Crime Survey* and the Federal Bureau of Investigation's *Uniform Crime Reports.*

The *National Crime Survey,* conducted under the auspices of the Law Enforcement

Assistance Administration, comprises a sample of 60,000 household, 50,000 business, and 135,000 personal interviews. Data from the interviews provide a basis for making national estimates of the extent and nature of crime in America.

The *Uniform Crime Reports* of the FBI are compiled from the monthly crime reports of local and state law enforcement agencies throughout the country. The *Uniform Crime Reports* are used to measure trends in criminal activity as well as the distribution of crime in the United States.

National Highway Traffic Safety Administration. Since 1975 the National Highway Traffic Safety Administration (NHTSA) has been using a computerized data base to analyze fatal motor vehicle crashes. Known as the Fatal Accident Reporting System (FARS), this program uses police accident reports, driver licensing files, death certificates, and reports from medical examiners to determine the elements that contributed to the fatalities.

Another data collection program used at the NHTSA is the National Accident Sampling System (NASS). Crash investigation teams at sites across the country collect detailed information about the people, vehicles, and environmental conditions involved in a representative sample of tow-away motor vehicle crashes; annually the teams investigate nearly 10,000 crashes. With this information researchers have been able to gain valuable information about the forces affecting both vehicles and passengers in a crash.

Local and state agencies. At the community level, agencies such as fire and rescue services, the police or sheriff's departments, and the board of health are involved in data collection about accident investigations. These organizations usually forward their information to state agencies, such as the state board of health, the division of vital statistics, the highway patrol, and the division of workers' compensation.

Ultimately the key to valid and reliable safety statistics lies with the individuals who are directly involved in providing safety services. Emergency medical technicians, paramedics, fire fighters, and law enforcement officers provide the initial input for what later becomes national statistics. Although it is a time-consuming and sometimes unpleasant task, filling out these data sheets and accident reports as completely and accurately as possible can have a significant impact on safety.

Systematic data collection is essential for planning, developing, and evaluating programs. By determining when, where, and how injuries occur and the types of injuries and their severity, local, state, and federal agencies can select and implement appropriate intervention strategies. This information can be used later to evaluate the effectiveness of the interventions.

In 1985 researchers in Colorado investigated the effectiveness of safety belts in one- and two-car crashes.[19] From a pool of 24,000 damaged vehicles, the investigators compared belted and unbelted front-seat passengers. The sample groups were matched in terms of crash severity, type of impact (front, side, rear), size of car, age, and sex. Analysis of the data showed a significant correlation between safety-belt use and reduced injury in motor vehicle accidents.

Because of the consistent data-collection practices of public safety and medical personnel, this study was able to provide detailed information about the efficacy of safety-belt usage. By the way, in 1987 Colorado passed a mandatory safety-belt law.

Classification of Accidents

There are many ways to categorize accidents to display statistical data. Most safety researchers follow the lead of the National Safety Council and use a two-step approach in organizing information. The first step separates accidents into four general classes: motor vehicle, work, home, and public, while the second step identifies specific causes of injury.

	Deaths	Change from 1988	Deaths per 100,000 Persons	Disabling Injuries[a]
All Classes[b]	94,500	–2%	38.1	9,000,000
Motor-vehicle	46,900	–4%	18.9	1,700,000
Public nonwork	42,800			1,500,000
Work	3,900			200,000
Home	200			([c])
Work	10,400	–4%	4.2	1,700,000
Nonmotor-vehicle	6,500			1,500,000
Motor-vehicle	3,900			200,000
Home	22,500	0%	9.1	3,400,000
Nonmotor-vehicle	22,300			3,400,000
Motor-vehicle	200			([c])
Public	19,000	+ 3%	7.7	2,400,000

Disabling Injuries[a] by Severity of Injury, 1989

Severity of Disabling Injury	TOTAL[b]	Motor-Vehicle	Work	Home	Public
All Disabling Injuries[a]	9,000,000	1,700,000	1,700,000	3,400,000	2,400,000
Permanent impairments	340,000	140,000	60,000	90,000	60,000
Temporary total disabilities	8,600,000	1,600,000	1,600,000	3,300,000	2,300,000

Source: National Safety Council estimates (rounded) based on data from the National Center for Health Statistics, state industrial commissions, state traffic authorities, state departments of health, insurance companies, industrial establishments and other sources. See glossary on page 105 for definitions.
[a]**Disabling beyond the day of accident.** Injuries are not reported on a national basis, so the totals shown are approximations based on ratios of disabling injuries to deaths developed from special studies. The totals are the best estimates for the current year; however, they should not be compared with totals shown in previous editions of *Accident Facts* to indicate year-to-year changes or trends.
[b]Deaths and injuries above for the four separate classes total more than national figures due to rounding and because some deaths and injuries are included in more than one class. For example, 3,900 work deaths involved motor vehicles and are in both the work and motor-vehicle totals; and 200 motor-vehicle deaths occurred on home premises and are in both home and motor-vehicle. The total of such duplication amounted to about 4,100 deaths and 200,000 injuries in 1989.   [c]Less than 10,000.

FIG. 2-4   Distribution of deaths and injuries for the four major classes of accidents, 1989.

(From National Safety Council: Accident facts, Chicago, 1990.)

Motor vehicle accidents. These accidents involve mechanically or electrically powered transport vehicles in motion on and off the highway.[13] This includes cars, trucks, buses, motorcycles, motorized bicycles, tractors, and any other machinery capable of traveling on highways. Pedestrian and bicycle collisions with motor vehicles are also included in this accident class.

Work-related accidents. Work-related accidents include those occupational injuries and illnesses incurred during the course of gainful employment. Motor vehicle accidents that occur while a person is on the job are included under both classifications.

Home accidents. Home accidents consist of deaths and injuries that occur in or around the home. Motor vehicle accidents that occur on private property are classified in both the home and motor vehicle categories.

Public accidents. Deaths and injuries that occur in buildings or places used by the general public are categorized as public accidents. Most sports, recreation, and major transportation accidents are included in this classification.

Figure 2-4 shows the distribution of deaths and injuries for the four major classes of accidents in 1989. From these data it can be seen that motor vehicle accidents account for almost half of all accidental deaths and permanently disabling injuries, whereas accidents in the home result in the greatest number of temporary disabilities.

The other method of accident classification, used by the National Safety Council, delineates specific incidents that cause deaths and injuries. This allows for a more detailed analysis than does grouping by class. The data can be further refined by grouping the specific types of accidents by age group. Fig. 1-1 categorizes how people died accidentally in 1989; information includes number of deaths, death rates by age group, and percent change from 1988. In the next section we will use these data to investigate changes in accident trends since 1903.

CHANGES IN THE ACCIDENT SCENE: 1903-1989

Since 1903 the accidental death rate has declined by 56% from 87.2 per 100,000 population to 38.1 in 1989.[19] In this 86-year period, death rates for home, work, and public accidents have decreased 68%, 81%, and 73%, respectively. Although the death rate for motor vehicles increased from 0.5 per 100,000 persons in 1906 to 18.9 per 100,000 in 1989, the motor vehicle death rate per 10,000 registered vehicles actually decreased by 93% (from 33.38 to 2.43 deaths per 10,000 vehicles).[13] This increased death rate is the result of significant increases in the number of vehicles, drivers, and miles driven. The vehicles have actually become safer to operate.

In the 1980s progress has been made in reducing accidental deaths. From 1979 to 1989 the number of accidental deaths decreased 10%, from 105,312 to 94,500. The death rate per 100,000 population declined by 19%, from 46.9 to 38.1.[13]

The four major classes of accidents (motor vehicle, home, work, and public) showed significant decreases in both number of deaths and death rates. Table 2-4 illustrates the distribution of deaths and death rates for the principal classes of accidental deaths since 1903.

Table 2-4   Principal classes of accidental deaths, 1903 to 1989

Year	TOTAL[a] Deaths	Rate[b]	Motor-vehicle Deaths	Rate[b]	Work Deaths	Rate[b]	Home Deaths	Rate[b]	Public nonmotor-vehicle Deaths	Rate[b]
1903	70,600	87.2	(c)		(c)		(c)		(c)	
1904	71,500	86.6	(c)		(c)		(c)		(c)	
1905	70,900	84.2	(c)		(c)		(c)		(c)	
1906	80,000	93.2	400	0.5	(c)		(c)		(c)	
1907	81,900	93.6	700	0.8	(c)		(c)		(c)	
1908	72,300	81.2	800	0.9	(c)		(c)		(c)	
1909	72,700	80.1	1,300	1.4	(c)		(c)		(c)	
1910	77,900	84.4	1,900	2.0	(c)		(c)		(c)	
1911	79,300	84.7	2,300	2.5	(c)		(c)		(c)	
1912	78,400	82.5	3,100	3.3	(c)		(c)		(c)	
1913	82,500	85.5	4,200	4.4	(c)		(c)		(c)	
1914	77,000	78.6	4,700	4.8	(c)		(c)		(c)	
1915	76,200	76.7	6,600	6.6	(c)		(c)		(c)	
1916	84,800	84.1	8,200	8.1	(c)		(c)		(c)	
1917	90,100	88.2	10,200	10.0	(c)		(c)		(c)	
1918	85,100	82.1	10,700	10.3	(c)		(c)		(c)	
1919	75,500	71.9	11,200	10.7	(c)		(c)		(c)	
1920	75,900	71.2	12,500	11.7	(c)		(c)		(c)	
1921	74,000	68.4	13,900	12.9	(c)		(c)		(c)	
1922	76,300	69.4	15,300	13.9	(c)		(c)		(c)	
1923	84,400	75.7	18,400	16.5	(c)		(c)		(c)	
1924	85,600	75.6	19,400	17.1	(c)		(c)		(c)	
1925	90,000	78.4	21,900	19.1	(c)		(c)		(c)	
1926	91,700	78.7	23,400	20.1	(c)		(c)		(c)	
1927	92,700	78.4	25,800	21.8	(c)		(c)		(c)	
1928	95,000	79.3	28,000	23.4	19,000	15.8	30,000	24.9	21,000	17.4
1929	98,200	80.8	31,200	25.7	20,000	16.4	30,000	24.6	20,000	16.4
1930	99,100	80.5	32,900	26.7	19,000	15.4	30,000	24.4	20,000	16.3
1931	97,300	78.5	33,700	27.2	17,500	14.1	29,000	23.4	20,000	16.1
1932	89,000	71.3	29,500	23.6	15,000	12.0	29,000	23.2	18,000	14.4

Year										
1933	90,932	72.4	31,363	25.0	14,500	11.6	29,500	23.6	18,500	14.7
1934	100,977	79.9	36,101	28.6	16,000	12.7	34,000	26.9	18,000	14.2
1935	99,773	78.4	36,369	28.6	16,500	13.0	32,000	25.2	18,000	14.2
1936	110,052	85.9	38,089	29.7	18,500	14.5	37,000	28.9	19,500	15.2
1937	105,205	81.7	39,643	30.8	19,000	14.8	32,000	24.8	18,000	14.0
1938	93,805	72.3	32,582	25.1	16,000	12.3	31,000	23.9	17,000	13.1
1939	92,623	70.8	32,386	24.7	15,500	11.8	31,000	23.7	16,000	12.2
1940	96,885	73.4	34,501	26.1	17,000	12.9	31,500	23.9	16,500	12.5
1941	101,513	76.3	39,969	30.0	18,000	13.5	30,000	22.5	16,500	12.4
1942	95,889	71.6	28,309	21.1	18,000	13.4	30,500	22.8	16,000	12.0
1943	99,038	73.8	23,823	17.8	17,500	13.0	33,500	25.0	17,000	12.7
1944	95,237	71.7	24,282	18.3	16,000	12.0	32,500	24.5	16,000	12.0
1945	95,918	72.4	28,076	21.2	16,500	12.5	33,500	25.3	16,000	12.1
1946	98,033	70.0	33,411	23.9	16,500	11.8	33,000	23.6	17,500	12.5
1947	99,579	69.4	32,697	22.8	17,000	11.9	34,500	24.1	18,000	12.6
1948 (5th Revn.)[d]	98,001	67.1	32,259	22.1	16,000	11.0	35,000	24.0	17,000	11.6
1948 (6th Revn.)[d]	93,000	63.7	32,259	22.1	16,000	11.0	31,000	21.2	16,000	11.0
1949	90,106	60.6	31,701	21.3	15,000	10.1	31,000	20.9	15,000	10.1
1950	91,249	60.3	34,763	23.0	15,500	10.2	29,000	19.2	15,000	9.9
1951	95,871	62.5	36,996	24.1	15,000	10.4	30,000	19.6	16,000	10.4
1952	96,172	61.8	37,794	24.3	15,000	9.6	30,500	19.6	16,000	10.3
1953	95,032	60.1	37,955	24.0	15,000	9.5	29,000	18.3	16,500	10.4
1954	90,032	55.9	35,586	22.1	14,000	8.7	28,000	17.4	15,500	9.6
1955	93,443	56.9	38,426	23.4	14,200	8.6	28,500	17.3	15,500	9.4
1956	94,780	56.6	39,628	23.7	14,300	8.5	28,000	16.7	16,000	9.6
1957	95,307	55.9	38,702	22.7	14,200	8.3	28,000	16.4	17,500	10.3
1958	90,604	52.3	36,981	21.3	13,300	7.7	26,500	15.3	16,500	9.5
1959	92,080	52.2	37,910	21.5	13,800	7.8	27,000	15.3	16,500	9.3
1960	93,806	52.1	38,137	21.2	13,800	7.7	28,000	15.6	17,000	9.4
1961	92,249	50.4	38,091	20.8	13,500	7.4	27,000	14.8	16,500	9.0

Source: From National Safety Council: Accident Facts. Chicago, 1990. Total and motor vehicle deaths, 1903-1932 based on National Center for Health Statistics death registration states; 1933-1948 (5th Revn.), 1949-1963, 1965-1987 are NCHS totals for the U.S. All other figures are National Safety Council estimates; 1989 preliminary, 1988 revised. [a]Duplications between Motor-vehicle, Work and Home are eliminated in the Total column. [b]Rates are deaths per 100,000 population. [c]Data insufficient to estimate yearly totals. [d]In 1948, a revision was made in the International list of causes of death. The first figures for 1948 are comparable with those for earlier years, the second with those for later years.

Table 2-4   Principal classes of accidental deaths, 1903 to 1989—cont'd.

Year	TOTAL[a] Deaths	Rate[b]	Motor-vehicle Deaths	Rate[b]	Work Deaths	Rate[b]	Home Deaths	Rate[b]	Public nonmotor-vehicle Deaths	Rate[b]
1962	97,139	52.3	40,804	22.0	13,700	7.4	28,500	15.3	17,000	9.2
1963	100,669	53.4	43,564	23.1	14,200	7.5	28,500	15.1	17,500	9.3
1964	105,000	54.9	47,700	25.0	14,200	7.4	28,000	14.6	18,500	9.7
1965	108,004	55.8	49,163	25.4	14,100	7.3	28,500	14.7	19,500	10.1
1966	113,563	58.1	53,041	27.1	14,500	7.4	29,500	15.1	20,000	10.2
1967	113,169	57.3	52,924	26.8	14,200	7.2	29,000	14.7	20,500	10.4
1968	114,864	57.6	54,862	27.5	14,300	7.2	28,000	14.0	21,500	10.8
1969	116,385	57.8	55,791	27.7	14,300	7.1	27,500	13.7	22,500	11.2
1970	114,638	56.2	54,633	26.8	13,800	6.8	27,000	13.2	23,500	11.5
1971	113,439	54.8	54,381	26.3	13,700	6.6	26,500	12.8	23,500	11.4
1972	115,448	55.2	56,278	26.9	14,000	6.7	26,500	12.7	23,500	11.2
1973	115,821	54.8	55,511	26.3	14,300	6.8	26,500	12.5	24,500	11.6
1974	104,622	49.0	46,402	21.8	13,500	6.3	26,000	12.2	23,000	10.8
1975	103,030	47.8	45,853	21.3	13,000	6.0	25,000	11.6	23,000	10.6
1976	100,761	46.3	47,038	21.6	12,500	5.7	24,000	11.0	21,500	10.0
1977	103,202	47.0	49,510	22.5	12,900	5.9	23,200	10.6	22,200	10.1
1978	105,561	47.5	52,411	23.6	13,100	5.9	22,800	10.3	22,000	9.9
1979	105,312	46.9	53,524	23.8	13,000	5.8	22,500	10.0	21,000	9.4
1980	105,718	46.5	53,172	23.4	13,200	5.8	22,800	10.0	21,300	9.4
1981	100,704	43.9	51,385	22.4	12,500	5.4	21,700	9.4	19,800	8.6
1982	94,082	40.6	45,779	19.7	11,900	5.1	21,200	9.1	19,500	8.4
1983	92,488	39.5	44,452	19.0	11,700	5.0	21,200	9.0	19,400	8.3
1984	92,911	39.3	46,263	19.6	11,500	4.9	21,200	9.0	18,300	7.7
1985	93,457	39.1	45,901	19.2	11,500	4.8	21,600	9.0	18,800	7.9
1986	95,277	39.5	47,865	19.9	11,100	4.6	21,700	9.0	18,700	7.8
1987	95,020	39.0	48,290	19.8	11,300	4.6	21,400	8.8	18,400	7.6
1988	96,500	39.3	48,900	19.9	10,800	4.4	22,500	9.2	18,500	7.5
1989	94,500	38.1	46,900	18.9	10,400	4.2	22,500	9.1	19,000	7.7
Changes										
1979 to 1989	−10%	−19%	−12%	−21%	−20%	−28%	0%	−9%	−10%	−18%
1988 to 1989	−2%	−3%	−4%	−5%	−4%	−5%	0%	−1%	3%	+3%

SOME MODERN APPROACHES TO ACCIDENT INVESTIGATION

The determination and correction of factors contributing to injury and illness are basic needs in the field of safety and health. Unless accident causes are found and remedied, there is little utility in collecting accident statistics.[15]

Before a detailed discussion of some of the modern approaches to accident investigation can be undertaken, it may be beneficial to review those factors that play a major role in accidents. As discussed in Chapter 1, there are four factors involved in the safe performance of an activity: (1) understanding the difficulty of the activity, (2) ability level of the performer, (3) immediate state of the performer, and (4) condition of the environment. If any of these cannot be controlled, an accident may result.

The following are examples of what it means to fail to control these factors:
1. Understanding the difficulty of the activity—inadequate knowledge to recognize and evaluate hazards
2. Ability level of the performer—insufficient skill or attempting skills beyond ability level
3. Immediate state of the performer—improper habits and attitudes leading to carelessness or risk taking
4. Condition of the environment—equipment failure, lack of safeguards

It might be appropriate to consider these four factors as components of a system. A **system** is an orderly arrangement of components that are interrelated and that act and interact to perform some task or function in a particular environment.[11] The main points to keep in mind are: (1) a system is defined in terms of a task or function and (2) each part of the system affects the others. As parts of a system, the components usually complement each other, but it is essential to recognize that a malfunction of any component can affect the other components and thus impair the performance of the task.[11]

Thinking of accidents in terms of malfunctions in a system can be traced to the aerospace industry. Because of the high reliability and precision of specifications demanded by this industry, it was necessary for engineers to locate and correct equipment problems as early as possible in the development of aircraft and missiles. As equipment became more complex and costly, it was no longer feasible to use repeated test flights to correct design errors. The result was the development of **systems safety analysis.** Using sophisticated analytical methods, engineers were able to predict where failures or malfunctions on aircraft were likely to occur. With this information, they were able to build in back-up systems and make design changes before the initial flight.

Systems safety involves the use of technical and managerial skills to identify and control hazards, thus reducing the potential for injury or damage. Anticipating and controlling hazards at the research and development stages of a project is the key, since the cost of retrofit or modifications is extremely high when a system is in production and fully operational. Once hazards are identified and evaluated, efforts are made to eliminate or control them to keep risks at a minimum.

The systems safety management program can be separated into four parts: (1)

design and engineering, (2) operational safety controls, (3) an emergency response plan in case of accidents, and (4) accident and incident investigations.[9, 11]

To demonstrate systems safety, let's consider the development of a new aircraft. Ideally this management program should function preventively; that is, during the design and engineering phase, foreseeable hazards are carefully explored. Parts and systems of the aircraft are subjected to stress until they fail. Known as "reliability testing," this process provides engineers with important information about the dependability of the components of the aircraft. If a component proves unreliable, it is either redesigned, modified, or a back-up is added to the system. The practice of using back-up components is called "redundancy."

In the second phase of systems safety, analysis focuses on hazards that may affect the actual operation of the system (that is, the aircraft). Engineers explore how components can work together to create a problem; for example, during the test firing of an aircraft engine, problems may arise from unexpected heat stress on certain components. This may mean redesign or additional back-up components.

In spite of the efforts put into design and development, no system is risk free. All hazards might not have been identified at the design and operational testing stages, or new hazards may occur after a system has become operational. To deal with such contingencies, safety managers as a rule include an emergency response plan for the system. In our aircraft example this emergency response plan might include a pilot ejection system, on-board fire extinguishers, a special braking system, or an additional landing-gear control mechanism.

The fourth phase of the systems safety program is the accident and incident investigation. In the event of a system failure, it will be necessary to determine the cause so that appropriate action can be taken to eliminate the possibility of a recurrence of the same or similar mishap. A key point to remember is that the purpose of an accident investigation is not to place blame; its function is to prevent additional system failures.

Since the development of systems safety analysis in the early 1960s, safety personnel in other disciplines, especially industry, have developed a variety of methods for safety analysis. These techniques are useful not only for identifying factors contributing to accidents, but also for identifying hazards before an accident occurs.

Failure Mode and Effects Safety Analysis

In the systems safety model known as **failure mode and effects safety analysis,** each component or factor is evaluated on how it will affect the overall system if it fails. A failure mode and effects form is developed, which lists all the parts that make up the particular piece of equipment. Each part or component is then analyzed with respect to how it might fail, the effect its failure would have on operation of the equipment, the seriousness of the hazard that might be created, and its frequency of failure. If the analysis indicates that a particular component is likely to fail or that its failure may create serious problems, design engineers may add a back-up component or system that will take over should the primary component fail. The advantage of failure mode and effects safety analysis is that it is relatively simple to use and provides an orderly examination of the hazardous situations in a system.[11]

Once the failure modes of the components in a system have been identified and their potential effects on the system assessed, engineers can make decisions about how the various components should be treated. To identify the most serious failure modes, critical item lists (CILs) are developed. A CIL that has been used in the aerospace industry lists the following classifications[16]:

1 Failure of component—loss of life or aircraft
1R Failure of both the component and its back-up—loss of life or aircraft
2 Failure of component—loss of mission, but the crew and aircraft would be saved
2R Failure of both the component and its back-up—loss of mission, but the crew and aircraft would be saved
3 Failure of the component would not lead to serious consequences

You may wonder why all critical components with a rating of 1 do not have a back-up component (the lower the number, the more critical the part; the letter *R* means there is a back-up part). Basically, there are two reasons: (1) it may not be feasible—a second set of wings is not going to be added to your plane; and (2) the first component is "fail-safe"; that is, the component is expected to last the lifetime of the craft—the probability of failure is nearly zero.

A critical item list alerts personnel quickly that a higher than normal level of care should be used with specific components.

Fault Tree Analysis

Fault tree analysis is an accident prevention/investigation model that reasons backward from a predetermined, undesirable event, tracking the sequence of events that could possibly lead to a system failure. Fault tree analysis is particularly useful in the early design phases of new systems but is equally useful in analyzing operational systems for desired and undesired outcomes.[11, 15] Fault tree analysis enables its user to consider combinations of events leading to a given outcome; this, in turn, can indicate a variety of alternatives for solving a problem. If a number of factors have the potential for causing an undesired event, mathematical calculations can be made to determine the factor or factors most likely to precipitate the event. With this information, safety personnel can determine where interventions should be applied first.

Developed by scientists at Bell Laboratories, fault tree analysis techniques were later refined at Boeing Aircraft; the company used them to analyze possible system malfunctions in the Minuteman missile. Once vulnerable parts or processes were identified, steps were taken to improve the missile system. Information from such analyses assisted engineers in making decisions about replacing components with more durable substitutes, developing back-up or redundant devices, and instituting preventive maintenance procedures.

Let's take a look at the fault tree methodology as it was applied to a plane crash at Los Angeles International Airport (LAX). On Friday evening February 1, 1991, a landing passenger jet (US Air flight 1439) slammed into the rear end of a small commuter plane (Sky West flight 5569) that was awaiting takeoff from the same runway. A total of 34 passengers and crew members from the two planes were killed in the incident.[14]

Upon initial examination, the cause of the crash was stated as air traffic controller error; the controller had allowed two planes on the runway at the same time. However, as a fault tree analysis was developed, a number of underlying problems in the air traffic control system appeared to have added significantly to the situation:

1. The tower position which the controller occupied on the night of the crash is one of the busiest at the airport. As early as 1988 the Federal Aviation Administration (FAA) had recommended that an assistant should be assigned to assist personnel at this position. This had not been done.

2. Just prior to the crash the air traffic controller had several problems involving additional aircraft under her supervision. An airliner from a foreign country required repeated instructions as it was making an approach to LAX. Additionally, a second commuter plane (Wings West flight 5006) taxiing on the ground at a location near the runway in question inadvertently disconnected communications with the controller in

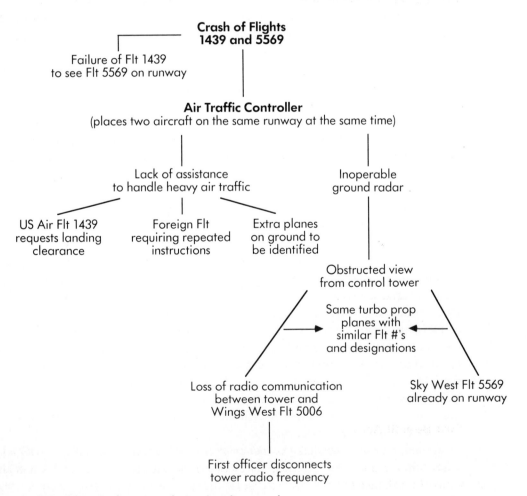

FIG. 2-5   Fault tree analysis of a plane crash.

the tower. During this critical time period, she had to attempt to reestablish contact with flight 5006, identify two other planes on the ground near the runway, and then give final clearance to flight 1439. In the confusion, Sky West flight 5569 had been told to taxi into takeoff position on the runway where flight 1439 was landing.

3. Radar used to identify planes taxiing on the ground was not operational on the night of the crash.

4. Light poles near the tower somewhat obstructed the controller's view of the runway on which the crash occurred.

5. The crew of the landing jetliner failed to see the commuter plane on the runway.

Fig. 2-5 illustrates events that were identified as underlying factors in this crash.

Management Oversight and Risk Tree

An analytical procedure that takes fault tree analysis one step further is known as **management oversight and risk tree (MORT)**. It is used to analyze accidents to determine basic and contributory causes; it is also used as an appraisal tool to evaluate existing safety programs. MORT analysis postulates that causes of an accident are attributable not only to inadequate performance, but also to a less than adequate management system.[5,7] Especially important is the management decision making that affects design, installation, maintenance, and operational practices as well as employee training in the industrial setting.[7]

Once the MORT analysis has identified a cause for an accident, a second step involves an evaluation of the management system and how it may have contributed to the accident. In a MORT investigation of foundry accidents, it was discovered that four workers had received second- and third-degree burns of the leg within a 2-week period. The initial examination indicated that injuries occurred when workers improperly ladled molten iron into molds (excessive run-off from the molds spilled down the workers' boots or onto their pants). Although protective Nomex leggings were available, none of the injured workers wore them.

Further investigation revealed that none of the workers had been trained to handle molten iron. Furthermore, only one of the workers knew of the availability of protective leggings, and she did not wear them because they only came in men's sizes. Ultimately, the post-accident investigation indicated that there had been less than adequate management support in training, supervision, and provision of safety gear. It was also determined that because the supervisors were not trained in basic emergency care, two of the injuries resulted in long-term disabilities. By using MORT analysis this company was able to identify its management weaknesses and correct them before more serious consequences resulted.

Cost-Benefit Analysis

Although cost-benefit analysis is not an actual method of accident investigation, it has become a key factor in the development of industrial safety codes and standards. In **cost-benefit analysis** the cost of changes made to increase safety are compared to the costs of accidents or illnesses resulting from exposure to uncorrected hazardous situations. If the gain in performance or safety proves to be too small to justify the cost, an otherwise desirable system or system modification may be ruled out.

The hard hat, a relatively low-cost item, has had significant influence on the construction industry. At a cost of $10 to $15 each, these devices provide maximum protection for minimal financial output—especially considering the average compensation for head injury cases is $2,945.[13]

Although it is a relatively expensive piece of equipment, $1200 per unit, the self-contained breathing apparatus (SCBA) has become standard gear for fire fighters. Most fire departments require all personnel entering a fire-involved structure to be equipped with SCBAs. Again, the cost benefit becomes quite obvious when one considers that the average cost per case for respiratory system injuries is $20,467.[17] (This high cost is the result of the disproportionate number of deaths seen in cases involving respiratory-system injuries.)

While it may be a valid way of comparing the performance of safety equipment versus cost, cost-benefit should never be the primary consideration in making decisions concerning human life.

Hazard Analysis

Hazard analysis is the identification of hazards before an accident occurs. It assesses the degree of risk in a system using quantitative measures. W. T. Fine has developed a formula for hazard evaluation[15]:

$$R = C \times E \times P$$

where R = risk score, C = potential consequences, E = exposure, and P = probability of occurrence.

Potential consequences (C) are divided according to severity into six levels, with values ranging from 100 (catastrophes) to 1 (minor cuts). Exposure (E) has six classes (from continuous or daily to remotely possible), with scores ranging from 10 to 0.1 (these numbers represent levels of exposure). The final category, probability, also has six classifications, from most likely (10) to almost impossible (0.1).

The risk score is used to compare two or more hazardous situations. Hazards with a potential for causing serious harm, but with a very low frequency of occurrence, can be detected quickly by this method.

Computer Profiles

One of the problems that has limited the effectiveness of accident investigation techniques has been an inability to show accident sequences where there are multiple contributing factors. A relatively new method is the computer profile.

The **computer profile** is a computer-generated sentence made up of several injury factors strung together in a strict format, using connecting phrases that make the sentence intelligible and show the relationship between the factors.[24] Safety personnel record such data as accident type, activity, part of body injured, and nature of injury.

Using programmed phrases such as *while, injury,* and *resulting in,* the computer takes the data and produces a sentence. An example of a profile would be the following sentence: "Struck by glass while carrying trash bag injuring leg resulting in laceration." The profiles can be expanded by programming the computer to yield more detailed information.

After data have been collected on a number of accidents, the computer can search through the profiles, enabling the safety researcher to determine how many accidents with a given combination of characteristics have occurred. The process is known as "trend analysis." If a particular sequence of events repeatedly leads to the same injury, the safety specialist would then have the opportunity to develop methodologies to interrupt the sequence, thus preventing the accidents and resulting injuries.

A variation of computer profiling is the critical incident technique. This accident research procedure is used most commonly in the reporting of unsafe acts or conditions (for example, air traffic control "near-miss" incidents). Evidence supports a significant correlation between observed unsafe behaviors and injury-producing situations; the critical incident technique can be useful in identifying hazards and developing preventive strategies.[9]

Through the use of systems engineering and computerization, the safety specialist of the 1990s has the ability to quickly and accurately identify the major hazards and contributing factors involved in a broad spectrum of accidents. With this information safety personnel are able to devote more time to the development of educational strategies and preventive measures in the field of safety.

When Systems Safety Breaks Down

Two factors affecting the decision-making process in any systems safety analysis program are cost effectiveness and timeliness of system operation.[11] If a product cannot be made cost effective, it will quickly disappear from the marketplace. Additionally, if that product or system cannot be operated or scheduled on a regular basis, it will receive minimal use and consequently show little profit for its developers.

In the systems safety model, hazards are identified, evaluated, and either eliminated or controlled to keep risk at a minimum. However, in the real world, considerable pressures are often placed on engineers and safety personnel concerning cost effectiveness and timeliness of system operation. Nowhere is this better illustrated than in the space shuttle Challenger accident of January 25, 1986.

The flight of the space shuttle Challenger (mission 51-L) began at 11:30 A.M. and ended 73 seconds later in an explosion of hydrogen and oxygen that fatally injured its seven crew members and destroyed the vehicle.[16] This was the twenty-fifth mission since the initial flight of space shuttle Columbia in March 1980 (Fig. 2-6).

Within hours after this disaster, evidence pointed to a failure of the right solid rocket booster (SRB), specifically in the area of the aft field joint. Solid rocket boosters assist the shuttle's main engines during lift-off. An SRB consists of four sections of solid fuel propellant connected at three junctures: the forward, center, and

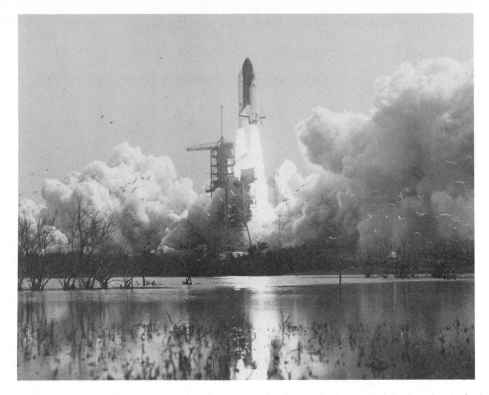

FIG. 2-6   Take-off of a space shuttle. Notice the large, dark external fuel tank to which the shuttle is attached; to the left and right of the external fuel tank are the solid rocket boosters.

(Courtesy National Aeronautics and Space Administration.)

aft field joints. Photographic and computer graphic analysis of the right SRB at the time of ignition identified a series of "puffs" of smoke coming from the aft field joint.

After several months, the presidential commission investigating the shuttle accident concluded that the cause of the Challenger explosion was the failure of the aft joint between the two lower segments of the right solid rocket booster. The failure was the result of the destruction of the seals known as "O-rings," which are intended to prevent hot gases from leaking through the joint during the propellant burn of the rocket booster.[16] The escaping hot gases burned through the SRB and the external tank that carried liquid oxygen and hydrogen to fuel the shuttle's main engines. The bottom of the solid rocket booster tore loose from its mooring to the external tank. This action allowed the SRB to swing out and puncture the top of the external tank. The ensuing mixture of liquid hydrogen and oxygen created the explosive burn that destroyed the space shuttle Challenger.

With the cause of the accident having been pinpointed to the failure of the O-rings, a detailed investigation was launched to determine just what caused their failure.

Analyses indicated a number of factors that could have contributed to the failure of the O-rings:

1. Temperature: At the time of the launch the air temperature was 36°F; 15 degrees lower than the next coldest, previous launch. Previous testing had indicated that the resiliency of the composition rubber O-rings could be affected by cold, inhibiting the O-rings' ability to properly seal the joints of the booster segments.

2. Composition of the O-rings: Not only can the composition rubber O-rings be affected by temperature, they can also be deformed by compression at lift-off, further impeding their ability to fill the gaps between the booster segments.

3. Effects of booster section reusability: Solid rocket boosters were designed for repeated use on shuttle missions, making them more cost effective. However, significant changes in the diameters of booster segments after a number of uses could affect the ability of the O-rings to seal the joints properly.

As the presidential commission's investigation continued, it was found that these critical O-ring deficiencies had existed for quite some time. It first became evident on the second shuttle flight in 1981, when significant erosion of an O-ring was discovered during a postflight examination. The National Aeronautics and Space Administration (NASA) had originally categorized the O-rings as a "criticality 1R" item, since it was theorized that the back-up O-ring would provide adequate protection, if the primary O-ring failed. (See p. 43 for a discussion of critical items lists.) However, it was found that the secondary O-rings would not always seal properly; thus in 1982, O-rings became a "criticality 1" item. This meant that the failure of the primary O-ring seal could lead to the destruction of both the crew and the shuttle. For future shuttle flights to continue, a waiver from NASA headquarters was necessary; the waiver was documented in 1983 and the shuttle missions resumed. During the next 3 years, partial failures of the primary and secondary O-rings occurred during five missions—before the Challenger accident.

The presidential commission concluded that a contributing cause of the shuttle accident was a serious flaw in the decision-making process of NASA personnel responsible for the mission. Although the successive O-ring failures indicated that a serious and potentially disastrous situation was developing, the warning was ignored. As one commission member stated, "NASA personnel accepted escalating risk apparently because they got away with it last time."[16]

Neither NASA nor the solid rocket booster manufacturer, Morton Thiokol, attempted to develop a new seal, even though the initial design seemed to be inadequate. Joint seal failure became an acceptable flight risk at a time when considerable pressure was being placed on the shuttle program to become a timely and cost-efficient operation.

As shuttle managers came to believe that the space missions were a routine operation, safety, reliability, and quality assurance programs were reduced. This error in judgment compounded the situation by forcing fewer individuals to monitor more operations in a highly experimental system. Decreasing attention to systems safety was, ultimately, NASA's biggest mistake.

After the presidential commission's final report, NASA established a new Office of Safety, Reliability, and Quality Assurance which is responsible for reporting and documenting problems, problem resolution, and trends associated with flight safety. NASA engineers also initiated a review of all critical item lists to identify the components that were to be improved before the next shuttle mission to ensure the highest degree of flight safety.

On September 29, 1988, the space shuttle *Discovery* was successfully launched after a 2-year period of redesign by NASA engineers. Three features have been added to increase the safety of the solid rocket boosters. At each field joint on the solid rocket boosters, a metal lip has been added to lock the sections tightly together. A third O-ring has been added to the two already located at each joint. And heating units have been incorporated into the design to keep O-ring temperatures at a minimum of 75°F, thus ensuring their ability to properly seal the joints of each SRB segment.[18]

As flights continue through the 1990s, NASA engineers and managers will carefully monitor the shuttle's progress. Crew safety will remain their ultimate responsibility.

SUMMARY

Statistical data are used to determine problem areas, develop educational strategies in safety, and develop safer equipment and facilities. Descriptive statistics are used to present information concerning the characteristics of groups. Inferential statistics are used to make predictions and estimations about a large population by using data from a sample population.

An important decision for safety researchers is how to present statistical material in a clear and orderly fashion. Numerical methods of presentation include frequency distributions, percentages, and rates. The use of frequency distributions is an efficient way to present large amounts of data. This is accomplished by compiling the information in several ordered classes. Percentages convert the numbers to proportions and are used to illustrate changes over time.

Graphic methods such as the histogram, frequency polygon, and pie chart are used to present data in a readily understandable and usable form. The ease of viewing information with these methods enables the observer to make rapid comparisons of data.

Two factors must be considered when evaluating statistical material: validity and reliability of the data. *Validity* refers to the accuracy of the information. *Reliability* refers to how closely observations or reports match one another. Some of the more valid and reliable sources of safety statistics include the National Safety Council, the National Center for Health Statistics, and the National Criminal Justice Reference Service.

A reduction of accidental deaths would have a greater effect on the average life span of Americans than would cures for cancer or heart disease. With this in mind, safety researchers have developed a number of sophisticated analytical methods to investigate accidents.

Failure mode and effects safety analysis, fault tree analysis, and hazard analysis are analytic methods used to determine the causes of accidents and identify hazards that may lead to accidents. These methods are based on the systems approach. When one or more of the system's components fails, an accident or malfunction may result. As we proceed into the 1990s, systems research and computerization will play an important role in reducing accidents in America.

Key Terms

Computer profile   Shows the sequence of an accident that has multiple contributing factors.

Cost-benefit analysis   The cost of changes made to increase safety are compared to the costs of accidents or illnesses resulting from exposure to the uncorrected hazardous situation. (This is not an actual method of accident investigation.)

Descriptive statistics   Inform the reader about the characteristics of a particular group; a factual report of what has occurred.

Failure mode and effects safety analysis   Each component is evaluated on how it will affect the overall system should it fail.

Fault tree analysis   Used after an accident occurs; traces the initial cause or causes of an accident.

Frequency distributions   An efficient way of presenting a large amount of data by grouping them in several classes.

Hazard analysis   Involves the identification of hazards before an accident occurs.

Inferential statistics   Consist of estimations, generalizations, or predictions about a particular group.

Management oversight and risk tree (MORT)   An evaluation of a company's management system and how it may have contributed to an accident.

Percentage   A part of the whole expressed as a decimal.

Rates   Percentages based on a particular population; they are usually based on the figure per 100,000 population.

Reliability   A measure of how closely a series of observations of the same thing match one another.

Specific death rate   The number of deaths that occur in a given year per 100,000 persons in a particular population.

System   An orderly arrangement of components that are interrelated and that act and interact to perform some task or function in a particular environment.

Systems safety analysis   Techniques that identify the factors contributing to an accident and also identify major hazards before an accident occurs.

Validity   A measure of how closely the data corresponds to the actual state of affairs.

References

1. Broyles, R. W., and Lay, C. M.: Statistics in health administration, vol. 1, Rockville, Md., 1979, Aspen Systems Corp.
2. Centers for Disease Control: Premature mortality due to unintentional injuries—United States, Morbidity and Mortality Weekly Report 36(49), 1987.
3. Gelinas, C. G.: Computerized system tracks toxic vapor releases, National Safety News 131(4): 42, 1985.
4. Graitcer, P. L.: The development of state and local injury surveillance systems, Journal of Safety Research 18(4): 191-198, 1987.
5. Hickey, J. M.: MORT provides disciplined method of analyzing accidents, Research and Development Newsletter of the National Safety Council, Feb. 1978, p. 1.
6. Huchingson, R. D.: New horizons for human factors in design, New York, 1981, McGraw-Hill Book Co.

7. Johnson, R. D.: Simplifying M.O.R.T. for supervisors, National Safety News 130(3):71, 1984.

8. Mausner, J. S., and Bahn, A. K.: Epidemiology: an introductory text, Philadelphia, 1974, W. B. Saunders Co.

9. McCormick, E. J., and Sanders, M. S.: Human factors in engineering and design, ed. 5, New York, 1982, McGraw-Hill Book Co.

10. Mendenhall, W.: Introduction to probability and statistics, ed. 4, North Seltuate, Mass., 1975, Duxbury Press.

11. Moriarty, B., and Roland, H. E.: System safety engineering and management, New York, 1983, John Wiley & Sons, Inc.

12. National Safety Council: Accident facts—1986 ed., Chicago, Stock No. 021.65, 1986.

13. National Safety Council: Accident facts—1990 ed., Chicago, 1990.

14. Phillips, D.: Woes of modern aviation underlie crash in L.A., The Washington Post, Feb. 5, 1991, p. A-4.

15. Ramsey, J. D.: Identification of contributory factors in occupational injury, Journal of Safety Research, Dec. 1973, p. 260.

16. Report of the presidential commission on the space shuttle Challenger accident, vols. 1-5, Washington, D.C., 1986.

17. Rice, D. P., MacKenzie, E. J., and associates: Cost of injury in the United States: a report to congress, San Francisco, Calif., 1989, Institute for Health and Aging, University of California and Injury Prevention Center, The Johns Hopkins University.

18. Sawyer, K.: NASA plans to test-fire shuttle booster today, The Washington Post, Aug. 27, 1987, p. A-3.

19. The National Committee for Injury Prevention and Control: Injury prevention: meeting the challenge, American Journal of Preventive Medicine 5(3), 1989.

20. United States Consumer Product Safety Commission: The national electronic injury surveillance system (NEISS), Washington, D.C., 1986, U.S. Government Printing Office.

21. United States Department of Health and Human Services: Vital statistics report: final mortality statistics, 1989, Washington, D.C., 1990, U.S. Government Printing Office.

22. U.S. Department of Justice, Bureau of Justice Statistics: The risk of violent crime, Washington, D.C., 1986.

23. U.S. Department of Justice, Bureau of Justice Statistics: Violent crime in the United States, Washington, D.C., 1986.

24. Waring, A. E.: Computers in safety, National Safety and Health News 134(1):40, 1986.

Resource Organizations

Consumer Product Safety Commission
1111 Eighteenth Street N.W.
Washington, DC 20207

National Center for Health Statistics
3700 East-West Highway
Hyattsville, MD 20782

National Criminal Justice Reference Service
Box 6000
Rockville, MD 20850

National Injury Information Clearinghouse
Room 625
5401 Westbard Avenue
Washington, DC 20207

National Safety Management Society
3871 Piedmont Avenue
Oakland, CA 94611

Veterans of Safety
203 North Wabash Avenue, Suite 2206
Chicago, IL 60601

CHAPTER 2

Applying What You Have Learned

1. Cite examples of descriptive and inferential statistics that could have been used in the investigation of the Bhopal, India toxic chemical release.

a.)   Descriptive statistics: _____

_____

b.)   Inferential statistics: _____

_____

2. How would you apply the four steps of a systems safety management program during construction of a nuclear power plant?

a.)   Design and engineering: _____

_____

b.)   Operational safety controls: _____

_____

c.)   Emergency response plan: _____

_____

d.)   Accident and incident investigations: _____

_____

3. Using a cost-benefit analysis strategy, determine the feasibility of hiring a full-time weight room supervisor for your university's recreation center.   _____

_____

_____

_____

_____

_____

3 When An Emergency Occurs

Strategies that will most effectively and most immediately reduce injury losses require a community or societal approach.

The Trauma Foundation: Report of the Injury Prevention and Health Policy Colloquium

Regardless of the precautions one takes, a breakdown is always possible in the performance of a given activity, resulting in injury or property damage. Should an emergency arise, would you know what to do or whom to call? The first person to reach the scene of an emergency should be able to assess the victims' conditions, contact the proper authorities, and give the appropriate emergency care until help arrives. In this chapter we will discuss some of the basic guidelines for responding to an emergency.

BASIC GUIDELINES FOR THE FIRST RESPONDER

Since the passage of the Highway Safety Act in 1966, the United States Department of Transportation has been actively involved in the updating of emergency medical services throughout the country. Sophisticated organizational structures of emergency care have been developed in most states; these include trauma centers, special systems of patient transport, and paramedic or advanced life-support training for personnel.

No matter how sophisticated the system becomes, it must be activated by persons in the general public. It has become increasingly important for the lay person, or first responder, to be able to recognize an emergency situation and to know how to activate emergency medical service systems; that is, to contact the appropriate authorities such as ambulance services and fire and police departments.

The **first responder** is the person who, after arriving at the scene of an emergency, initiates care or assistance for the victim or victims.* The emergency situation may include illness, injury, or property damage, resulting from an accident or criminal action.

The first person to arrive at the emergency scene has three basic responsibilities:

1. To assess the situation, including the victim's condition
2. To render emergency care (if appropriately trained)
3. To activate the emergency medical service system

In some instances, the action of the first responder may be limited because the situation can be effectively handled by the victims or their families. Other cases may require the rescuer to take a broad range of actions. Probably the most important actions taken by the first responder are assessment or evaluation of the emergency and contacting the proper authorities. These actions may be as simple as noticing suspicious people in your neighborhood and contacting the police; they may include evaluating the injuries of an auto accident victim, giving first aid, and calling rescue personnel.

Perhaps the most important function of the first responder is to alert the personnel who can best provide assistance at the emergency site. However, before doing this, the first responder must make a number of quick observations:

1. What has happened?
2. Are there any injuries?
3. If so, what are they?
4. What emergency care procedures should be used with the victims?

The best way to answer these questions is to use a rapid evaluation process known as the "cursory exam." A first responder can complete this process in less than 2 minutes. With information from the cursory exam, he or she can give authorities an accurate picture of the emergency. This allows them to respond more rapidly and with the appropriate equipment and personnel.

The box on pp. 58-62 outlines the basic steps that should be taken by a first responder.

Contacting the Proper Authorities

Having obtained information at the scene about the kind of emergency, the number of persons involved, and their conditions, the first responder must decide whom to call for further assistance.

Knowing whom to call in an emergency can save valuable time, and may be the difference between victim survival and nonsurvival. The process for activating emergency services varies across the United States. In many areas a single phone number

---

*Although this is not a first aid text, we strongly feel that the basic emergency care training offered by the American Red Cross, the American Heart Association, the National Safety Council, and the U.S. Department of Transportation's First Responder Training Program is essential for everyone. All assessment and emergency care procedures described in this text follow the guidelines of the above organizations.

is used to reach a variety of emergency services. Most major metropolitan areas use the 911 number for contacting police, fire, and rescue services. All calls on the 911 line go to a central dispatcher who determines what emergency service is needed. It is hoped that one day 911 will be the only number needed to activate emergency services anywhere in the country.

At present, not all localities use the 911 system. Some communities have different telephone numbers for fire, police, and ambulance services, whereas others use a single telephone number (not 911) for all emergency services. When people move to a new community, they should familiarize themselves with the local system for contacting emergency authorities. To aid in this process, many communities provide stickers which list emergency numbers and which can be affixed to the telephone or to surfaces near the phone. Once the decision has been made to activate the emergency system and the proper authorities have been contacted, the next step is to communicate pertinent information to emergency personnel.

Making an emergency call. The following details should be supplied when making an emergency phone call:

1. Give your name and the exact location of the incident. This information is essential to activate the system.

2. Describe the problem, how many people were involved, and your assessment of their conditions. Indicate any treatment you may have administered.

3. Give the dispatcher the telephone number from which you are calling. This will allow people at the emergency center to call back if they need more information.

4. Do not hang up until the emergency personnel do. This is more likely to ensure that all information has been correctly recorded.

A number of major metropolitan areas now have **Enhanced 911**, a computerized phone system that automatically provides the addresses of callers to emergency operations personnel. When an emergency dispatcher answers the phone, he or she sees the address of the caller on a video display screen. This enables emergency personnel to respond more rapidly and accurately.

The system has been further refined by the development of computerized street maps. Some fire and police departments now have on-board video display terminals in all emergency vehicles. When a fire or police unit is notified of an emergency, personnel can punch the address into the computer and a detailed street map will appear on the video display. This saves valuable minutes in response time.

Legal Liability

A recent review of court cases found that no certified first responder who used established procedures for treatment of an ill or injured person has ever been successfully sued. Nevertheless, people are reluctant to offer help at an emergency scene because they are afraid of being sued, when, in fact, such suits are rare. The key to protection for a first responder is that he or she act in a reasonably prudent manner. This can be accomplished if the person follows established treatment procedures listed in emergency care manuals such as those of the American Red Cross and does

Text continued on p. 63.

The Cursory Exam

Information From the Scene

After arriving at the emergency scene, you need to carefully check the area to determine what has happened. This is known as "looking for the mechanism of injury." Skid marks may indicate that a person was the victim of a hit-and-run accident. The presence of a ladder may indicate the victim has fallen. Torn clothing or emptied contents of a wallet or purse may indicate a robbery or assault.

Witnesses can give valuable information. They may be able to describe how the incident occurred, whether the victim or victims have been moved from their original positions, or whether anyone else was involved.

Before attempting to work with any victims, the rescuer needs to make sure the area is free of hazards such as downed power lines, a vehicle with the motor still running, or a mugger looking for other victims. If the hazard endangers your life, wait for emergency personnel who have the appropriate equipment to make a safe rescue. Each year many would-be rescuers lose their lives when they touch downed electrical lines, are overcome by toxic fumes and smoke, or are hit by motor vehicles while attempting to provide assistance.

Illness/Injury Assessment

Unless it is necessary to move victims for safety reasons, assess the extent of their injuries in the position in which you find them.

If you find the victim of a motor vehicle accident still in his car, examine him where he is sitting or lying. It is unwise to move the victim unless there is a danger of fire or the possibility that another vehicle might strike the car. Rescue personnel are more skilled at extricating and moving victims and have equipment specially designed for this purpose. Consequently, they should take that responsibility, not the first responder.

The actual cursory exam of the victim should take approximately 90 seconds and proceed in a head-to-foot direction. The assessment consists of the following steps:

Patient response. Determine responsiveness by talking to the patient or gently shaking and tapping him on the shoulders. Unresponsiveness or confusion in the victim may indicate a possible head injury. The examination is made easier if the victim is coherent and can speak (Fig. 3-1,A).

Determining responsiveness, checking breathing and pulse

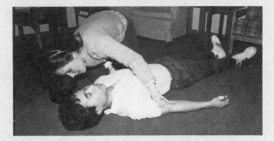

FIG. 3-1 A, Talk to the victim while gently shaking his shoulders. Be sure to hold the arms down firmly; an incoherent victim may unintentionally strike the rescuer.

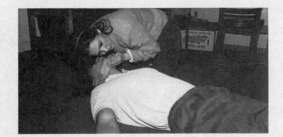

FIG. 3-1 B, Open the airway by using the head tilt–chin lift method. (Look, listen, and feel for respiratory movement.)

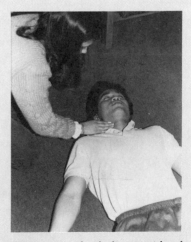

FIG. 3-1 C, Check the carotid pulse.

Airway, breathing, and circulation. Check breathing by hyperextending the head and neck to open the airway; then look, listen, and feel for respiratory movement. While tilting the head back using the chin-lift method (Fig. 3-1, B), the rescuer looks at the chest and abdomen of the victim for signs of respiratory movement. At the same time, with her ear directly over the victim's nose and mouth, the first responder listens for signs of breathing. Even if a victim's breathing is weak, the first responder will be able to feel the victim's expelled breath with her ear.

After checking breathing, palpate the victim's carotid pulse; this can be done easily from this position (Fig. 3-1, C). (When we use the words *palpation* or *palpate* in our discussion of the cursory exam, we are referring to a process of touching with light fingertip pressure.)

A lack of respiration or pulse is a true emergency and resuscitative efforts should be initiated—if you know how to perform them. If you do not possess these skills, emergency personnel must be contacted immediately. When breathing and pulse are present, the examination can continue.

Check for severe bleeding. Any significant blood loss (clothing soaked with blood or pooling of blood around the victim) must be controlled immediately. The average adult has 5 to 6 quarts of blood in his or her circulatory system. An adult may lose a pint of blood with little or no effect; however, the loss of a quart of blood or approximately 20% of the body's blood supply is considered serious.

Examination of the head area. Examination of the head includes observations of the eyes, ears, nose, and mouth. If the victim is conscious, observe the pupils. If they are enlarged or dilated, this may indicate shock. If the pupils are unequal in size, a head injury is likely. Do not attempt to examine the eyes of an unconscious person.

Check the mouth for possible trauma or bleeding. Burns around the mouth and strong odors coming from the oral cavity may indicate ingestion of a poison. While examining the mouth, look for possible obstructions.

In the examination of the ears and nose, the rescuer is looking for blood or cerebrospinal fluid discharge. The appearance of this type of fluid may indicate a head injury.

Thoroughly check the head and scalp area for lumps or depressions that may be the result of a head injury. At the same time, check the cervical vertebrae to determine whether there are any deformities in the neck. A deformity in this region may indicate a fracture or dislocation of the cervical spine (see Figs. 3-1, D and E).

Examination of the head area

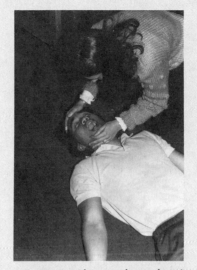

FIG. 3-1 D, Observe the oral cavity.

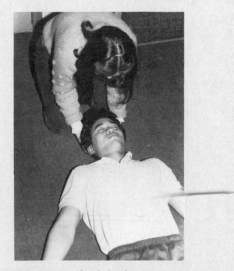

FIG. 3-1 E, Check for lumps or depressions in the skull and examine the scalp and cervical vertebrae.

Continued.

The Cursory Exam—cont'd

Examination of the thorax, arms, and abdomen. The thorax is the part of the body between the neck and diaphragm and is encased by the ribs.[4] Feel the clavicles (collarbones) and sternum (breastbone) for any deformities. Quickly palpate the area of the rib cage for lumps or deformities. A further test of the rib area is to push in gently on both sides of the rib cage. Because broken bone ends scraping together make a grating sound known as "crepitus," this is an indication that ribs have been fractured. To check the back and thoracic spine, the rescuer should move one hand from the base of the neck downward and the other from the small of the back upward. In this manner, most of the vertebrae can be examined with limited movement of the victim.

Both arms should be examined for obvious deformities and swelling. If the victim is conscious, ask him to move his arms, hands, and fingers. Also check the victim's grip strength and ability to push or pull with his arms. Weakness may indicate some kind of neurological damage.

The abdomen may be divided into quadrants for the purpose of examination. The navel should be considered the dividing line or midpoint of the quadrants. As you gently feel each of the quadrants, check for abnormal masses or abdominal rigidity. These conditions indicate serious internal injury. Again, if the patient is conscious, he will be able to tell you where it hurts and how much pain he feels (see Figs. 3-1, F to J).

While examining the thorax, arms, and abdomen, check for a Medic Alert tag (a necklace or bracelet that contains important medical information about its wearer).

Examination of the pelvic girdle and lower extremities. The pelvic girdle is examined in much the same way as the rib cage. Steady inward compression of the hip and pelvic area will allow the rescuer to notice any instability in this region. Crepitus from this inward pressure would also denote possible fracture damage.

Each leg should be examined for deformities and swelling. If the patient is conscious, ask him to move and bend each leg if possible. Also check for leg strength by allowing him to push or pull with his legs against your hands. Weakness in the lower extremities may indicate neurological damage. If the patient is unconscious, a simple check for possible spinal damage is to prick the sole of the foot with a sharp object. A lack of reflex movement in the foot may indicate a spinal injury. Figs. 3-1, K to M illustrate these body survey procedures.

Examination of the thorax, arms, and abdomen.

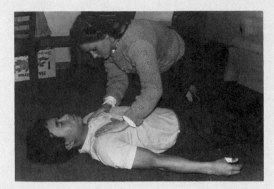

FIG. 3-1 F, Check the shoulders and collarbones for deformities.

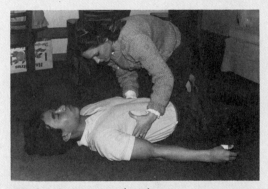

FIG. 3-1 G, Examine the ribs.

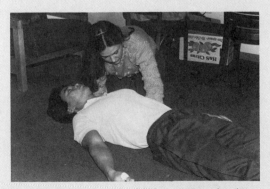

FIG. 3-1 H, Check the back and spinal column.

Examination of the pelvic girdle and lower extremities

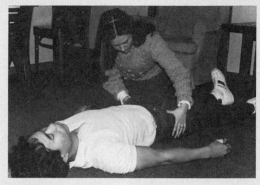

FIG. 3-1 K, Check for instability of the pelvic girdle.

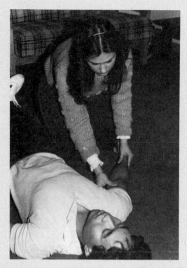

FIG. 3-1 I, Check for swelling or deformity in the arms.

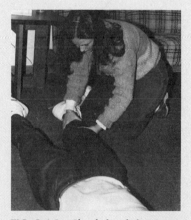

FIG. 3-1 L, Check for deformity or swelling in the legs.

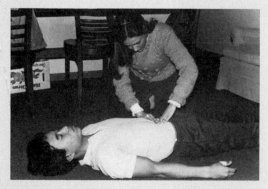

FIG. 3-1 J, Palpate the abdomen for abnormal masses or rigidity.

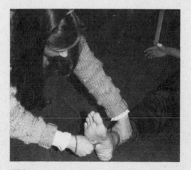

FIG. 3-1 M, Use a sharp object (here a housekey) to check for reflex movement of the foot.

Continued.

The Cursory Exam—cont'd

Review of the Cursory Exam

Following is a list of the basic steps that should be taken by a first responder using the cursory exam at the scene of an emergency:

1. After arriving at the emergency scene, carefully look over the area to determine what has happened.

2. After locating victims, begin assessment of injuries. Do not move victims unless there is a life-threatening situation.

3. Determine the victim's level of responsiveness or state of consciousness.

4. Open the airway and look, listen, and feel for respiratory movement.

5. Check the carotid pulse to determine cardiac function.

6. Inspect the area around the victim for noticeable blood loss.

7. Examine the head region: skull, eyes, ears, nose, mouth, and neck.
   a. Eyes—check for dilated or unequal pupils.
   b. Ears and nose—check for blood or cerebrospinal fluid discharge.
   c. Mouth—check for bleeding and obstructions.
   d. Skull—feel for depressions or lumps.
   e. Neck—check for deformities in cervical spine.

8. Examine thorax, arms, and abdomen.
   a. Thorax—palpate or feel for lumps or deformities.
      (1) Gently push on rib cage and listen for crepitus.
      (2) Check for deformities in the spinal column.
   b. Arms—examine for obvious deformities or swelling. If victim is conscious, check grip strength and arm movement.
   c. Abdomen—palpate for abnormal masses or rigidity.

9. Examine pelvic girdle and lower extremities.
   a. Pelvic girdle—while applying gentle pressure, listen for crepitus and observe for instability.
   b. Lower extremities—examine for deformities or swelling. If victim is conscious, check movement and leg strength. Stimulate soles of the feet to test for possible spinal damage.

**As you continue through the succeeding chapters in this text, a number of medical emergencies will be addressed. To assist you in gaining a better understanding of what you can do in these situations, key treatment protocols and emergency care procedures have been described and illustrated in Appendix A, p. 461.

not attempt to administer treatment beyond his or her level of skill. If a rescuer invents his or her own procedures for treating a problem, negligence might be proved.

To assist persons willing to help others in times of need, most states have enacted **Good Samaritan laws.** (See the box below.) These laws were originally designed to protect medical personnel (for example, doctors, ambulance personnel, and nurses) who stopped at an emergency and gave assistance free of charge. Recently these laws have been amended to protect the lay person who stops to assist in an emergency.

Basically, the Good Samaritan law states that no one who attempts to aid the victim of an emergency can be held liable for increasing the victim's injuries, provided the rescuer acted in a reasonable manner, did not charge for services rendered, and did not intentionally or willfully attempt to increase the victim's injuries.

The following are general guidelines for the first responder:

1. Although the general public is under no legal obligation to assist an injured person, there is a moral or humanitarian obligation to the community that transcends legality. If you were in trouble or hurt, wouldn't you want someone to stop and give you a hand? The only time a lay person is legally obliged to offer assistance is when he or she has been directly responsible for the injury-causing situation. In most states the party responsible for an automobile accident is required to stay at the scene and render aid, if possible.

Public Law No. 447 (H.1719.)*

An act to amend IC 1971, 34-4-12 concerning the rendering of first aid or emergency care at scenes of accidents or emergencies.

Be it enacted by the General Assembly of the State of Indiana.

Section 1. IC 1971, 34-4-12-1 (formerly Acts 1963, c.319, s.1) is amended to read as follows: Sec. 1. Any person, who in good faith gratuitously renders emergency care at the scene of an accident or emergency care to the victim thereof, shall not be liable for any civil damages for any personal injury as a result of any act or omission by such person in rendering the emergency care or as a result of any act or failure to act to provide or arrange for further medical treatment or care for the injured person, except acts or omissions amounting to gross negligence or willful or wanton misconduct.

Section 2. No act or omission of any person who has successfully completed a course of training in cardiopulmonary resuscitation according to the standards recommended by the Division of Medical Sciences, National Academy of Sciences, National Research Council, while attempting to administer cardiopulmonary resuscitation, without pecuniary charge, to any person who is an apparent victim of acute cardiopulmonary insufficiency shall impose any liability upon the person so attempting the resuscitation: Provided, however, that this chapter shall not apply to acts or omissions amounting to gross negligence or willful or wanton misconduct.

---

*Good Samaritan laws of the State of Indiana

2. In certain occupations (police, fire fighters, emergency medical technicians, physicians, nurses, or paramedics), whether the individual is on or off duty, he or she must administer emergency care to the public. Teachers are also legally obliged to render first aid to students in the school setting. (The legal obligations of teachers and coaches will be addressed in Chapter 11.)

3. Once a rescuer has voluntarily started care, he or she should not leave the scene or stop care until a qualified and responsible person (for example, ambulance personnel) relieves him or her. An exception to this rule is when there is a lone rescuer who must briefly leave the scene to call for additional assistance.

4. The rescuer should follow recognized emergency care procedures and should never attempt treatments that are above his or her level of ability.

5. The first responder should never force treatment on anyone except in the case of a life-threatening emergency (cardiac arrest, severe bleeding, poisoning). In an emergency where a victim is unconscious or there is a significant risk of death, the law assumes that the patient would agree to treatment. This is known as **implied consent.**

The law will go out of its way to protect the first responder who follows the above guidelines and does his or her best under the circumstances. The legal system, after all, attempts to reflect the thinking and morality of the community.

HELPERS AND THEIR RESPONSIBILITIES

Not only is it essential to know how to evaluate an emergency and how to call for help, it is as important to know whom to call. A study of rescue services in Cambridge, Massachusetts found that as many as 25% of the persons who called for help had delayed for at least 15 minutes. The major reasons for these delays were either not knowing what to do or being unsure of whom to call.[15] Given the importance of rapid intervention in a potential crisis, the causes of lengthy delays in decision making are of particular interest. Confusion about the seriousness of the emergency, the appropriate action to take, and reluctance to use emergency services unnecessarily have been identified as significant factors that contribute to these delays.

Several steps were suggested that could facilitate the public's decision making in regard to contacting emergency service personnel. One approach, addressed earlier in this chapter, was the installation of a single, direct, highly publicized emergency telephone number. A second approach, is the use of detailed public education programs to inform the community about available emergency personnel and the services they render.

Law Enforcement: Local, State, and Federal

Why is a description of police agencies included in a safety text? Because safety entails those efforts made to ensure personal security and protection of property from deliberate and nondeliberate acts of violence or destruction.

The two agencies that most people think of when law enforcement is mentioned are **city police** and **county sheriffs' departments.** City or municipal police officers are responsible for enforcing the laws of the city and state within the geographical confines of the city. However, the city police officer has authority anywhere in the state and beyond state lines, if he is in pursuit of a felon.

Although sheriff's department officers have jurisdictional rights in cities, their major responsibility is in the unincorporated areas of the county. As with city officers, the sheriff's deputies have authority statewide. Duties of most county sheriffs' departments include providing bailiffs for the courts, maintaining county jail facilities, and transporting prisoners. In certain instances these officers will be responsible for enforcing health and safety, building, and professional codes as well.

Not only do police officers enforce the law, they may also be called upon to render emergency care at the scene of an accident or, from time to time, psychological counseling in a family or domestic dispute. If you live within the city limits, it is a good idea to have the city police number posted in a prominent place near the phone. If you are involved in an accident or are the victim of a crime, the city police will be the primary responders. If you are outside the city limits, you will use the number for the county sheriff's department.

At the state level, either the **state police** or the **highway patrol** is the major law enforcement agency. The primary responsibility of these agencies is to enforce the vehicle codes of the state and to investigate accidents occurring on state roads and interstate highways. Because state police officers may have enforcement responsibilities in a number of adjacent counties, they often work closely with county sheriffs' departments. It is not uncommon to have both state troopers and county police responding to a highway accident.

Most federal agencies such as the Federal Bureau of Investigation (FBI), Secret Service, Drug Enforcement Administration, and Customs Service have specifically outlined responsibilities; only in rare cases would any of these organizations be in a position to act as first responders at a crime scene. Their work is more investigative in nature and closely follows federal rather than state or local guidelines.

A federal agency that may become involved in the enforcement of state and local codes is the United States Marshal's Office. The major responsibilities of deputy marshals are to transport prisoners to and from federal courts and prisons, provide protection for witnesses at federal trials and for visiting officials from other nations, and to act as bailiffs in federal courts.[14] However, U.S. marshals may enforce local or state codes when they have been violated on federal property lying within the jurisdiction of the specific locality.

In terms of providing personal protection and immediate victim assistance to the public, municipal police, county sheriffs' departments, and the state police or highway patrol are usually the agencies involved.

Fire Protection Services

Many people have a rather narrow view of the function of local **fire protection services.** Although it requires positive and often dramatic action, fire fighting is only one of the roles of fire service personnel. Other important functions of fire departments include inspection of public buildings and residential dwellings, enforcement of building and fire codes, fire prevention education and public relations, and fire investigation.

Building inspections and fire codes. In their inspections of public facilities and buildings under construction, fire service personnel concentrate on two areas: (1) design and installation violations and (2) the use of hazardous materials, processes, or machinery in the finished structure. Buildings are generally inspected on a priority basis, with target properties (those structures that present special hazards) receiving the most attention. Oil and chemical plants, schools, hotels, and nursing homes would be considered target properties. Violations of the building and fire codes may result in fines or possibly the closing of a building that has major deficiencies.

The inspection of residential dwellings is usually extended to the community as a courtesy. Unlike public building inspections, where violations must be corrected immediately, home inspections are carried out without threat to the owner. Although fire inspectors suggest ways to correct fire hazards, it is left to the discretion of the homeowner to correct the problem.

Fire prevention education and public relations. A large part of fire prevention education and public relations is to develop public awareness and secure community cooperation in maintaining safe conditions. An inspection program offered to home-owners is an excellent means of establishing a rapport between fire service personnel and the community. The fire department public relations officer can enhance the image of the department by carefully explaining the responsibilities and duties of fire fighters to the public.

Once the public becomes familiar with the role of the fire department in the community, fire service personnel can concentrate on their primary duty—to prevent loss of life and property from fire. Fire prevention education has resulted in a measurable decrease in fire losses and in greater safety.

Fire investigation. Although fire investigation is primarily the responsibility of the state fire marshal's office, it is not uncommon for local authorities to do much of this work and data collection after a fire. Fire investigation is the basis from which methods of fire prevention and protection are developed.

These investigations are the primary means of arson detection. Arson investigation has become highly specialized and requires long hours of training for the fire personnel who work in this area; the equipment used by arson investigators is very technical and complex.

Fire investigation also plays an important role in determining fire damage. An assessment of fire damage by the investigating officer can help to ensure that a homeowner receives an equitable insurance settlement. By accurately estimating fire losses, the investigating personnel can also help to hold the line on insurance costs in the community.

Today's fire fighters inspect buildings and must, accordingly, have some knowledge of engineering principles and building design. They educate the public about fire prevention and must, therefore, have a background in teaching methodology. Finally, they are investigators who must have a thorough knowledge of hazardous materials, fire ignition, patterns of spread, and damage estimation.

Emergency Medical and Rescue Services

Before 1966, prehospital emergency medical care was a haphazard operation in most states. Services were provided by private corporations, funeral directors, hospitals, volunteer organizations, and local governments. There was little coordination or standardization of emergency medical services from community to community. Many sections of the country were dependent on ambulance services that provided, almost exclusively, patient transportation with little or no victim-care capability.

The Highway Safety Act of 1966 requires states to have a highway safety program developed with uniform standards set by the United States Department of Transportation. The act includes a section entitled "Emergency medical services," which established minimum federal standards for personnel training, equipment, communications, and operational coordination of ambulance services.[18]

From this legislation developed the **emergency medical technician (EMT)** training program. An EMT is a paraprofessional emergency specialist trained to provide life-sustaining care and transportation for patients outside the hospital setting. The training consists of approximately 80 to 100 hours of classroom instruction, demonstrations, and in-hospital emergency-room training.

The EMT training stresses six major areas of skill development: (1) cardiopulmonary resuscitation, (2) patient assessment, (3) mechanical aids used in treating breathing difficulties, (4) splinting, (5) bandaging, and (6) patient transport.[5] These measures are called "basic life support skills" because they are used to maintain or stabilize the patient's condition.

Since the passage of the Highway Safety Act, medical researchers have become aware of the importance of rapid identification and evaluation of emergency patients. In most cases an emergency patient receives initial evaluation and treatment from an EMT. Rarely is a physician the first person to work with an ill or injured individual in an emergency setting; therefore, the EMT's ability to evaluate the patient and stabilize his or her condition can often be the difference between life and death.

A further development in prehospital emergency care has been the introduction of paramedic service. **Paramedics** are emergency specialists qualified to deliver advanced life support in an emergency situation. Advanced life support has been defined as care given at the scene of an accident or illness, during transport, or at the hospital, which is more advanced than that usually rendered by an emergency medical technician. Specific skills performed by paramedics that are beyond the scope of EMT training are (1) defibrillation, (2) endotracheal intubation, (3) administration of appropriate medications, (4) cardiac monitoring, and (5) intravenous therapy.[8] Paramedic instruction consists of anywhere from 150 to as many as 1000 hours of training in addition to previous EMT certification.

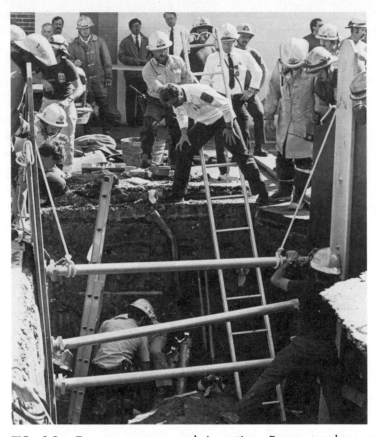

FIG. 3-2   Emergency personnel in action. Rescue workers spent nearly 2 hours removing the two victims of this construction cave-in. Notice how they reinforced the excavation site to prevent further shifting of the soil.

(Courtesy Fairfax County Fire and Rescue Department, Fairfax, Va.)

The paramedic is an extension of the physician in the field. Through the use of telemetry equipment and two-way radio contact with paramedics, the emergency-room physician (at the hospital) is able to make a diagnosis and prescribe definitive therapy for the patient at the scene. The paramedic carries out the physician's orders. Under certain conditions, such as cardiac arrest, immediate action is required, and the paramedic is allowed to perform a number of advanced life-support skills before contacting the emergency physician. Recent studies show that as many as 20% of the deaths resulting from cardiac arrest could be prevented if the patient received prompt emergency care from well-trained medical specialists.[20]

The third member of the emergency medical and rescue team is the rescue or extrication specialist. Although they are likely to have received EMT training, their major function is not patient care, but seeing that emergency medical personnel can gain access to the patient. It may be as simple as opening a door, or as difficult as cutting off the roof of a vehicle and bending the steering column forward to gain access to the victim. After emergency treatment has been initiated by an EMT or paramedic, the next concern of the rescue specialist is removal of the victim to a more stable location. A knowledge of mechanics and experience in using the specialty tools of rescue work are essential to protect the victim from further injury (Fig. 3-2). In most cases these specialists are associated with a fire department because many of the tools used at an accident site can also be used at the scene of a fire.

The emergency medical and rescue team consists of EMTs, paramedics, and fire rescue specialists. All three groups are often associated with volunteer and paid fire departments. The ambulances and rescue vehicles are stationed at firehouses throughout the district they cover. Another method of personnel and vehicle placement consists of stationing EMTs and paramedics at local hospitals, while the rescue crews continue to operate from the firehouses.

SUMMARY

Even in the safest enviroments, there is a chance that someone may be injured. Prevention is an important aspect of safety; however, it is also important for an individual to know what to do in an emergency.

The public is not legally obliged to help persons in distress; it is a moral obligation that transcends legality. Most states have enacted "Good Samaritan laws" to protect first responders from legal liability. The only exception is when negligence or willful misconduct has occurred on the part of the rescuer.

In an emergency, one of the first things a rescuer should do is evaluate the situation; this includes determining what has happened as well as assessing injuries or property damage. With this information the first responder can decide whether assistance is needed; it is important for the rescuer to know whom to call and how to report concisely what has happened.

The three services most often called in an emergency are the police, fire, and emergency medical and rescue services. These organizations have specific responsibilities in the community.

The most widely used law enforcement agencies are municipal police, county sheriffs' departments, and the state police or highway patrol.

Fire department personnel do more than fight fires. They are actively involved in fire prevention through activities such as building inspections, fire education programs, and fire investigation.

Emergency medical and rescue services have vastly improved in the past 25 years. Certification and regulation of personnel and services have increased the standard of care. Emergency medical technicians are first responders who evaluate the situation and provide basic life support. Paramedics are highly trained medical specialists who can provide a higher level of care than EMTs. The third member of this team is the rescue or extrication specialist whose responsibility is to obtain access to the patient so that EMTs and paramedics can initiate treatment.

With information from this chapter, you should have a better understanding of what to do in an emergency situation and whom to call for assistance.

Key Terms

City police and **county sheriffs' departments**   Responsible for enforcing the laws of the city and state within the geographical confines of their respective jurisdictions.

Emergency medical technician (EMT)   A paraprofessional emergency specialist trained to provide life-sustaining care and transportation for patients outside the hospital setting.

Fire protection services   Include firefighting, building inspection, enforcement of fire codes, fire prevention education, and fire investigation.

First responder   The person who, after arriving at the scene of an emergency, initiates care or assistance for the victim or victims. This person should assess the situation (including the victim's condition), render emergency care (if appropriately trained), and activate the emergency medical service system.

Good Samaritan laws   These laws protect the lay person who stops and assists in an emergency.

Paramedics   Emergency specialists qualified to deliver advanced life support in an emergency situation; this includes defibrillation, endotracheal intubation, administration of appropriate medications, cardiac monitoring, and intravenous therapy.

State police or **highway patrol**   Primary responsibilities are to enforce the state vehicle code and investigate accidents occurring on state roads and interstate highways.

References

1. Fairfax County Fire and Rescue Department: Fairfax County emergency operations plan, Fairfax, Va., 1986.
2. Hafen, B. Q.: First aid for health emergencies, ed. 3, St. Paul, 1985, West Publishing Co.
3. Hafen, B. Q., and Karren, K. J.: First aid and emergency care workbook, ed. 4, Englewood, Colo., 1990, Morton Publishing Co.
4. Hafen, B. Q., and Karren, K. J.: First responder: a skills approach, ed. 2, Englewood, Colo., 1986, Morton Publishing Co.
5. Hafen, B. Q., and Karren, K. J.: Prehospital emergency care and crisis intervention, ed. 2, Englewood, Colo., 1986, Morton Publishing Co.
6. Herron, R. T., and Wilson, J.: Health and safety: getting the picture, Medscope 3(1):2, 1984.
7. Indiana Emergency Medical Services Commission: EMT training information, Indianapolis, 1986, Indiana State Board of Health Printing Office.
8. Indiana General Assembly: The Indiana advanced life support and paramedic act, House Bill No. 2057, March 27, 1975.
9. Indiana General Assembly, Public law no. 447: immunity—rendering emergency first aid, House Bill No. 1719, 1971, 1973.
10. Kaiser, R. A.: Liability and law in recreation, parks, and sports, Englewood Cliffs, N.J., 1986, Prentice-Hall, Inc.
11. Lahey, J. W.: The changing face of disaster, National Safety News, April 1985, p. 39.
12. Lewis, G., and Appenzeller, H., editors: Successful sport management, Charlottesville, Va., 1985, The Michie Co. Law Publishing.
13. National Safety Council: Unit first aid kits, National Safety and Health News, Jan. 1986, p. 53.
14. Swaton, J. N., and Morgan, L.: Administration of justice: an introduction, ed. 2, New York, 1980, Van Nostrand Reinhold Co., Inc.
15. The Trauma Foundation: Report of the 1985 injury prevention and health policy colloquium, San Francisco, June 6-8, 1985.
16. U.S. Coast Guard: Boating statistics: 1988, COMDPUB P16754.1, Washington, D.C., 1989, U.S. Government Printing Office.
17. U.S. Department of Transportation: Emergency medical services: first responder training course, Washington, D.C., 1984, U.S. Government Printing Office.

18. U.S. Department of Transportation: Highway safety program manual no. 11: emergency medical services, Washington, D.C., 1974, U.S. Government Printing Office.
19. U.S. Department of Transportation, Materials Transportation Bureau, Research and Special Programs Administration: Hazardous materials: 1980 emergency response guidebook, D.O.T. P 5800.2, Washington, D.C., 1980, U.S. Government Printing Office.
20. Virginia Department of Health: Virginia's emergency medical services, Richmond, 1980.

Resource Organizations

American Law Enforcement Officers
Association
1000 Connecticut Avenue N.W., Suite 9
Washington, D.C. 20036

International Association of Firefighters
1750 New York Avenue N.W.
Washington, D.C. 20006

International Association of Women Police
P.O. Box 7635
Kansas City, MO 64128

International Fire Service Training
Association
Fire Protection Publications
Oklahoma State University
Stillwater, OK 74078

International Rescue and Emergency Care
Association
8107 Ensign Drive
Bloomington, MN 55438

International Society of Fire Service
Instructors
P.O. Box 88
Hopkinton, MA 01748

National Association of Emergency Medical
Technicians
P.O. Box 334
Newton Highlands, MA 02161

National Association for Search and Rescue
P.O. Box 2123
LaJolla, CA 92038

National Registry of Emergency Medical
Technicians
P.O. Box 29233
Columbus, OH 43229

Chapter 3

Applying What You Have Learned

1. To obtain hands-on experience with the Cursory Exam, use the following skills checklist as you perform this procedure on a classmate.

    a.)   Survey the scene ☐

    b.)   Determine level of responsiveness ☐

    c.)   Check breathing ☐

    d.)   Check pulse ☐

    e.)   Look for noticeable blood loss ☐

    f.)   Examine head region ☐

    g.)   Examine neck ☐   back ☐

    h.)   Examine chest ☐   arms ☐   abdomen ☐

    i.)   Examine pelvic girdle ☐   lower extremities ☐

2. You have witnessed a shooting in front of your townhouse at 2235 Simms Court. The victim is an elderly male, bleeding heavily from the right shoulder. List the actual steps of making a call and giving emergency personnel the information.

_____

_____

_____

_____

_____

_____

_____

3. List three examples when the Good Samaritan law would not protect a first responder.

    a.) _____

    b.) _____

    c.) _____

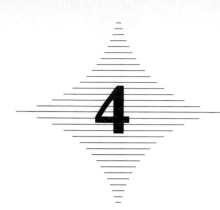

4 Home Safety

Given the fact that people drink in the home environment and that they feel more or less secure at home, it may well be that the involvement of alcohol in serious home accidents is as strong as it is in motor vehicle injuries and deaths—perhaps even stronger.

National Institute of Alcohol Abuse and Alcoholism: Alcohol health and research world

In 1989 22,500 persons were killed in home accidents and another 3.4 million suffered disabling injuries, some 90,000 of which resulted in permanent impairment.[18] It is estimated that another 21 million people receive minor injuries annually in home accidents. This means that approximately 1 person in 12 is injured in a home accident during the year. When such things as wage loss, medical expenses, and property damage are included in the home accident picture, the annual cost to the nation is conservatively estimated at $18 billion.

A major part of one's life is spent in and around the home setting. Young children spend nearly 90% of their time at home. Throughout the school years one spends less and less time in the home environment. During the working years, the amount of time spent at home stabilizes; and with ensuing age, most people spend more of their nonworking hours in the home. In their retirement years, most people have gone full circle and again are spending 90% or more of their time at home.

As defined by the National Safety Council, "home is a dwelling and its premises within the property lines, including in addition to the usual single-family dwellings and apartment houses, duplex dwellings, boarding and room houses and seasonal cottages."[18] Although barracks, dormitories, and fraternity or sorority houses are not included in this standard definition of a home, most of the information included in this chapter is highly applicable to college and university students regardless of where they may live.

In this chapter we will attempt to investigate the major accidents that occur in the home and some options for preventing or reducing the severity of damage from such accidents.

SO YOU WANT TO HAVE A PLACE OF YOUR OWN!

Whether it's new or old, whether you're buying or renting, taking possession of a house or moving into an apartment or townhouse brings with it many responsibilities.

Before that first piece of furniture is moved onto the premises, you should make some insurance protection arrangement. Most major insurance companies have a property and casualty division that offers various coverages for home and condominium owners as well as renters. A basic policy covers damage or losses resulting from fire; theft; vandalism; explosions; failure of electrical, plumbing, and heating systems; as well as a variety of weather conditions. Although standard policies are similar, there may be variations from state to state in specific coverages and premiums. For those who live in areas which are prone to earthquake or flood damage, special insurance must be purchased.

Renter's Insurance

For college and university students, their first experience in truly independent living is often when they move into a rented apartment or house. The building's owner is responsible for the structure and its surrounding grounds; however, the renter is responsible for protecting such valuables as clothing and furniture. Renter's insurance policies are designed to protect personal belongings. Coverages include personal property, personal liability, medical payments to others, and damage to others' property.

Each unrelated person living in an apartment should have a separate renter's policy. Most insurance companies will not issue a policy to one person until it has been confirmed that all roommates have some type of personal property coverage. This practice ensures that others living in the apartment will not attempt to make a false claim on someone else's policy when personal belongings have been destroyed or stolen.

However, before purchasing a renter's policy, the student should check with his or her parents about their policy. Students who are receiving financial support from their parents for school and housing may be covered by the family's policy. If this is the case, there is no need for a student to purchase a separate policy.

Students living in dormitories, fraternity houses, or sorority houses should be aware that organizations operating these facilities are not responsible for personal items that may be stolen or damaged. Again, it is advisable to check your parents' policy to determine whether personal belongings will be insured at school. If not, then it may be wise to contact the family's insurance agent and investigate alternative ways to insure personal valuables.

In the following sections we will discuss the various coverages in the renter's policy.

Personal property. The major item of concern for any renter is the coverage for the contents of the structure. This includes clothing, furniture, appliances, and other **personal property.** The contents of a rental unit may be insured up to the limits you set. In certain instances, endorsements may be added to the policy to cover special items such as jewels, furs, and antiques.

Personal property protection extends outside the boundaries of an apartment when a person is traveling or vacationing. The personal property that is taken on a trip usually will be covered up to 10% of the total personal property value of a renter's policy. For example, an individual whose personal property coverage is $20,000 will be insured for at least $2000 when traveling or vacationing.

To ensure that you can identify all of your personal property, if it ever is destroyed or stolen, make a videotape of your belongings. Go from room to room and include everything in the apartment. When you have finished the tape, store it in a bank safety deposit box or keep it at a relative's house.

Loss of use. If your residence becomes untenable as a result of an insured loss such as a fire or tornado, the insurance company will pay for **loss of use**—the cost (up to 20% of the personal property coverage) of living elsewhere while your rental unit is being repaired. For example, if you have a $20,000 renter's policy and your apartment is destroyed by fire, additional living expenses will be covered up to $4000.

Personal property and loss-of-use coverages are subject to a **deductible fee** when a claim is made. The deductible ranges from $50 to $250 or more, depending on the policy. When a claim is filed, the renter will pay the deductible amount and then the insurance company will pay the remainder up to the limits of the policy. Depending on how old the lost or stolen personal property is, the insurance company will deduct an additional amount from your claim; this is known as ''**depreciation**.''

Personal liability. The **personal liability** feature of a policy protects renters whose actions have resulted in injury to others. It also protects renters when someone is hurt as a result of unsafe conditions on their premises. The minimum amount of personal liability coverage is $25,000; however, most insurance agents feel that $100,000 is the minimum for which an individual should be covered. The maximum amount of coverage offered is $5 million. This type of endorsement may be suggested for people who have swimming pools, hot tubs, dogs, horses, or similar attractive nuisances that have the potential to produce serious or fatal injuries. It is known as ''catastrophe liability insurance.''[25]

Medical payments to others. Another standard feature of most policies is the provision of **medical payments to others**—coverage for persons injured while on your property or because of your actions. This clause differs from the liability clause in that medical payments do not usually involve litigation. If a neighbor slips on your kitchen floor and breaks her leg, your medical payment endorsement will take care of this, regardless of who was at fault. However, if she decides to sue you because she was disabled from the fall, your liability policy would come into play.

Goodwill coverage. The final feature of most policies is known as **goodwill coverage.** It pays for damage to the property of others for which you are responsible. If you were at a party and spilled a drink that stained the host's carpet, your renter's policy would cover the damage up to a certain maximum, usually $250.

Homeowner's Insurance

Insurance coverage for the homeowner is similar to that provided for the renter, with one major variation. Homeowners are also responsible for insuring the structure of their residence. The **structural protection endorsement** will cover the costs of repairing or rebuilding a home that has been damaged. Other structures on your property such as detached garages and sheds are also covered by this endorsement. In addition, most homeowner's policies have inflation clauses that protect homes as they appreciate in value.

Condominium Insurance

Unlike homeowner's insurance, the standard condominium insurance policy does not protect the building you live in, outside your interior walls. Because all condominium-unit owners jointly own the building in which they live, the association or management firm that represents this group usually has a separate policy to protect the building from property damage and liability claims. Generally, a part of the monthly condominium fee of each unit owner will be used to pay for this insurance. Other coverages in the condominium policy are similar to those found in renter's and homeowner's policies.

In some condominium developments all unit owners may be assessed a fee to pay for damages to common properties such as club houses, swimming pools, or landscaped grounds. A condo policy generally covers these charges. This is known as "**loss assessment coverage.**"[4]

Special Options

Even the most comprehensive policies may not adequately cover certain valuables that you have. In the basic homeowner's, condominium, or renter's policy there are limits to the amount of coverage that can be obtained for certain items such as jewelry, cameras, collector's items, guns, silverware, and works of art. However, an endorsement can be added to the policy that will cover these items for their current cash value. Known as a **scheduled personal property endorsement,** it allows specific articles to be listed or scheduled with the insurance company so that there will be an official record of the descriptions and values of this property.

Another valuable supplement to most policies is the **replacement cost value endorsement.** Normally, lost or damaged personal property is replaced on the basis of current replacement cost of the item, minus depreciation. With this clause the policy holder is entitled to reimbursement at the full replacement cost of the item, less deductible. Nothing will be deducted for depreciation of the items that were lost or damaged. As an example, if a person lost a 5-year-old television set in a burglary, he would be awarded the value to replace the television at today's cost. If he did not have the replacement cost value endorsement, his settlement would equal the cost to replace the television minus a depreciation factor. This would force the policy holder to use a significant amount of his or her own money to replace the television.

Depending on individual needs, there are numerous endorsements that can be added to a standard policy to ensure adequate financial coverage. With today's escalating inflation, insurance is not a luxury item; it is a necessity for one's personal protection.

FALLS: A PROBLEM OF AGE

Of the 22,500 home-related deaths in 1989, approximately 6600 of them resulted from falls; 5500 or 83% of the deaths resulting from falls involved people over 65 years of age.[18]

Those over 65 make up about 11% of the U.S. population; however, they are involved in 21% of all falls. Of the estimated 1 million falls that occur in any given year, the elderly account for over 200,000 of them.

Children under 5 years of age constitute a second group that also seems especially susceptible to falls. Although they represent only 7% of the population, young children account for nearly 15% of all falls—roughly 150,000 incidents per year.[22]

However, unlike elderly fall victims, few young children die from falls. In 1989 only 80 children under 5 years of age died as a result of falls. The difference is that older individuals are unable to absorb as much physical trauma as the young. Young people are more resilient—their skeletal structures are cartilaginous and flexible. It will take a relatively great force to break their bones.

A problem affecting thousands of individuals 65 and older, especially women, is osteoporosis. This condition results when calcium is lost from the body with age, and bony structures tend to become thinner and more brittle.[17] Consequently, relatively minor forces can break these weakened bones. A very common and often serious injury that occurs when the elderly fall is the fractured hip. The damage results when a person lands on his or her side, and the head of the femur (the long bone in the upper leg which fits into the hip socket) breaks. In some cases where an older person suffers from osteoporosis, the head of the femur can spontaneously fracture and thus cause a fall. Small children who fall will seldom sustain a similar injury; often they suffer no more than bruises.

The young are also more readily able to recover from injury than the elderly. The recuperative powers of the elderly tend to be somewhat slower. It is not uncommon for an older individual to develop respiratory difficulties while in the hospital recovering from a fracture of the femur or hip. Often they do not die from injuries from the fall but from complications that arise during the recovery period.

Why do young children and the elderly have more trouble with falls than other age groups? The neuromuscular system of children under 5 years of age is just beginning to develop. Their lack of coordination and inability to perceive distances is the reason that young children may have so much trouble negotiating stairs or running across a room without falling. Additionally, a significant portion of their body weight is concentrated in the upper torso and head region, making them somewhat top-heavy.

For the elderly fall victim, the aging process has taken its toll. With increasing age, visual acuity and depth perception may be seriously affected. Physical responses become slower and one's balance and coordination may not be what they once were. Unlike younger individuals, the elderly cannot react quickly enough when they start to slip or fall. If a person beginning to lose balance can grab something, the fall may be broken or it may never occur.

Another important factor that must be considered in any discussion of falls in the elderly is drug use. It is generally accepted that older people have more diseases, take more medications, and have more drug-related side effects. Many of these individuals take four or more different medications every day. The widespread use of sedatives, tranquilizers, and high-blood-pressure medications has been associated with increased incidences of dizziness, loss of coordination, and falls in older Americans.[28]

Stairways

The U.S. Consumer Product Safety Commission estimates that more than 750,000 people require emergency-room treatment each year for injuries involving falls on stairways. Factors involved in these accidents include obscured vision, poor lighting conditions, obstacles on the stairs, slippery tread surface, and running on or near the stairway. Any one or a combination of these factors may contribute to a fall. In any investigation of stairway accidents, three areas that should be discussed are design, use, and maintenance of stairways.

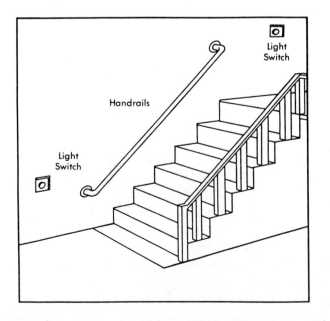

FIG. 4-1 Stairs should have light switches at top and bottom and handrails on both sides.

Courtesy U.S. Consumer Product Safety Commission.

Stairway design in homes is fairly standard. Contractors and builders often follow the guidelines established by the Building Officials and Code Administrators International (BOCA), an organization comprised of leaders in the construction industry and the field of environmental management. Many states have adopted the BOCA guidelines and use them as standards for their own building codes.

Because accident potential is greater when descending stairs and because most people are right-handed, it is recommended that handrails be placed on the right side of each descending flight of stairs. Ideally, all stairways should have handrails on both sides; however, most building codes require only one (Fig. 4-1).

Open stairways that rise more than 30 inches above the floor must have a guardrail, and the vertical supports for the guardrail should be not more than 5 inches apart.[37] This design specification becomes extremely important for families with small children. The close proximity of the supports prevents small children from falling through them to the floor.

The dimensions of each step or riser contribute significantly to the sensation of steepness one encounters on stairways. BOCA guidelines suggest that the maximum height of steps be no more than 8.25 inches, while the tread width of steps should be at least 10 inches.

Steps that are exceptionally high or that have a narrow tread width increase a person's chances of tripping or completely missing a step. Among older persons, there is a gradual loss of depth perception with age. This reduces the accuracy with which a person will be able to detect the precise location of each tread edge as he goes up or down stairs. Improper lighting conditions on stairways that may cause shadows or excessive glare will further aggravate this condition and increase the likelihood of a fall.[1]

One other specification in the design of stairs is that each tread have a nosing or effective projection of at least 1 inch. This small extension of each stair tread allows for a more equal distribution of a person's weight when ascending or descending a stairway. Anything that reduces the size of this lip or extension, such as carpeting, reduces the size of the step and can contribute to a loss of balance.

Often the improper use of a stairway can contribute to an accident. It is neither a storage area nor an art gallery. Families frequently use the basement stairs as a storage center for shoes, buckets, tool boxes, brooms, and mops (Fig. 4-2). Pictures, diplomas, and craft displays can add a decorative touch to a stairway wall, but these can be highly distracting, to the point of affecting one's sense of balance. If you decorate a stairway wall, place these materials on the same side as the stairway railing so that visitors can maintain a point of balance as they look.

The U.S. Consumer Product Safety Commission recommends the following for the reduction of stairway accidents:[28, 31]

1. Avoid slippery wax finishes on stairs.
2. Carpeting on stairs should be avoided since it can become very slick in spots where there is a high amount of traffic. In certain cases, a longer fiber carpet such as a shag may cause heels to catch, creating a sudden traction situation, thus leading to a fall.

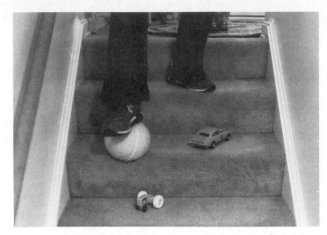

FIG. 4-2 Is this a common occurrence in your home?

3. Stair coverings that supply the greatest slip resistance with uniformity of traction are: rubber treads, abrasive strips, and skid-resistant paints.

4. Avoid placing small rugs near stairs.

5. Place lights at the top and bottom of stairways to eliminate shadows that may appear on stairs.

6. See that handrails and stairs terminate at the same point, since the rail is the primary indication for persons with poor vision that a stairway is ending.

7. Whether or not one has visual difficulties, it is of utmost importance that a person maintain a clear field of vision when carrying materials up or down stairs.

Floors and Walkway Surfaces

Annually over 600,000 falls occur on floors and walkways.[13] Most of them are the result of unexpected, sudden changes in the adherence characteristics of these surfaces.

The development of shoe and flooring materials that offer the same slip resistance or "equivalent adherence" to surfaces under a variety of conditions could significantly reduce slips and falls. The term **equivalent adherence** implies that an optimal level of slip resistance must strike a balance between slipperiness and excessive gripping.

In the home, falls on level surfaces occur in numerous places and result in a wide range of injuries. Statistics on household injuries have consistently shown that the bathroom is one of the most hazardous areas in the home. Many of the accidents occurring here are linked to falls in bathtubs and showers. Each year these structures are involved in nearly 70,000 injuries serious enough to be treated in hospital emergency rooms.

The following examples illustrate a number of factors that must be controlled if falls and their resulting injuries are to be reduced:

As Mary was washing her hair in the shower, she slipped on the soapy film that covered the floor of the bathtub. The towel rack that she grabbed broke under the force of her weight. Mary consequently fell through the glass tub enclosure and suffered severe lacerations on her face, right arm, and hand.

Six-year-old Jimmy was running through the living room on his way outside to play when his waffle-soled shoes caught on the shag carpet. The sudden excessive gripping of the shoes caused him to fall forward into the storm door. As he fell, the glass broke and lacerated his stomach, causing internal bleeding.

These case histories are examples of surface traction problems in the home. The ideal solution would be to eliminate the traction problems, because that could prevent many falls. Most floor-related accidents occur on slippery surfaces, so we will discuss that problem first. Spilled water in such places as the bathroom, kitchen, or laundry room forms a thin layer between a person's foot and the floor. The water, in effect, becomes a lubricant and does not allow friction to occur. Agents such as mud, oil, soap, and wax have similar lubricating effects on floors and other nonporous surfaces such as bathtubs and showers.

However, slipperiness is only part of the problem. Don't forget the element of surprise. Often people fall on the wet kitchen floor because they didn't expect it to be wet. If a person expects an area to be slippery, he is much less likely to fall, because he will be prepared to react to this condition.

Consequently falls may be prevented in two ways. People must first be educated about situations that may lead to slippery conditions; then they can develop measures to correct the slippery conditions.

1. Water spilled on a tile or hardwood floor will act as a lubricant.
2. Areas of the home where water is often spilled on the floor are the kitchen, laundry room, bathroom, and entranceways.
3. Liquid- and paste-wax residues are very slippery before drying.
4. Oil, grease, or mud on a garage floor can form a slick lubricant film.
5. A soap water mixture will create an extremely slippery residue on tub surfaces.

With this information, a person can then take the necessary steps to prevent these situations.

1. When water is spilled on the floor, it should be wiped up immediately.
2. Nonskid mats should be placed in areas that are frequently damp, such as the bathroom or entranceways.
3. Any time you wash or wax the floor, block off the room until the area is completely dry.
4. Absorbent chemicals should be used to soak up oil and grease spills in the garage or basement.
5. To make your footing more secure in the bathtub, install rough-surfaced adhesive strips. Many shower stalls and tubs are now manufactured with slip-resistant surfaces.

Although they occur less frequently than falls related to slippery conditions, falls resulting from excessive traction conditions can also lead to serious injuries, such as the case with young Jimmy. In recent years the popularity of running shoes as casual footwear has presented further problems. Many of the more popular styles have small rubber extensions or cleats that provide traction when a person is running on dirt paths or grassy areas. People wearing these shoes indoors must be sure to pick up their feet when walking. A person with a shuffling gait will constantly be catching the cleats of the shoes in thick-piled carpeting. Caution must be taken as to how and where one walks.

Even the most diligent preventive measures will not eliminate all falls. An alternative is the reduction of the severity of injuries when a person does fall. As in the cases of Mary and Jimmy, more than 90,000 people are injured each year when they fall into or through glass doors and windows. The type of glass with which they come in contact contributes significantly to the severity of the injuries they receive.

Falling against a window or door that contains ordinary plate glass can create a life-threatening situation, because it breaks into large, daggerlike pieces that can cut and pierce the body. However, a similar fall into a window or door made with the newer safety glazing materials will result in little or no injury.

Safety Glazing

The U.S. Consumer Product Safety Commission has recognized the injury hazards associated with ordinary glass. It has developed a mandatory safety standard requiring the use of safety glazing materials in sliding glass doors, entrance doors, and bath and shower enclosures. Safety glazing materials are also required in the replacement of these products in existing homes and buildings.

The three types of safety glazing materials are as follows:

1. **Tempered glass:** This type of glass is heated and then cooled in a special way to make it much stronger than ordinary glass. On impact, it crumbles into small pieces that minimize the chance of injury.

2. **Laminated glass:** In the production of this material, two layers of ordinary glass are bonded together with a layer of plastic. If this glass is broken, the pieces generally stick to the plastic and do not shatter.

3. **Rigid plastic:** This glazing material is made from one or more layers of heated plastic. Unlike glass, this material is relatively easy to scratch, thus marring its surface and distorting vision through it.

Of the three types of safety glazing, tempered glass is the least expensive and most widely used in the home. Its one disadvantage is that it cannot be cut but must be purchased in the exact size you need. Whatever your choice, you can always identify safety glazing by a permanent label at one of the corners that identifies the manufacturer and the type of material.

A final word on safety glass: Safety glazing materials can prevent many serious injuries, because they are usually more impact resistant and do not break into large, jagged pieces. If you have small children, it is a good idea to replace ordinary glass in those locations in the home that are subject to frequent accidental human impact, i.e., the windows in the playroom, recreation room, family room; bath/shower doors; and storm doors.

Ladders

Although not as numerous as stairway accidents or falls on level surfaces, falls from ladders account for over 90,000 injuries yearly.[40] A fall from even a low ladder can mean a painful and incapacitating injury.

Major considerations in the safe use of ladders include the type of work for which the ladder will be used, its proper positioning, and the skill of its user. The following examples illustrate what can happen when these factors are not taken into consideration:

> *A 63-year-old man suffered a fractured skull and fractured right leg when he fell from a stepladder while climbing to the roof of his home. Because the ladder was too short, he placed it on a small table and then leaned it against the side of the house.*
>
> *A 34-year-old woman suffered multiple fractures of both arms as the ladder she was climbing began to slide away from the house on wet grass. She had failed to secure the ladder in the wet, soft ground.*
>
> *A 19-year-old house painter suffered pelvic fractures and internal injuries when he fell from the top of an extension ladder. Before his fall, he was seen leaning from the left side of the ladder with only his right hand and foot in contact with the ladder.*

Taking proper precautions with ladders begins with proper selection. A ladder should be long enough for any use to which it might be put. Remember, however, that the length of a ladder is not the same as its usable length. The top three rungs of a straight or extension ladder should not be used, while the top platform and top step of a stepladder should not be used for supporting one's weight. Most ladders have maximum load ratings that include the user plus materials. They range from type III light-duty ladders with a maximum load of 200 pounds to type I heavy-duty ladders with a maximum capacity of 250 pounds.[40]

Before each use, a ladder should be inspected for wear and damage. This is especially true if it has been stored for a long time. If you have a wooden ladder, be careful to examine the rungs for rotting or splitting. Never paint a wooden ladder; the paint can hide cracks and other defects. Examine your metal ladder for stress marks— that is, any bending or warping in the rungs or side rails.

Once you have determined that the ladder is functional, proper positioning is the next step. Fig. 4-3 illustrates the proper placement of a straight or extension ladder. To position the ladder properly, place it against the wall so that the distance between the wall and the base of the ladder is *one fourth* of the ladder's working length. Because ladder rungs are normally 1 foot apart, this distance is easy to compute. If the ladder is to be used for getting onto a roof, at least three rungs should extend beyond the edge of the roof.

Before you climb the ladder, make sure that its base is secured. Ground under the ladder should be flat and firm. If the ground is soft or uneven, no one should climb

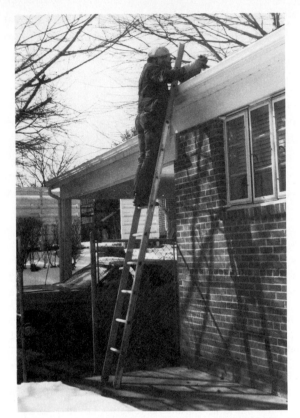

FIG. 4-3   Proper positioning of a straight ladder. Remember, the distance between the wall and the base of the ladder is one fourth of the ladder's working length.

the ladder until it has been firmly anchored in the ground. A good practice would be to have a helper hold the bottom of the ladder.

When working on the ladder, some key points to remember are:

1. Face the ladder and use both hands when climbing or descending. Tools and equipment you may need can be carried in your pockets or attached to your belt. To lower or raise larger items such as buckets, use a rope as a safe alternative.

2. Do not lean too far to the side while working. A good general guide is to keep your body centered between the rails of the ladder. Rather than leaning farther out to reach a particular spot, get down and move the ladder.

3. When working with electrical tools or near power lines, use a dry wooden or nonconductive fiberglass ladder. If this cannot be done, use extreme caution when operating from the metal ladder. Numerous fatalities occur each year when metal ladders contact power lines.

Many of these suggestions apply equally to the use of the stepladder (Fig. 4-4). Some of the specific points worth mentioning are:

1. Erect a stepladder only on a flat surface. Never use it as you would a straight ladder.

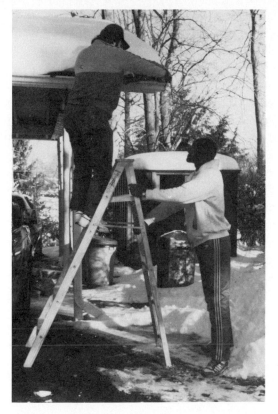

FIG. 4-4   Notice that the legs of this stepladder are in a fully extended and locked position. He is standing on the second step from the top of the ladder, the highest recommended standing level.

2. Before you start to climb, make sure that its legs are fully extended and locked into position. The stability of a stepladder can be checked by standing on the first step from the bottom and twisting the ladder. If it feels unsteady, choose another ladder.
3. Do not stand on the ladder's top, top step, or bucket shelf for support.
4. Regardless of the type of ladder, never leave it unattended when it is in a raised position. Remember, you would be legally liable if someone were hurt because of the ladder.

Childhood Falls and Related Injuries

Children of all ages fall and hurt themselves from time to time. Falls are part of growing up, and luckily most aren't serious. However, some falls can cause severe damage, such as head injuries.

Even at 4 or 5 months of age, children are very active. They are capable of rolling over and moving in various directions. As they get older, they quickly learn to climb and explore, yet have little concept of the risks involved.

In recent years the U.S. Consumer Product Safety Commission has identified a number of devices that are involved in child falls. Cradles, high chairs, walkers, bassinets, and shopping carts are just a few of the support structures that have been implicated. Most of these falls resulted when safety devices were not used or the children were left unsupervised.[40]

A second problem involving a variety of household and nursery products is that of entrapment. In these incidents, children's bodies become wedged or caught in the structural components of cribs, crib toys, beds, toy chests, baby gates, playpens, and drapery cords. Often the child's head and neck become caught, leading to suffocation or strangulation. In the past 10 years, nearly 400 such fatalities have been reported to the U.S. Consumer Product Safety Commission. Most of the victims were under 2 years of age, with those aged 6 to 12 months being at greatest risk. At this stage of development, children become increasingly mobile and learn to push up, pull up, stand, and even walk. However, if they become entangled in cords hanging from crib toys and draperies, or they become entrapped by mattresses, toy chest lids, or even something as simple as a plastic garbage bag, they often lack the coordination or strength to extricate themselves from these potentially hazardous situations.[40]

An example of this entrapment hazard can be illustrated by the older, accordion-style baby gates. When put in place at the top of a stairway, these gates have V-shaped and diamond-shaped openings in which children can get their heads trapped (Fig. 4-5, A). In contrast, mesh-style baby gates have no openings large enough for a child's head and thus do not present a strangulation hazard (Fig. 4-5, B). Although the accordion-style baby gates are no longer manufactured and sold in the United

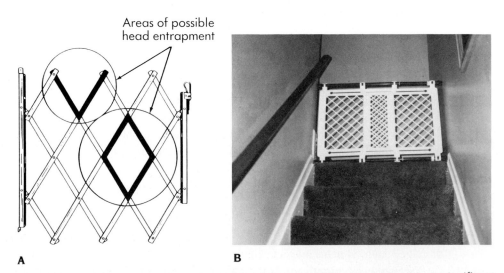

A **B**

FIG. 4-5 A, This baby gate with its diamond-shaped openings presents a significant entrapment hazard for small children. **B,** This mesh-style baby gate does not present a strangulation hazard.

Courtesy of U.S. Consumer Product Safety Commission.

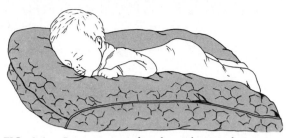

FIG. 4-6   Do not use infant bean-bag cushions.

States as a result of a voluntary standard developed by the Juvenile Products Man-ufacturers Association and the CPSC, it is estimated that at least 10 million of these potentially hazardous products are still in use. If you have friends using this type of baby gate, have them get rid of it or buy them one of the newer and safer mesh-style gates.

A nursery product that has been identified recently as a suffocation hazard for young infants (under 6 months of age) is the infant bean-bag cushion. These fabric covered, polystyrene pellet-filled cushions have been associated with at least 40 deaths in the last 2 years.[23] The deaths occurred when infants were left to sleep on the cushions and then were later found in a face-down position. Because of the design of the product, it would be hard for a small child to keep his face away from the fabric once he had rolled onto his stomach.

Since mid-1990 there has been a national campaign to recall the more than 1 million infant cushions that were sold between 1986 and 1990. At this time only about 12% of these devices have been returned. If you know someone who has an infant bean-bag cushion, urge them to return the product to the place of purchase for a refund (Fig. 4-6).

Even household chairs can present hazards for the very young. A number of children have been killed when they became wedged between the footrest and the chair seat of a recliner. After parents or grandparents left the chair in the tilt-back position and went into another room, the child got into the opening between the footrest and the chair seat. As the child leaned on the foot support, it collapsed downward into its original position, causing strangulation.[40]

To reduce the risk of children's falls and entrapment injuries, the following basic precautions should be taken:
1. Always use both the waist and crotch straps that are provided on high chairs, baby swings, and baby carriers.
2. Never leave infants on waterbeds, adult, or youth beds. They can become en-trapped between the mattress and wall or bed frame and suffocate (Fig. 4-7, A).
3. If you have stairs, always use a safety gate when children are in the home. When they are upstairs, use a gate at the top of the steps to prevent a long tumble. If they are downstairs, put the gate at the base of the steps; children will inevitably try to crawl up the stairs, given the opportunity.

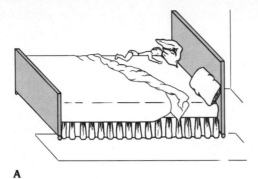

A

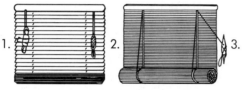

To keep cords out of the reach of children,
use these devices:

1. Clamp or clothes pin   2. Tie the cord to itself

3. Cleat   4. Tie-down device

B

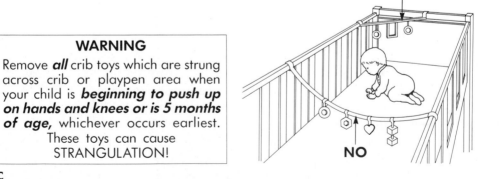

WARNING

Remove **all** crib toys which are strung across crib or playpen area when your child is **beginning to push up on hands and knees or is 5 months of age,** whichever occurs earliest. These toys can cause STRANGULATION!

C

FIG. 4-7 A, Infants should not be left on adult or youth beds. **B,** Keep cords away from your little one. **C,** Remove hanging crib toys by the time your child is 5 months old.

Courtesy of U.S. Consumer Product Safety Commission.

4. If your nursery equipment is more than 10 years old, be sure to check with the local pediatric center to be sure that these items meet current safety requirements and are in good repair, or call the CPSC Hotline at 1-800-638-2772.

5. Keep cords from blinds or draperies out of the reach of children (Fig. 4-7, B).

6. Remove all hanging crib toys when your child is beginning to push up on hands and knees or is 5 months of age (Fig. 4-7, C).

7. When you have children, there is no substitute for close supervision!

DOING IT YOURSELF

Power tools used in the home offer an efficient and economical means of building, maintaining, or repairing items around the home. However, some of the features of this equipment (sharp, rapidly moving parts, and electrical current) can make them extremely dangerous if they are defective, in poor repair, or misused. Figures released by the National Injury Information Clearinghouse indicate that chain saws and power saws account for over 70,000 injuries annually; electric home-workshop tools (excluding power and chain saws) account for 30,000 injuries; and power mowers and hedge trimmers cause nearly 60,000 injuries.[35] If we include accidents involving manual tools such as hammers, screwdrivers, rakes, saws, and staplers, it is necessary to add another 100,000 persons to the injury list.

Chain and Power Saws

Gasoline and electric chain saws, often used to clear land of trees or cut firewood, present a cutting hazard because of their sharp, rapidly moving chains. Contact with the chain is the primary cause of most injuries, which often include severe lacerations or amputations. In Appendix A (p. 461-471), we have discussed emergency procedures for controlling bleeding.

The most serious hazard associated with chain saw use is kickback (the sudden violent backward and upward rotation of the saw toward its operator).[38] Kickback generally occurs when the saw chain around the tip of the guide bar touches an object such as a nearby log or branch (Fig. 4-8). It can also occur when the wood being cut closes in and pinches the saw chain or when the chain contacts an unusually hard piece of wood. Because kickback results in such a sudden and violent movement, it is not unusual for the moving saw chain to come into contact with the operator.

Ron was cutting logs for his new wood stove when the tip of his chain saw hit an adjacent log and kicked back into his face. As it cut across his cheek and forehead, he reached up to regain control of the saw, and in so doing, severely lacerated three fingers of his left hand.

Ron was relatively lucky in that little facial scarring remains and he has regained almost complete mobility in his fingers. Each year many others who are not so lucky receive permanently disabling injuries.

While kickback is associated with more severe injuries, it is not the only hazard

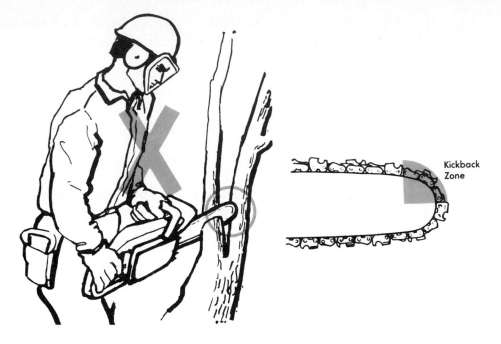

FIG. 4-8 Avoid contacting any object with the tip of the guide bar.
Courtesy of U.S. Consumer Product Safety Commission.

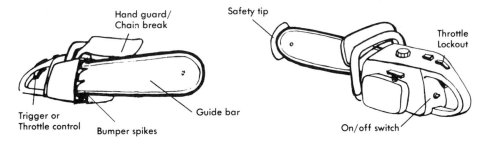

FIG. 4-9 Check for features such as these when you shop to find a saw that is easy and safe to use.
Courtesy of U.S. Consumer Product Safety Commission.

involved with chain saws. A variety of nonkickback incidents cause the majority of injuries. They include the following:[42]

1. Skating and bouncing: Most of these cases occur when a person is holding a branch in one hand and the chain saw in the other. Instead of cutting into the wood, the saw skates or bounces along the surface of the branch until it cuts into the victim's hand.

2. Follow-through: In these cases the saw cuts through the wood more quickly than expected and continues into the victim's leg.

3. Operator changing positions: These incidents involve inadvertent contact with the moving chain while the victim is reaching for another log, walking with an idling chain saw, or changing the positioning of the saw.

4. Loss of balance: Frequently, in cutting operations, a branch or log may fall near the chain saw operator or strike him, causing a loss of balance and consequent contact with the moving chain.

Other injuries involve pieces of wood that may fly up and hit the operator in the face and electrical shocks when power cords are severed, insulation on electric chain saws fails, or the saw comes into contact with electrical wires.

The following suggestions from the U.S. Consumer Product Safety Commission and the National Safety Council concern the purchase and safe use of chain saws:[38]

1. Test the saw to see if the chain stops immediately after the trigger is released. If the chain continues to move, the saw should not be used until it has been repaired.

2. Buy a saw that you can easily control. Always hold the chain saw firmly with two hands, keeping the left arm straight to prevent the blade from bouncing back toward you.

3. Make sure an electric chain saw is insulated against shock by double-insulation or three-prong grounded plugs.

4. New chain saws have a variety of safety features which reduce the risk of kickback. When shopping for a chain saw, check for these features: hand guard/chain brake, low-kickback chains and guide bars, and tip guards (Fig. 4-9).

5. Keep your work area clear of other branches and objects that may present a kickback hazard and avoid cutting limbs above midchest height.

6. When making a cut, stand to the side of the chain saw so that it does not touch your body on the follow-through. This stance will also offer protection in case of kickback (Fig. 4-10).

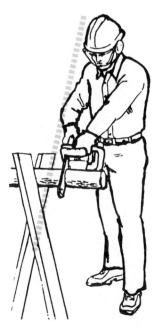

FIG. 4-10 You should stand to the side of the cut so that the saw does not touch your body on the follow-through.
Courtesy of U.S. Consumer Product Safety Commission.

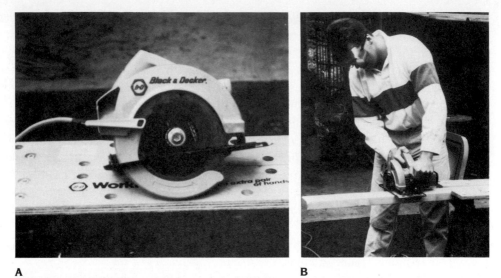

A   B

FIG. 4-11 A, Notice the blade guard on this portable power saw.   **B,** In this position the operator will be able to keep the saw under control.

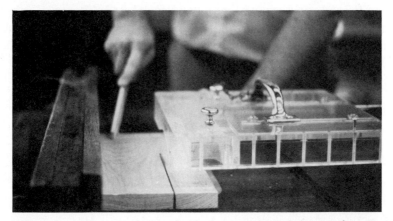

FIG. 4-12 The use of a push block or push stick keeps the operator's hands a safe distance from the cutting blades. The clear plastic guard protects him from flying debris.

7. Wear sturdy shoes, heavy trousers, sure-grip gloves, a safety visor or goggles, hearing protection, and a hard hat when cutting wood.

8. Never let the saw run unattended. When walking with the saw, shut off the motor. And keep children away from the work area at all times.

In recent years there has been good news about chain saws. A 1989 study by the CPSC reported a reduction of nearly 20,000 chain saw injuries per year since the introduction of low kickback safety features in 1985.[42] It is not surprising to find that the biggest reduction was in kickback injuries. Other injury incidents resulting from skating and bouncing, inadvertent contact, and loss of balance showed a decline as well. It is likely that this greater general safety awareness was a result of the significant publicity given to kickback hazards in the mid and late 1980s.

Power saws, both portable and table models, present many of the same dangers as chain saws. Contact with the blade causes most power saw injuries. Portable saw injuries occur when the blade guard has been removed or it fails to return after the completion of a cut and the operator brushes against the blade; the saw kicks back when it hits a knot in the wood; the blade continues rotating after the trigger is released; or there is faulty electrical insulation of the device. Injuries with stationary saws result when an operator fails to use a push stick and his fingers or hands hit the moving blade. In some cases wood will be thrown toward the operator when kickback occurs with stationary equipment.

When using a power saw remember the following[29]:
1. Keep blade guards and safety devices in place at all times (Fig. 4-11).
2. When making a straight cut with a stationary saw, always use a push block (Fig. 4-12).
3. Do not force the cut; the saw operates at its own speed.
4. Before cleaning around it or attempting to repair it, make sure that your saw is unplugged.
5. To prevent the possibility of a shock, do not use the saw in a damp or wet area.

Electrical Home Workshop Tools

Electrically powered home tools include drills, sanders, routers, lathes, grinders, planers, and soldering guns. The most frequently used item is the electric drill, which accounts for nearly one third of the injuries involving this group of products.[40]

A leading cause of injuries is contact with the blade, bit, or other sharp revolving surface of a power tool. Too often people who are injured using this equipment have broken the most important workshop rule: Safety first. They have either failed to use a safety device such as a push block or they have removed guards from equipment.

Cutting or drilling tools that hit embedded nails or screws may suddenly kick back or break off, exposing the user's hands to the moving parts. When operating one of these high-speed tools, do not exert undue pressure on the device. Let the machine do the work while you guide its progress.

Another cause of injuries is contact with flying particles such as sawdust, wood, or metal chips. When operating one of these devices, wear safety glasses or goggles to protect the eyes from fragments (Fig. 4-13). The National Society for the Prevention of Blindness reports that an estimated 41% of the 1 million people with vision impairments caused by eye injuries suffered the damage in the home. Of these home eye injuries, it is further estimated that 90% could have been prevented with eye protection.

An additional hazard associated with any household electrical appliance is the possibility of serious shock or electrocution. Poor insulation, defective wiring, or frayed electrical cords can bring the user into contact with the flow of electricity—and, in effect, the victim becomes a part of the electric circuit. In a well-insulated tool

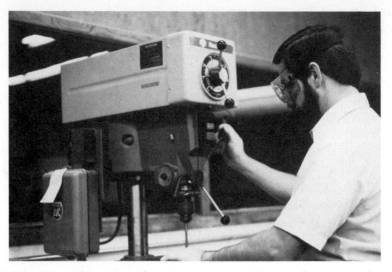

FIG. 4-13 Whenever you operate power equipment that can produce particles of wood or metal, wear eye protection.

there exists only one pathway for electric current to travel. Normally current travels from an electrical outlet through the positive or ''hot'' wire of a power cord to an appliance's motor. The current then returns to the outlet through the neutral or ''ground'' wire in the cord. However, if there is a break in the insulation, either inside the tool or on the appliance's power cord, there will be a leakage of current known as a ground fault. A person touching the damaged cord or ''electrically hot'' tool may provide another pathway to ground for the electric current. Depending on a variety of conditions, users may receive no more than a mild tingling sensation when they use such tools or they may be electrocuted. Let's take a look at some of those conditions that create this danger.

The severity of damage to the body is related to the amount and duration of the electrical current that a person receives. The higher the current, the lower the resistance, and the longer the shock, the greater the damage to the individual. For our purposes *resistance* refers to the resistance of human skin; the higher the resistance of the skin, the lower the electrical current one receives. Skin resistance depends to a great extent on the moisture present; wet skin is about 100 times less resistant to an electric current than dry skin. For example, 110 to 120 volts AC (voltages found in most homes in North America) can produce 1 mA (milliampere) of current through dry skin, 110 mA through perspiring skin, and 750 mA to skin submerged in water. Currents in excess of 18 mA can contract the chest muscles so that breathing is stopped during the shock. If the current persists, collapse, unconsciousness, and death follow in a matter of minutes. Currents of 100 to 200 mA are the values most likely to produce ventricular fibrillation when applied to the exterior of the body.[34] In ventricular fibrillation, heart muscle fibers contract in a rapid, uncoordinated manner and do not effectively pump oxygenated blood. If this condition—known as cardiac arrest—is not immediately corrected, death will occur in 4 to 6 minutes. In Appendix A (pp. 461-471), you will find a discussion of the emergency care procedures used in a cardiac arrest incident.

As one can see, there are significant dangers when working with electrical tools around water, especially in such areas of the home as the bathroom, kitchen, or garden. However, even when working conditions are dry, inadequate grounding or poor insulation of equipment may lead to serious consequences.

To reduce the risk of electrocution or serious shock from power tools, the following alternatives should be considered:

1. Three prong grounded plug: Today most power tools on the market have this safety feature. If there is leaking current, wiring in the power cord and the third prong act as a ground to draw off current (Fig. 4-14). Always insert a three-prong plug into a three-prong socket. It is safer to have your wall outlets rewired to accept three-prong plugs than to use two-prong adapters. However, if you must use an adapter, attach the pigtail wire to the screw holding the faceplate of the wall socket. If this is not done, the three-prong plug will be of no benefit as a ground.

2. Double insulation: Two separate layers of nonconductive materials are placed around the motors and contact points of power tools to prevent current leakage. In tools that generate high internal temperatures, the primary insulation often breaks down after extended use, and this second layer of insulation provides continued protection. Double insulation is a great advance, but it is not effective for appliances immersed in water or soaked in rain.

3. Ground fault circuit interrupter (GFCI): This device monitors how much electricity goes into an appliance and how much comes out. If there is a leak or ground fault, the GFCI cuts power to the appliance immediately. GFCIs can be installed in outlets or in circuit breakers. They can detect leakage levels as low as 5 mA. These fast-acting circuit breakers will rapidly stop current flow to the tool and the operator will

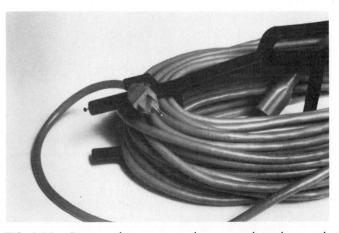

FIG. 4-14   Be sure that power tools you purchase have a three-prong plug.

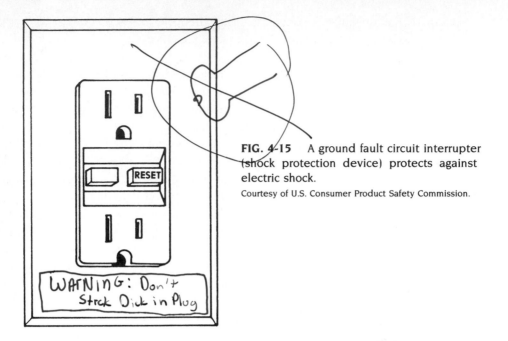

FIG. 4-15 A ground fault circuit interrupter (shock protection device) protects against electric shock.

Courtesy of U.S. Consumer Product Safety Commission.

have received, at most, a mild shock. It has been estimated by Underwriters Laboratories (UL) that as many as 81% of home electrocutions could be prevented if GFCIs were used (Fig. 4-15).

Two new safety devices that are likely to receive widespread usage in the 1990s are the Appliance Leakage Current Interrupter (ALCI) and the Immersion Detection Circuit Interrupter (IDCI). Like the GFCI, these products detect current leakage and cut off power to an electrical appliance; however, unlike GFCIs, which are installed in outlets, ALCIs and IDCIs are built into small appliances and can be used in any outlet. This makes them very effective for usage in all portable appliances such as hair dryers, curling irons, and hand-held electrical tools.

Because they have been found to work especially well with electrical appliances that come into contact with water, ACLIs or IDCIs have been placed on all hair dryers and portable bathtub spas that have been manufactured since January 1, 1991. The next time you purchase one of these electrical appliances, be sure to check that it has an ALCI or IDCI.

Power Mowers and Hedge Trimmers

Two of the most widely used lawn and garden tools are power mowers and hedge trimmers. Both of these devices save the homeowner a great deal of time and effort. However, any equipment that has cutting blades operating at high speeds offers a certain potential for injury. Most of the injuries involving power mowers (68%) occur when a person's hand or foot contacts the whirling blade. Another 20% result from objects thrown by the blades. In the case of power hedge trimmers, over 90% of persons receiving emergency-room treatment for injuries had come into contact with moving blades. Severe lacerations or amputations of extremities are the primary injuries in power mower and hedge trimmer accidents.

Contact with the rotating blade of a power mower often occurs when the victim is clearing the discharge chute of grass clippings, especially when the grass is wet; when the victim attempts to adjust the machine without shutting it off; or when the victim's foot slips under the blade housing. Bystanders may be injured when objects such as rocks, twigs, and pieces of metal are propelled at high velocity from discharge chutes located in back or on the side of the mower.

The fast-moving cutting teeth of a hedge trimmer do their damage when people fail to control the trimmer's movement. This may occur when a person attempts to change hand positions while the trimmer is running or tries to operate the machine with one hand while holding branches away from the cutting blade with the other. Another danger to consider with electric hedge trimmers is the potential for shock or electrocution.

To provide maximum safety for those using power mowers and hedge trimmers, two factors must be considered: the type of equipment to buy and how to properly use these power tools. Before you purchase a power mower, ask the dealer the following questions[2]:

1. Does the mower have a blade guard to prevent hands and feet from coming into contact with the rotating blade?

2. Is there a "deadman control" on it? (A deadman control is a bar or handle that must be held in place to operate the blade. If the control is released, the engine may or may not keep running, but the blade must stop within 3 seconds.)

3. Is the grass discharge chute aimed downward, and does it have a shield to prevent objects from being thrown at high velocities? (See Fig. 4-16.)

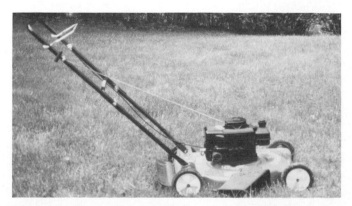

FIG. 4-16 Notice the rear blade guard, grass discharge chute, and deadman control on this new mower.

After purchasing the mower, be sure to read the owner's manual so that you will be familiar with its operation. Before you cut the lawn, a quick survey of the area can help you to eliminate such hazards as rocks, cans, twigs, and other objects that can be thrown by the blades. It is also important to change into proper clothing before you cut the grass; wear work shoes or boots and close-fitting slacks and shirts. If your foot were to come into contact with the mower blade, the thicker work shoe would afford you some amount of protection. Sneakers, sandals, or bare feet offer absolutely no protection. Tightly fitting slacks and shirts reduce the risk of clothing becoming entangled in moving machine parts.

To ensure safe operation of the mower consider the following:

1. Never mow a wet lawn. Slips on wet grass increase one's chances of coming into contact with the blade. Wet grass also has a tendency to clog blades and discharge chutes; this condition, in turn, tempts many people to clear the machine without shutting it down.

2. If you have to unclog or adjust the machine, always shut it off and disconnect the spark plug wire. A slight rotation of the blade could start the engine if the plug wire remains connected.

3. Keep people away from the area you are mowing to reduce the possibility of injury to bystanders from thrown objects.

4. When you refuel the mower, be sure that the engine is cool so that unseen gasoline vapors cannot be ignited.

When purchasing a power hedge trimmer, the safety-conscious shopper will check the distance between the cutting teeth. They should not be wide enough for anyone to put a finger between them. The safer hedge trimmers have two handles for easier maneuverability and pressure-sensitive switches that immediately shut them off when finger pressure is removed. Because most hedge trimmers are electrically powered, they should be double insulated or have a three-prong grounded plug (Fig. 4-17).

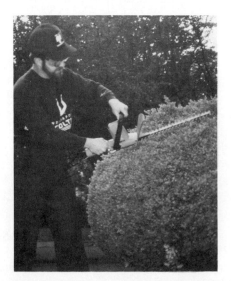

FIG. 4-17 Use both hands to maneuver this device; that is why it has two handles.

As with any power tool, always read the operating instructions before you attempt to use your hedge trimmer. Remember, the key to safe operation of this device is to keep your hands away from the cutting blades. When you are trimming that hedge or shrubbery, be sure to work from a sturdy surface and never attempt to hold back branches with one hand while guiding the device with the other hand. The only way to operate safely is to keep both hands on the tool.

According to studies conducted by the U.S. Consumer Product Safety Commission, power mower injuries and injury rates have decreased nearly 40% over the past 10 years. This significant decline in injuries has been attributed to the development of the 1982 mandatory standard which requires all new mowers to have deadman controls, blade guards, and downward-aimed discharge chutes. It is estimated that these product design changes have prevented more than 80,000 injuries at a cost savings of $700 million.[2]

Manual Workshop Tools

As mentioned earlier in this chapter, manually operated tools account for slightly more than 100,000 of the injuries each year requiring emergency-room treatment. Five tools associated with the majority of these injuries are hammers, axes, wrenches, pliers, and screwdrivers.

With each of these tools there are basic guidelines that one should follow. The common nail or claw hammer is involved in over 40% of these injuries. Chipping of the hammer face causes both the greatest number of hammer-related injuries and the most serious problems—for example, eye injuries from flying pieces of metal. If you are going to use a hammer, wear safety goggles or safety glasses. Remember that a household hammer should be used only for driving or removing nails; it is not made for use with other steel tools such as chisels or wedges. A variety of other hammers should be used when working on masonry or metal products.

With the increased number of wood stoves used in the home, more people are buying hatchets, axes, and mauls to chop kindling, clear small trees, and split wood. Any of these sharp-bladed cutting instruments can do serious damage when improperly used. A hatchet is often used to cut and trim small branches or to chop kindling. Because of its short handle, there is a danger of hitting yourself in the leg or foot as you follow through with the tool. Whenever possible one should be in a kneeling position when using a hatchet so that if you miss, the blade will hit the ground, not your leg.

Axes can be used for felling small-diameter trees and chopping them into sections for firewood; however, they should not be used as splitting tools. To split wood into smaller sections, a wood maul or a splitting wedge and sledge hammer should be used because they are heavier, thicker, and can provide a greater splitting force. When an ax is used to split wood, it can easily be deflected into a person's foot or leg. Goggles or safety glasses should always be used to protect one's eyes from flying wood chips.

Even pliers, wrenches, and screwdrivers can lead to painful injuries if they are not used correctly. Whenever you are using a pair of pliers or a wrench to loosen or tighten a bolt or nut, always pull the device toward you, never push it. And never use a length of pipe over a wrench to increase leverage; get a bigger wrench to do the job properly. The same holds true for a screwdriver; make sure a screwdriver blade is the proper size for the screw slot that it must fit. Never use a screwdriver as you would a chisel or punch!

What About The Kitchen?

Although they are not considered power tools, electrical kitchen appliances present hazards similar to those of many power tools. The U.S. Consumer Product Safety Commission estimates that more than 10,000 persons are treated in hospital emergency rooms every year for injuries associated with electric blenders, mixers, garbage disposals, meat and food grinders, choppers, slicers, and food processors.[35]

As Dan was disposing of the garbage, he accidently dropped a spoon into the disposal. Without thinking, he reached into the device to remove the spoon. His resulting injuries included the loss of three fingers and part of his thumb.

Cheri was mixing frozen strawberry daiquiris in a blender. The ice at the top of the blender was not being mixed with the rest of the ingredients, so Cheri used her fingers to push the ice closer to the blades. When her fingers contacted the blades, the tip of her right index finger was amputated (Fig. 4-18).

Contact with blades, beaters, or cutting edges is a major cause of injuries associated with kitchen appliances. A moment of inattentiveness can bring tragic results. Lack of knowledge concerning the hazards of these devices is a major contributor in the accident sequence. The importance of reading the manufacturer's instructions carefully for proper use and maintenance cannot be emphasized enough.

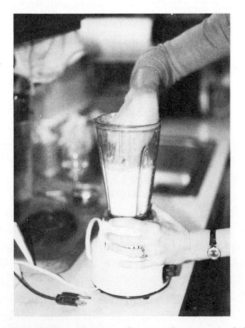

FIG. 4-18 Never make an adjustment while the appliance is in operation or plugged in.

The following measures should be taken for the safe handling of these appliances:
1. Make sure all parts are connected tightly before operating.
2. Do not adjust parts or insert utensils into blades of mixers, blenders, or grinders while the motor is on or the power cord is plugged in.
3. Keep fingers and hands away from the blades of operating appliances, and always use the safety equipment that comes with these devices.
4. Owners of processors with chutes that feed sliced or shredded food into a separate bowl should never attempt to unclog the chute while the appliance is running or plugged in.

Since these kitchen appliances are powered by electricity, avoiding wet conditions is a primary concern for safe operation. Never immerse the motor housing in water when you are cleaning it after use. Try to avoid handling the appliance with wet hands or when standing on a wet or damp floor. When you are operating this equipment near the sink, make sure the sink has no water standing in it.

Although great technological strides have been made by manufacturers to ease the work load in the home, these time-saving devices do have their costs. As with all of the power tools mentioned in this chapter, kitchen appliances require your undivided attention if they are to be used safely.

POISONS IN THE HOME: A THREAT TO THE YOUNG

Any substance that negatively affects body tissues and organ functions can be considered a **poison.** Some poisons may slightly irritate skin tissue, whereas others may lead to cardiorespiratory failure. Not all poisons are harmful in every case. Certain drugs and medications that are normally beneficial and safe become poisonous only when they are taken in excessive dosages or when they are taken in combination with another substance. For instance, aspirin is a widely used and highly effective analgesic with relatively few side effects; however, when it is taken in large amounts, it may inhibit respiratory function and ultimately lead to death. The same holds true for the often-prescribed tranquilizing agent diazepam (Valium). It is an effective anxiety- and tension-relieving agent when taken in the prescribed dosage. However, when diazepam is combined with a depressant such as alcohol, its effects are multiplied to the point that respiration and heartbeat stop and death occurs.

Medications aren't the only poisons; there are cleaning agents, insecticides, petroleum products, toxic plants, and a variety of fumes, gases, and vapors. Poisons may be in solid, liquid, or gaseous form, and they can enter the body in a number of ways. Depending on the poisonous substance, routes of entry include oral ingestion, inhalation, injection, and absorption through the skin.

Each year over 4000 people die as the result of accidental poisoning in the home; an additional 6000 persons use poisoning as their method of suicide. Nearly 2 million persons are involved in nonfatal poisonings yearly. Studies by the American Association of Poison Control Centers indicate that children under 5 years of age account for 60% of all poisoning cases and that adults (those 18 and older) are involved in only

24% of the cases. They further indicate that more than 80% of all poisonings occur in the home.[16, 18]

The implications for home safety are clear:

1. Parents of young children must learn to recognize and correct poisoning hazards in the home.

2. They must be prepared to recognize signs and symptoms of poisoning and administer proper emergency care if the need arises.

Child-Proofing Your Home

Anyone who says that rearing children is not a full-time job obviously has never had a child. To be successful in this task requires constant parental awareness. The rapid development of children forces parents to expect the unexpected. Today she may be crawling, but in a very short time she'll be walking and climbing. Childhood is not only an age of rapid growth and development, it is also a time of investigation. What does your 18-month-old do when he picks something up? More often than not, a small child's reaction is to put it in his mouth for a ''taste test.'' His sense of taste is not yet fully developed, and consequently he may swallow relatively large quantities of substances that would not be palatable to an older child or adult. Also a number of these poisonous substances have a sweet, lemon or cherry odor that attracts children.

A tragic example of what can happen in a very short period of time is the case of 2-year-old Bobby.

When Bobby's mother went to answer the telephone, Bobby picked up and drank a cup of liquid drain cleaner that his mother had left on the corner of the bathroom sink. He died 12 days later in the intensive care unit at a university medical center. Ironically, the call that Bobby's mother answered was a wrong number!

If anything can be learned from such a tragedy, it is that it's impossible to watch a child every minute. Don't depend on close supervision alone to protect your child from poisoning hazards. Children can move very quickly; and even if you are in the same room, the child may be able to act before you can react.

No matter how attractive a hazardous product may be, children usually cannot be poisoned if they can't get their hands on the poison. Therefore, one key to poison prevention in the home is keeping all medicines and hazardous substances locked up when not in use. With slight modifications, locks can be installed on most cabinets. An alternative is to install safety latches on drawers and cabinets (Fig. 4-19); however, older children may be able to manipulate devices and gain entry to the hazardous materials inside.

Many serious poisonings occur while a toxic substance is actually being used. If you are interrupted while using the product, take it with you. Do not leave the furniture polish on the coffee table within reach of your toddler when you go into the front room to answer the door.

Keep all hazardous products in their original containers, and never store them in cups, soda bottles, or other containers normally associated with food storage.

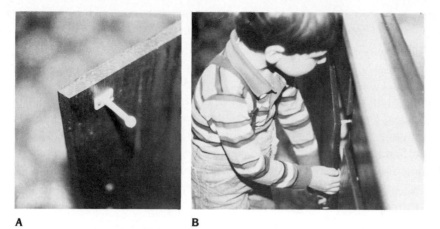

FIG. 4-19   A, This flexible plastic latch must be depressed before the cabinet door can be opened.   **B,** Safety latches keep inquisitive fingers away from poisonous products.

Since children often imitate adults, especially their parents, avoid taking medications in a child's presence. If your child is receiving a medication, never suggest that it is candy; refer to the medicine by its proper name. Even vitamins in large amounts can have toxic effects, so use the same approach in giving them to children as you would a medication.

A wide variety of drugs and hazardous household products are now required to be packaged in containers with safety closures that are very difficult for most children to open. The Poison Prevention Packaging Act of 1970 requires that numerous over-the-counter (OTC) drugs be sold in containers with child-resistant closures. This legislation was directed primarily at manufacturers of aspirin and aspirin substitutes, because these products were commonly associated with poisoning fatalities in children under 5 years of age. In the 20 years since this action was taken, aspirin deaths in children have declined from 140 a year to fewer than 10 in 1990. Several factors have led to the decline of aspirin poisoning: child-resistant caps, increased consumer awareness, and the voluntary limiting of the contents of children's aspirin containers (fewer pills in each bottle) by manufacturers. The packaging of other over-the-counter medications in blister or strip packs has also made it more difficult for a child to swallow a lot of pills at once.

Although the Poison Prevention Packaging Act has been a step in the right direction in terms of OTC medications, there are still some problems. Not all OTC medicines must be packaged in child-resistant containers; an amendment to this act allows manufacturers to use ordinary caps on at least one size of container for a given product. If you have children, examine the medication to ensure that it has a child-resistant cap before you make a purchase.

In 1974 the Poison Prevention Packaging Act was revised to include the use of safety caps on all prescription drugs. Today all prescribed medications are put in containers with child-resistant closures unless the patient specifically requests an easy-to-open container. Another revision of this act requires that caustic or corrosive household products or products that contain petroleum distillates must have child-resistant caps, and there must be some type of warning concerning the products' contents. These products include furniture polishes, charcoal lighter fluids, cleaning agents, drain and bathroom bowl cleaners, detergents, and certain insecticides and pesticides. However, the regulations allow manufacturers a great deal of latitude in interpreting what must be done to protect the public. A word to the wise: To protect oneself and one's children, the consumer must become aware of the many chemical hazards in the home and learn to take appropriate actions for the safe handling and storage of these products. Following are a number of poisonous products frequently found in the home:

Bathroom

Aspirin and over-the-counter medicines
Cosmetics
Drain cleaners
Hair preparations
Nail polish and remover
Perfumes and colognes
Prescription medications
Room deodorizers
Toilet bowl cleaners
Vitamins and minerals

Kitchen

Ammonia
Bleach
Detergents
Disinfectants
Drain cleaners
Flavoring extracts
Furniture polish
Insecticides and pesticides
Oven cleaner

Bedroom

After shave
Aspirin
Cosmetics
Perfume
Sleeping pills
Tranquilizers

Garage or basement

Antifreeze
Fertilizers
Gasoline
Herbicides
Kerosene
Lye
Paint thinners
Paint and varnish
Pesticides
Polishes and waxes
Rust remover
Turpentine

Poisoning Emergencies: Some Basic Guidelines

Regardless of the preventive measures that may be taken, there is always the possibility of accidental poisoning if hazardous substances are used in and around the home. Although orally ingested poisons are most often the culprits in poisoning emergencies, we must also discuss other situations, such as the inhalation of toxic gases, insect bites, and the absorption of toxic materials through the skin. In the following sections we will discuss signs and symptoms that most often occur in a poisoning emergency and the first aid procedures used in treating the victim.

With any poisoning situation there are several major points to remember:
1. If a person takes enough of anything, it can be detrimental to one's health.

2. The longer a poison remains in a person's system, the greater the chance for serious injury or death.

3. The sooner a rescuer can recognize the problem and give treatment, the greater the chances of recovery.

4. Never delay in seeking medical aid, even if you are unsure as to whether a poisoning has occurred. This is especially true in the case of young children who may not be able to communicate clearly or are afraid to do so.

Orally ingested poisons: corrosives versus noncorrosives. When discussing the recognition and treatment of oral poisonings, we refer to two types: noncorrosive poisons and corrosive poisons. By far the most common type is a **noncorrosive poison,** which includes prescription and nonprescription drugs. A **corrosive poison** is generally an acid, alkali, or a petroleum product. They are so named because they burn and inflame tissues immediately upon contact. Mucous tissues lining the mouth, esophagus, and intestinal tract are especially susceptible to the action of corrosive poisons.

Identifying the problem. Over 80% of orally ingested poisons are noncorrosives; the majority of these are medications. If you suspect that a poisoning has occurred, there are specific signs to help you determine whether it was a corrosive or noncorrosive product. If the person is conscious, ask him to tell you what he took. If it is a very small child, have him show you what he swallowed. Difficulty with swallowing or breathing, burns in and around the mouth, and peculiar odors on the breath are usually indicators that a corrosive poison has been ingested. Quickly survey such areas as the bathroom, garage, kitchen, or bedroom for any empty or open containers. They can be of value to poison control personnel in identifying the poison and the correct treatment. Once you have determined whether or not the poison is corrosive, definitive treatment can be started.

If the victim is unconscious, both identifying the poison and treating him become somewhat more complicated. However, you must do basically the same thing: (1) Look around for open containers, (2) observe for burns around the mouth and (3) check for peculiar odors. For any unconscious individual, pay particular attention to respiratory movement: Is the person having difficulty breathing? Loss of consciousness and breathing difficulty denote a life-threatening situation that requires immediate action by the rescuer, regardless of the type of poisoning. This would include maintaining cardiorespiratory function of the victim and calling for an ambulance or rescue personnel as soon as possible. *Never attempt to give fluids to an unconscious or stuporous victim of poisoning.*

Initial treatment. In any type of poisoning, call the local poison control center, your physician, or the rescue squad and report what has happened in as calm a manner as possible:

1. Identify yourself, your location, and phone number.

2. Identify the victim by name, age, and sex.

3. If you were able to identify the poison, tell the poison center its name and ingredients and give them an estimate of how much was ingested.

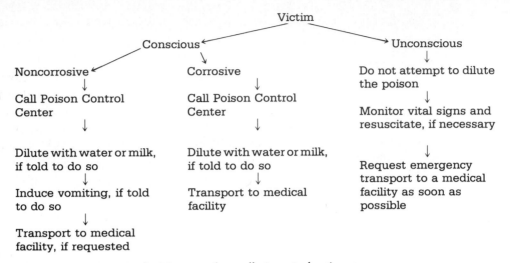

FIG. 4-20   Treatment decision tree for orally ingested poisons.

4. If you cannot do this, describe the patient's symptoms.

5. Listen and carefully follow the instructions given you.

6. Do not hang up until the emergency personnel do.

If the victim eventually goes to the hospital, take bottles, packages, or vomited materials with you, because they may provide additional information concerning identification of the poison and emergency treatment.

Noncorrosive poisons. If after the initial call to the poison control center it is determined that the substance ingested is noncorrosive, further procedures generally focus on diluting and/or getting the material out of the body.

In approximately half of the orally ingested poisoning cases handled by poison control centers, the initial therapy provided is the dilution of the poison with one or two glasses of water or milk. Dilution weakens the concentration of the poison and slows down its rate of absorption into the blood stream.

Depending on the type of poison and the quantity ingested, it may be necessary to rapidly remove it from the stomach. The quickest and easiest way to remove a noncorrosive poison is to get the victim to vomit. The best method is to give the patient syrup of ipecac, a commercially prepared emetic. An **emetic** is a substance that causes vomiting. One tablespoon of this preparation for children (or 2 tablespoons for adults) with one or two glasses of water usually induces vomiting in 10 to 15 minutes. When vomiting occurs, a sample of the vomitus should be retained and taken to the hospital for possible analysis.

In many cases the poison control center may be close enough that attempting to induce vomiting at home may not be necessary. Less time will be wasted if the patient is quickly transported to the treatment center. In other situations it may not be necessary to induce vomiting, if only a small amount of the noncorrosive substance was ingested. Poison control personnel may suggest that a parent closely monitor the child for the next 8 to 12 hours. The parents are instructed to call back if they notice a change in the child's condition. Be sure to call the center before attempting any major interventions.

Corrosive poisons. *Do not induce vomiting!* Remember, corrosive poisons will severely irritate and burn the mucous tissues lining the digestive system, including the mouth, esophagus, and stomach. Vomiting will cause the poison to come into contact with these tissues repeatedly, thus increasing the chances of further damage. With petroleum products, there is another danger when a person vomits. Petroleum distillates such as gasoline, kerosene, and turpentine can cause chemical pneumonia; and when people vomit, it is not uncommon for them to aspirate some of this material into the lungs.

Because care must be taken not to induce vomiting, do not try to force the victim to drink fluids. In many cases the damage has occurred rapidly and it may be impossible for the victim to swallow. Poison control centers will usually request that the patient be transported to a medical facility as soon as possible.

Fig. 4-20 is designed to help you to handle an emergency involving the oral ingestion of a poison.

Protective Packaging

The deaths of seven Chicago area residents in September and October of 1982 illustrated the ease with which over-the-counter (OTC) products could be contaminated with a poisonous substance. The victims died after ingesting Extra-Strength Tylenol capsules that contained lethal amounts of potassium cyanide. In ensuing weeks, other serious injuries resulting from the use of products that had been adulterated with a poison were reported around the country.

These tragic events elicited a quick response from the federal government and manufacturers of OTC drugs. On November 5, 1982, the U.S. Food and Drug Administration announced requirements for the **tamper-resistant packaging** of all over-the-counter drug products. These regulations require OTC drug containers to have an indicator or barrier to entry that provides consumers with visible evidence that a package has been tampered with or opened (Fig. 4-21).

Methods of tamper-resistant packaging include the following:[41]

1. Film wrappers: A transparent plastic film is wrapped securely around the container. The film must be cut or torn to open the container.

2. Bubble packs: Containers or medications are mounted on cardboard and sealed by a hard plastic covering.

3. Tape seals: Plastic, paper, or foil bands seal the union of the cap and container. The seal must be cut or torn to open the container and remove its contents.

4. Breakable caps: A portion of these metal or plastic caps breaks away when the container is opened.

5. Sealed tubes or bottles: The mouth of the container is covered with a thin plastic or metal coating which must be punctured before the contents can be removed.

6. Sealed cartons: The product is placed in a cardboard carton and all flaps are

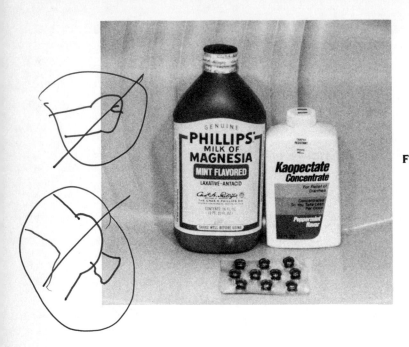

FIG. 4-21   Tamper-resistant packaging.

secured with an adhesive. To remove the product, the carton must be visibly damaged.

In addition to tamper-resistant packaging, the Food and Drug Administration has required that containers carry labeling statements that caution against the purchase of a product if its particular tamper-resistant feature is missing. By alerting consumers to the type of protective packaging being used, labeling statements allow them to detect tampering more easily.**

Although these federal packaging requirements can reduce the potential for tampering, they cannot totally eliminate it. In March of 1991 two deaths and several serious poisoning injuries resulted when packages of "Sudafed 12-Hour" capsules were adulterated with cyanide in the Seattle-Tacoma, Washington, area. Investigations of these incidents indicated that there was visible evidence of tampering; however, consumers failed to notice.[7]

A likely step to be taken by pharmaceutical manufacturers will be the elimination of all over-the-counter medicines in capsule form. Today most companies produce their products as pills or caplets. Unlike capsules, pills and caplets cannot be easily adulterated.

Inhaled Poisons

In its most recent report of yearly accidental inhalation poisoning deaths, the National Center for Health Statistics indicated that more than three fourths of the 900

**Words to the wise: Before you purchase medications at the drugstore or food at your supermarket, take a brief moment to inspect the containers in which they are packaged. If there are signs of tampering, return the product to the store manager; don't leave it on the shelf for someone else to pick up.

deaths reported were the result of carbon monoxide poisoning.[18] The majority of the carbon monoxide deaths occurred in the home setting. Motor vehicle exhaust gas accounted for the greatest number of deaths, while other deaths resulted from incomplete combustion involving furnaces, cooking stoves, and faulty ventilating systems.

Methane, the major component of natural gas, was associated with slightly more than 100 of the poisoning deaths. The remainder of the gas fatalities were caused by a wide range of industrial gases such as chlorine, sulfur dioxide, ammonia, and numerous chemical solvents.

As with most accidents, it would be much simpler to prevent a poisoning. If the following recommendations were carried out, there would be a significant decrease in gas poisoning deaths:

1. Never operate a motor vehicle in an enclosed garage. Take the extra 30 seconds and raise the garage door before you start the car in the morning. If you need to tune up the car, leave the garage door open while you do the job or purchase a special hose that carries exhaust gases to the outside.

2. A yearly inspection of the furnace and ductwork in the home by a certified heating and cooling specialist can reduce the chances of furnace malfunction or the development of gas leaks in the ventilating system.

3. Never use charcoal in an enclosed area such as a garage, barn, or the back of a pickup truck with a camper top on it. Large amounts of carbon monoxide are produced when charcoal burns, and any enclosed area will allow the gas to become concentrated.

4. When working around toxic fumes, follow the safety procedures that have been developed by the manufacturers of the product you are using. Use the buddy system when working with or near toxic gases. If you are overcome by vapors, there will be someone who can call for assistance.

Carbon monoxide (CO) is a colorless, odorless, and tasteless gas that results from the incomplete combustion of any carbon-containing fuel. The burning of fuels such as gasoline, kerosene, wood, coal, and charcoal produce varying amounts of carbon monoxide. Because it is relatively undetectable, poisoning may occur without one's realizing what is happening.

Death from CO intoxication results from the displacement of oxygen from red blood cells (RBCs) in the body. Hemoglobin, the oxygen-carrying component in red blood cells, has a much greater affinity for carbon monoxide than it does for oxygen (O_2). If a room contains concentrations of both CO and O_2, the red blood cells will more readily accept the carbon monoxide molecules. As the CO level in the blood increases, the O_2 level will decrease and tissues will begin to die. Nerve tissue, especially the brain, must have a constant supply of oxygenated blood. If the O_2 level in the blood continues to drop, centers in the brain controlling respiratory and cardiac function will shut down and death will occur rapidly.

The onset of symptoms may be very gradual. As the concentration of CO in the blood starts to rise, the victim may become dizzy and complain of a headache. He or she will become lethargic and have difficulty moving. With a continued elevation of

CO blood levels, the victim loses consciousness and, if the condition is not corrected, death will ensue.

Even relatively small amounts of CO can affect brain function, especially coordination and reaction time. In congested city traffic, drivers of motor vehicles have been found to have CO blood levels that well exceeded the point at which symptoms of carbon monoxide poisoning begin to occur. It has been suggested that many rush-hour traffic accidents are the result of CO intoxication.

Although most gas poisonings, including those in the home, are associated with carbon monoxide, other products such as cleaning agents and solvents, chlorine, and methane may be involved in home poisonings. Chlorine leaks can occur around some large home swimming pools. This irritant gas, used for water purification, causes acute respiratory-tract irritation when inhaled. The same holds true for many home cleaning agents such as oven cleaners (Easy-Off, Mr. Muscle, Dow) and drain cleaners (Drano). Fumes from these products will react with mucous linings in the throat and respiratory tract and cause severe irritation. Extended exposure to these vapors could seriously damage the respiratory passages.

Two cleaning agents commonly found in the home that require special mention are household bleach (such as Clorox) and ammonia. Separately, they are used to clean a variety of surfaces around the house. However, if they are combined, these same agents produce an irritating gas known as chloramine. This compound causes burning of the eyes, severe coughing, and sometimes nausea and vomiting. Generally symptoms are of short duration if one gets away from the fumes and rinses the eyes with water.

However, a more dangerous reaction occurs if one mixes bleach with acids such as those found in toilet bowl cleaners (generally hydrochloric acid, HCl). When these two products are mixed, chlorine gas is formed; it is more toxic than chloramine. Each year a small number of people die or receive serious lung damage when they inadvertently mix these two products and are overcome by the fumes.

Another word to the wise: Always read the label and directions before you use a product. On every container of ammonia and toilet bowl cleaner is a specific warning that it should never be mixed with chlorine bleach. So pay attention: *Read all labels!*

Methane, a tasteless, odorless, and colorless gas, is the principal constituent of natural gas that is widely used throughout the United States and Canada for heating and cooking. Although it is not an irritant like chlorine, ammonia, or sodium hydroxide vapors, methane can become deadly in several ways. In a closed house or apartment, methane gas from a leaking stove or furnace will replace oxygen in the dwelling and lead to asphyxiation of those inside. That is why gas companies add odor-producing substances to pipeline gas. When your gas pilot light goes out, it is usually very easy to smell the leaking gas. However, from time to time, people do not detect the gas odor for various reasons and they are asphyxiated while they sleep.

Although it is not germane to the issue of poisoning as such, the other reason that methane is a deadly gas is that it is highly explosive. A spark from a light switch, a match, or a lighted cigarette is sufficient to ignite the methane gas concentrations that can build up in a closed structure. If you are having problems with your gas appliances or you consistently smell gas in the home, call your gas company and get it checked out.

Emergency care procedures. In any gaseous poisoning, the initial concern of rescuers is to remove the victim from the affected environment and get him or her into fresh air. Care must be taken by the rescuer not to become a victim as well. If the fumes are too strong or irritating as you first enter an enclosed area, proceed no further. Instead, immediately contact the fire department and request assistance. Rescue personnel will have breathing apparatus and protective equipment that will allow them to remove the victim quickly.

EMTs or paramedics will be able to ventilate the patient's lungs with high concentrations of oxygen—standard protocol for most inhalation poisonings. Even when victims quickly recover and seem very alert, they should still be taken to a medical facility for a thorough examination. This reduces the chances of a patient's having a delayed reaction to the poison.

Poisons Absorbed Through the Skin: Contact Poisons

What is O,O-diethyl 2-isopropyl-6-methyl-4-pyrimidinyl-phosphorothioate? It is a major ingredient in a number of well-known insecticides and has been shown to produce liver and brain damage in humans. Its trade name is Diazinon, and it is only one of a multitude of highly toxic chemicals, called **contact poisons,** that can be readily absorbed through the skin. Ant and roach preparations, garden sprays, and rodenticides (rat poisons) likewise contain toxic substances that may be absorbed through the skin and into the circulatory system. Depending on the agent that has been absorbed by the victim, signs and symptoms range from nausea and vomiting to severe internal bleeding, convulsions, and in some cases respiratory arrest.

The toxicity of these poisons depends on the amount of poison absorbed, the number of exposures, the size of the individual, and the current health status of the victim. Adults are generally affected during the application of the pesticide. They may either inhale fumes or accidentally spray the contents on their skin. When applying these chemicals one should wear a mask, gloves, a long-sleeved shirt, and slacks. This will significantly reduce a person's chances of contamination. Children may absorb these materials through their skin when they play in and around areas that have been freshly sprayed. The major concern for parents is to prevent children from orally ingesting pesticides. Never leave these chemicals in an open shed or garage; make sure they are in a locked cabinet when they are not being used.

Many of the corrosive substances we mentioned earlier in the discussions of orally ingested and inhaled poisons are also known to damage skin tissues on contact. Although they are not generally absorbed into the bloodstream, as is the case with pesticides, corrosives may cause extensive skin or mucous membrane destruction unless removed from tissues immediately. Three corrosives that are frequently used in the home are bathroom bowl cleaners (hydrochloric acid), drain cleaners (sodium hydroxide), and oven cleaners (sodium hydroxide). The longer they are allowed to remain in contact with tissues, the greater will be the damage. It is not uncommon for these substances to produce blistering of the skin, the equivalent of a second-degree thermal burn. If these poisons are splashed into the eyes, major tissue destruction resulting in loss of sight is a very real possibility.

First aid for contact poisons. When one is contaminated with a corrosive contact poison, the immediate action is to remove clothing that may have been saturated and flush the affected skin with large quantities of water for 15 to 20 minutes or until the poison has been removed. If blistering occurs after this initial treatment, cover the damaged areas with sterile dressings soaked in cool water. This will protect the skin from further blistering and help to reduce the pain.

When exposed to a corrosive substance, the eyes should be irrigated with copious quantities of water for approximately 30 minutes. Do not allow the victim to rub his eyes after the injury. It may be necessary to cover the damaged eye or eyes with a protective dressing. Transport the victim to a hospital emergency room as soon as possible.

There is a slight variation in the emergency procedure for noncorrosive contact poisonings. Remove contaminated clothing and flush the skin with large quantities of water. Then wash the skin with soap to remove residues. (This step is not included for corrosive contact poisonings, since soap—which is an alkaline substance—may aggravate the situation.) Unless the victim is exhibiting immediate symptoms, take the time to call a poison control center before you transport the person to a medical facility; it may not be necessary to do this.

Contact With Poisonous Plants

A number of poisonous plants around the house are capable of causing severe itching, burning, and swelling of skin tissues on contact. Probably the most common of these are poison ivy, poison oak, and poison sumac. A sensitizing agent (urushiol) produced by these plants can cause severe itching and blister formation on the skin of susceptible individuals. It is basically an allergic reaction, with symptoms occurring from 1 to 10 days after contact. Some people are highly susceptible to this plant poisoning, whereas others seem to be naturally immune. People may develop a poison ivy rash without having come into direct contact with the plant, since urushiol can be transferred from shoes, gloves, clothing, or from material being burned in the yard.

If you suspect that you have come into contact with poison ivy, oak, or sumac, flushing the skin with large quantities of water may be effective in removing the contaminant if done promptly. Over-the-counter medications have a minimal effect on this condition. Preparations that keep the skin relatively dry seem to provide the greatest relief. Most cases will clear up with little or no treatment in a week or two. For individuals who are highly susceptible to these irritants, the corticosteroids, which are antiinflammatory agents, seem to be highly effective in reducing tissue swelling and relieving itching. However, since they are prescription medications, the corticosteroids, must be obtained through a physician.

Two popular indoor plants that have been implicated frequently in poisoning cases involving children under age 5 are philodendron and dieffenbachia (also know as

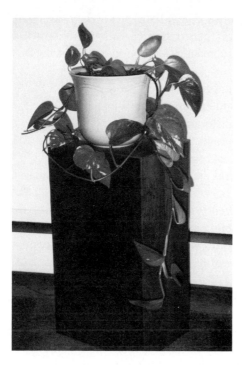

FIG. 4-22 When small children chew on the leaves of these plants, calcium oxalate crystals become imbedded in the tissues of the tongue and mouth, causing inflammation and swelling.

elephant's ear and dumbcane) (Fig. 4-22). Both of them contain calcium oxalate crystals, which can cause inflammation of skin and mucous tissues. These crystals are found in plant leaves and sap. Small children will chew on the leaves, and the calcium oxalate crystals will imbed in tissues of the tongue and mouth, resulting in severe pain and swelling. Occasionally, swelling of the tongue may cause respiratory difficulty. When little ones pull leaves from these plants, the crystal-containing sap may contact skin tissue on the hands leading to swelling of the fingers, or the child will put his fingers in his mouth and transfer the calcium oxalate to his tongue.

There is no specific antidote for this poison. If skin tissues are affected, irrigation of the area with water will help to remove the sap and crystals from the skin. Application of cold washcloths dipped in ice water will alleviate pain and reduce swelling. If the calcium oxalate crystals have come into contact with the child's tongue or mouth, give him a popsicle or small chips of ice to eat. The cold from these products has an anesthetic effect and will soothe the pain. At the same time, the popsicle or ice treatment will reduce swelling in the tongue and mouth area and prevent possible airway blockage. If the swelling does not begin to subside, it is advisable to take the child to an emergency room where further treatment can be given.

Injected Poisons: The Problem With Insects

Have you ever been bitten or stung by an insect while working around the house or yard? If so, you could have been the victim of an **injected poison.** Many insects produce enzymes that are used to kill or digest their prey. They are equipped with teeth, snouts, and stingers capable of penetrating a variety of tissues, including human skin. Physiological changes and reactions to the injection of these substances vary from person to person.

The National Center for Health Statistics reports that each year 50 to 100 people die as the result of allergic reactions to insect stings. While most of us would have minimal reactions to stings from insects, there are certain individuals who are highly sensitive to the enzymes produced by them. It is estimated that as many as 11 million Americans are allergic to insect bites and stings.[9]

The real culprits in the insect world are honeybees, wasps, hornets, and yellow jackets. They are from the order Hymenoptera, which includes those insects with fine, membrane-like wings. A sensitized individual who receives a sting from one of these insects may suffer a severe reaction known as anaphylactic shock. In **anaphylactic shock** the victim's blood vessels dilate rapidly, resulting in an extreme drop in blood pressure and an inadequate flow of oxygenated blood to the organs of the body. This is often accompanied by swelling of the trachea and bronchial tissues, leading to severe respiratory distress. If the conditions are not immediately corrected, the victim may die within 20 to 30 minutes after the sting.

Another reaction may be the occurrence of hives (large red welts that appear over the skin surface). Victims are often very uncomfortable, since hives are associated with intense itching. Once a person has suffered this type of reaction to an insect bite or sting, future reactions may yield more serious consequences.

Treatment of insect bites and stings. Depending on the level of severity of the sting, various actions may be taken. If the victim has no history of reaction to insect stings, probably the only thing that would be helpful is the application of cold packs to the affected area to reduce swelling and relieve pain.

If hives or generalized swelling over a large area of the body occurs, observe the victim for further signs of difficulty. It may be necessary to go to the family physician or a nearby emergency room to obtain an antihistamine to reduce the swelling and itching.

For cases in which the victim begins to exhibit signs of distress such as breathing difficulty (shortness of breath, wheezing), nausea, dizziness, and loss of consciousness, immediate action is needed. Until paramedics or EMTs arrive, your major goal is to maintain the victim's respiratory and circulatory functions. (See Appendix A pp. 461-471)

For persons who have been diagnosed as allergic to insect stings, there is a prescription first aid kit that may be obtained from a physician. The kit contains several premeasured doses of epinephrine, which can be administered at the first signs of an anaphylactic reaction. The epinephrine serves to constrict blood vessels and thus maintain the victim's blood pressure; it also increases activity of the heart, which in turn maintains adequate circulation of oxygenated blood. These kits also contain antihistamine tablets and an aerosol spray, which alleviate tissue swelling and aid breathing. Summer recreation areas such as schools, playgrounds, golf courses, and swimming pools should have these kits available, and personnel should know how to use them.

A relatively new advance for persons who have been diagnosed as allergic to insect stings is a program of immunization. Over a 2-month period, the allergic patient receives increasingly larger doses of the insect venom (up to about twice the strength of an average sting). Maintenance doses are then given at specified intervals throughout the year to continue the level of protection.

AIRWAY OBSTRUCTION

Dexter J. White was celebrating his seventy-sixth birthday in fine style. He was with his favorite nephews, Jimmy and Richard, and their families. And he was eating his favorite meal, a charcoal-broiled T-bone steak, corn-on-the-cob, and ice-cold beer. Midway through the meal, Uncle Dexter suddenly became very quiet and had a startled look on his face. As Jimmy looked up, he asked Uncle Dexter if he was okay. When Dexter didn't reply, Jim got up quickly and asked his uncle if he was choking. Hearing no reply, he immediately began using emergency procedures he had learned at work to relieve an obstructed airway. Within seconds a large piece of steak popped from his uncle's mouth, and he started to breath again. Dexter J. White would live to celebrate many more birthdays, thanks to the quick actions of his nephew.

D. J. White was a lucky man; however, each year 2000 others are not so lucky. They die as the result of airway obstructions. Although it can happen to anyone, two groups that seem most susceptible to this problem are the very young (children under 4 years of age) and older adults (those 65 and older). The latter group accounts for over half of all obstruction deaths.

In children, it seems that everything they pick up has to go in the mouth for a "taste test." Whether it is a piece of candy, a coin, or a button, the first stop is the mouth. Since the mouth is one of the most important sources of sensory input, children explore their world by bringing things into their mouths for manipulation and exploration. It is not surprising that nearly half of all toy-related deaths involve the aspiration of balloons, small balls and marbles, small toys, and parts of toys.[15]

For older Americans, a lack of teeth is often the problem; additionally, ill-fitting dentures can hinder rather than help in chewing food. Alcohol consumption seems to play a significant role in choking incidents by slowing down reflexes, desensitizing the back of the throat, and affecting one's judgment of the size of pieces of food to be eaten.

Most airway obstruction emergencies result when a large piece of food lodges deeply in the throat, blocking the tracheal opening and cutting off the oxygen supply to the lungs. However, in some instances a small foreign body may be sucked deeply into the trachea, causing it to spasm and contract tightly around the object, which also blocks the oxygen supply to the lungs. The death of well-known playwright Tennessee Williams, who died in February 1983, was attributed to this type of airway obstruction. He accidentally inhaled the cap from a bottle of nasal spray, and it went deeply into the trachea. Similar deaths have occurred with small children who have inhaled objects such as peanuts, popcorn, whistles, and marbles. Although they are relatively small objects, the irritation to the trachea causes it to contract tightly around them.

The best way to handle airway obstruction is to prevent it. Some of the key points one should remember include the following:

1. Do not put foreign objects in your mouth or hold them in your teeth. (People will place small caps from bottles of cologne, nasal sprays, and eye drops in their mouths while they have their hands full; sudden inhalation can draw one of these caps directly into the trachea.)

2. Closely watch small children to make sure they do not place foreign objects in their mouths, and do not allow them to run while eating.

3. When you purchase toys for children, be sure that they are appropriate for the age group for which you are buying. Read the warning labels on the packages.

4. Denture wearers should take special care to cut food into smaller pieces and chew thoroughly.

5. Avoid talking and laughing while chewing and swallowing food.

6. Be especially observant if some of your friends have had too much to drink and then decide to have something to eat.

Emergency Procedures

Because the airway can be either partially or completely obstructed, symptoms will vary. In the case of a partial obstruction, the victim will have some air exchange; heavy, forceful coughing is generally what occurs. Restrain yourself and do not start slapping the victim on the back; this may actually drive the obstruction deeper, causing a complete blockage. The coughing of the victim and the forceful exhalation of air usually brings the obstruction out, thus making the situation self-correcting.

If the victim continues having difficulty and coughing becomes shallow or you notice high-pitched noises each time he attempts to inhale, the obstruction may be getting worse. This situation or a complete obstruction warrants immediate attention. A classic sign of complete airway obstruction is the inability to speak, because air cannot be expelled over the vocal cords to produce sound. Other signs of complete obstruction may include a sudden look of alarm on the face of the victim, straining of muscles in the neck and face as he attempts to breathe, or he may use the universal sign of choking, clutching the throat with his hand.

Once a rescuer recognizes these signs of respiratory-tract obstruction, treatment should be attempted immediately. First aid procedures for airway obstruction are illustrated on pp. 461-471 to in Appendix A.

SUMMARY

Although the home is considered by most of us to be a haven from the hassles and dangers of everyday life, it is not always the protective environment we think it is. Each of us needs some form of insurance protection for those situations that cannot be prevented, whether it is homeowner's, condominium, or renter's insurance.

In proportion to other age groups, the elderly and the very young seem especially susceptible to falls. The elderly seem especially vulnerable, accounting for over 80% of the deaths resulting from falls. Their inability to absorb physical trauma and their lack of recuperative powers play a major role.

There are a variety of fall hazards in and around the home, including stairways, floors and walkway surfaces, and ladders. Probably the biggest contributor to falls is the unsuspected slippery or high-traction area that may appear on a stair or walkway surface. It is not the slipperiness of a surface that causes the problem; it is the lack of uniformity of traction.

Although not as numerous as other fall accidents, falls from ladders account for over 90,000 injuries yearly. Major considerations in the safe use of ladders include the type of work for which the device will be used, its proper positioning, and the skill of its user.

With today's escalating costs, more people are performing maintenance and doing repair work around the house. No longer is it uncommon to find homeowners who own a wide assortment of power tools. Some of the features of these tools (sharp, rapidly moving parts) can make them extremely dangerous.

Since most of this equipment is electrically powered, an additional hazard is the possibility of serious shock or electrocution. Three-prong grounded plugs, double insulation, and ground fault circuit interrupters are just three of the effective methods that have been developed to control electrical hazards.

Chain saws, power mowers, and power hedge trimmers save homeowners a great deal of time and effort. However, any equipment that has cutting blades operating at high speeds presents a certain potential for injury. The key to safe operation of these devices is to keep all body parts (especially hands and feet) away from the cutting blades.

Electric kitchen appliances present many of the same hazards that are found in power tools. Contact with sharp and fast-moving blades, beaters, and cutting edges is a major cause of injuries associated with kitchen appliances. Because they are powered electrically, kitchen devices also present shock hazards.

The National Safety Council indicates that more than 80% of the 2 million annual poisonings occur in the home, and that 60% of those poisonings involve children under the age of 5. Medications, cleaning agents, insecticides, petroleum products, toxic plants, and a variety of fumes, gases, and vapors constitute the principal culprits. Depending on the poisonous substance, routes of entry include oral ingestion, inhalation, injection, and absorption through the skin.

It is impossible to watch growing children every minute—they often act before you can react. The implications are clear: (1) Parents of young children must learn to recognize and correct poisoning hazards in the home, and (2) they must be prepared to recognize signs and symptoms of poisoning and to administer proper emergency care if the need arises.

More than 75% of deaths from inhaled poisons are the result of carbon monoxide ingestion. Motor vehicle exhaust gas and fumes from malfunctioning heating systems account for the majority of these deaths.

More and more we are finding chemical components in a broad spectrum of household products that can be absorbed through the skin or mucous membranes and severely damage tissues and organ systems. Certain plants in and around the house can also irritate skin and mucous membranes on contact.

Another form of poisoning is through injection of substances into the tissues. Around the home, especially in warmer weather, insect bites and stings can be a serious problem. It is estimated that as many as 11 million Americans are allergic to these insect stings.

Airway obstruction can happen to anyone, but children and the elderly are most at risk. The best way to handle the airway obstruction problem is to prevent it. Everyone should learn the emergency procedures to handle this life-threatening situation.

Key Terms

Anaphylactic shock   An extreme drop in blood pressure resulting in inadequate flow of oxygenated blood to body organs. If not corrected immediately, death can follow in 20 to 30 minutes.

Contact poison   Toxic or irritant substances that can be absorbed through the skin.

Corrosive poison   Usually acids, alkalies, and petroleum products that burn and inflame tissues immediately on contact.

Double insulation   Two separate layers of nonconductive materials are placed around motors and contact points of tools to prevent current leakage.

Emetic   A substance that causes vomiting.

Equivalent adherence   An optimal level of slip resistance so that there is a balance between slipperiness and excessive gripping.

Goodwill coverage   Payment for damage to the property of others for which you are responsible.

Ground fault circuit interrupter (GFCI)   A fast-acting circuit breaker that stops a current flow to an electric tool.

Injected poison   Allergy-causing enzymes that are delivered to tissues under the skin as a result of the bite of an insect.

Laminated glass   Two layers of ordinary glass are bonded together with a layer of plastic.

Loss of use   Insurance payment for temporary housing when your home becomes untenable as a result of an insured loss.

Medical payments to others   Payment for medical expenses resulting from a mishap on your premises or because of your actions.

Noncorrosive poison   Usually prescription and nonprescription drugs; they will not burn or inflame tissues when ingested.

Personal liability   Insurance coverage that protects the homeowner whose actions (or property) results in injury to others.

Personal property   Includes clothing, furniture, appliances, and other family possessions.

Poison   Any substance that negatively affects body tissues and/or organ function.

Replacement cost value endorsement   Lost or damaged personal property is replaced on the basis of current replacement cost.

Rigid plastic   Glazing material made from one or more layers of heated plastic.

Scheduled personal property endorsement   Specific articles of value are listed with an insurance company to insure these articles for their current cash value.

Structural protection endorsement   Insurance protection for rebuilding the existing structures of a home if damaged through natural disaster or disaster of human origin.

Tamper-resistant packaging   Provides consumers with visible evidence that a package has been opened.

Tempered glass   Glass that on impact crumbles into pieces, minimizing the chance of injury.

Three-prong grounded plug   The third prong acts to draw off possible leaking current.

References

1. Archea, J. C.: Environmental factors associated with stair accidents by the elderly, Clinics of Geriatric Medicine 1(3):555, 1985.
2. Blechschmidt, C.: Power lawnmower injuries, Washington, D.C., July 1990, U.S. Consumer Product Safety Commission.
3. Burke, B.: Child poisonings: the problem persists, Family Safety and Health 45(1):24, 1986.
4. Condominium insurance: Stock No. PAC-502, Holmdel, N.J., 1990, Prudential Insurance Co.
5. Gladden, M.: Safety bulletin no. 8: poisonous plants, Chicago, 1984, National Safety Council.
6. Gladden, M.: Safety bulletin no. 21: solid and liquid poisons in the home, Chicago, 1984, National Safety Council.
7. Gladwell, M.: Sudafed poisoning probe narrows, Washington Post, March 5, 1991, p. A-5.
8. Goodson, B., and Bronson, M.: Which toy for which child: a consumer's guide for selecting suitable toys, Washington, D.C., Sept. 1986, U.S. Consumer Product Safety Commission.
9. Hafen, B.Q., and Karren, K. J.: First aid and emergency care workbook, ed. 4, Englewood, Colo. 1990, Morton Publishing Co.
10. Homeowners insurance: Stock No. PAC-500, Holmdel, N.J., 1990, Prudential Insurance Co.
11. Horan, M.: Handling the hazards of getting older, Family Safety and Health 44 (1):16, 1985.
12. Jones, P., Roy, C., and Miller J. D.: Head injury in the elderly, Age and Aging 15(4):193, 1986.
13. Kelly, S. M.: Fall protection is worth the investment, National Safety and Health News 133(1):41, 1986.
14. Kramer, J.: Incidents involving death and brain damage associated with chests used to store toys, Washington, D.C., Nov. 1989, U.S. Consumer Product Safety Commission.
15. Kramer, J., and Tinsworth, D.: Toy-related deaths and injuries, Washington, D.C., Oct. 1990, U.S. Consumer Product Safety Commission.
16. Litovitz, T., Normann, S., and Veltri, J.: 1985 Annual report of the American Association of Poison Control Centers National Data Collection System, 4(5), Sept. 1985.
17. Melton, L. J., and Rigs, B. L.: Risk factors for injury after a fall, Clinics in Geriatric Medicine 1(3):525, 1985.
18. National Safety Council: Accident facts—1990 ed., Chicago, 1990.
19. National Safety Council: Power tool safety is in your hands, Family Safety and Health 45(1):4, Spring 1986.
20. National Safety Council: Chain saws are changing, Family Safety and Health 44(3):20, Fall 1985.
21. National Safety Council: Why electricity and water do not mix, Family Safety and Health 43(4):6, Winter 1984-1985.
22. Pater, R.: How to reduce falling injuries, National Safety and Health News 132(4):87, Oct. 1985.

23. Pavlich, A.: 1990 Holiday season—toy information, Washington, D.C., Nov. 1990, U.S. Consumer Product Safety Commission.
24. Pepper, S.: A physiological review of toys causing choking in children, Washington, D.C., Sept. 1989, U.S. Consumer Product Safety Commission.
25. Personal Catastrophe Liability Insurance: Stock No. PAC-504, Holmdel, N.J., 1990, Prudential Insurance Co.
26. Podolsky, D.: The not-so-safe refuge: unintentional injuries in the home and at play, Alcohol World and Health Research 9(4):24, Summer 1985.
27. Renters insurance: Stock No. PAC-501 EZ, Holmdel, N.J., 1990, Prudential Insurance Co.
28. Rousseau, P. C.: Falls in the elderly, Postgraduate Medicine 78(6):1985, pp. 87-88.
29. Srachta, B.: What you should know about: safeguarding machines, tools, and equipment, National Safety News 131(3):62, March 1985.
30. Tennant, H.: The most dangerous room in your house? Family Safety and Health 45(4):8, Winter 1986-1987.
31. Tideiksaar, R.: Geriatric falls in the home, Home Healthcare Nurse 4(2):14, 1985.
32. Tinsworth, D.: Analysis of choking-related hazards associated with children's products, Washington, D.C., Sept. 1989, U.S. Consumer Product Safety Commission.
33. Tinsworth, D.: Nursery product-related injury data, Washington, D.C., May 1989, U.S. Consumer Product Safety Commission.
34. U.S. Consumer Product Safety Commission: Consumer experience with ground fault circuit interrupters (GFCIs)—results of a national survey in June 1985; final report, Washington, D.C., 1986.
35. U.S. Consumer Product Safety Commission: 1989 product summary report—all products, Washington, D.C., 1990.
36. U.S. Consumer Product Safety Commission: Electric shock accidents involving hand-held electric hair dryers, Washington, D.C., 1985.
37. U.S. Consumer Product Safety Commission: Home safety checklist for older consumers, Washington, D.C., 1985.
38. U.S. Consumer Product Safety Commission, Chain saw safety: consumer information guide, Washington, D.C., 1984.
39. U.S. Consumer Product Safety Commission: Injuries associated with home workshop power tools: hazard analysis, Washington, D.C., 1981.
40. U.S. Consumer Product Safety Commission: Consumer product safety alerts, Washington, D.C.:
    (Dec. 1982) Electric home workshop tools (excluding power saws and chain saws).
    (Dec. 1982) Ladders.
    (Sept. 1985) High chairs.
    (Nov. 1985) Older consumers and stairway accidents.
    (July 1986) CPSC warns of strangulation with crib toys.
    (July 1987) Some baby gates are dangerous; others are safer.
    (July 1987) CPSC warns parents about child accidents in recliner chairs.
    (Aug. 1989) Parents warned about the danger of strangulation if children become entangled in window blind or drapery cords.
    (Nov. 1989) Over 200 infants died from entrapment/suffocation on beds since 1985.
    (March 1990) Falls from shopping carts cause head injuries to children.
    (March 1990) Children still suffocating with plastic bags.
41. U.S. Food and Drug Administration: Protective packaging regulations for OTC drugs and cosmetics, The Federal Registers, November 5, 1982.
42. Van Ty Smith, E., and McNamara, J.: Summary of the status report on chain saw related hazards since the revised voluntary standard, Washington, D.C., May 1989, U.S. Consumer Product Safety Commission.

Resource Organizations

American Association of Poison Control
Centers
c/o Dr. Gary Oderda
Maryland Poison Center
20 North Pine
Baltimore, MD 21201

American Pharmaceutical Association
2215 Constitution Avenue N.W.
Washington, DC 20037

Building Officials and Code Administrators
International
4051 West Flossmoor Road
Country Club Hills, IL 60477

Portable Power Equipment Manufacturers
Association
4720 Montgomery Lane, Suite 514
Bethesda, MD 20814

Consumers' Research
517 2nd Street N.E.
Washington, DC 20002

Consumers Union of United States
256 Washington Street
Mt. Vernon, NY 10553

Major Appliance Consumer Action Panel
20 North Wacker Drive
Chicago, IL 60606

National Association of Home Builders of
the United States
15th and M Streets N.W.
Washington, DC 20005

National Capital Poison Center
Georgetown University Hospital
3800 Reservoir Road N.W.
Washington, DC 20007

National Consumers League
815 15th Street N.W., Suite 516
Washington, DC 20005

National Poison Center Network
125 DeSoto Street
Pittsburgh, PA 15213

National Product Liability Council
600 New Hampshire Avenue N.W., Suite
920
Washington, DC 20037

Outdoor Power Equipment Institute
1901 L Street N.W., Suite 700
Washington, DC 20036

Pharmaceutical Manufacturers Association
1100 15th Street N.W.
Washington, DC 20005

Power Tool Institute
501 West Algonguin Road
Arlington Heights, IL 60005

Proprietary Association
1150 Connecticut Avenue N.W.
Washington, DC 20036

CHAPTER 4

Applying What You Have Learned

1. Make a list of the personal property you have at your apartment, dorm room, or fraternity/sorority house. With this information determine how much insurance you would need.

ITEM	COST
a.) Clothing	_____
b.) Stereo/TV/VCR	_____
c.) Athletic equipment	_____
d.) Jewelry	_____
e.) Furniture	_____
f.) Appliances	_____
g.) Artwork	_____
h.) Camera equipment	_____
i.) Guns	_____
j.) Computer equipment	_____
k.) Other	_____
Total	_____

2. Look through the products in your medicine chest, in the cabinets beneath the bathroom and kitchen sinks, and in other storage areas where you might have medicines, cosmetics, or cleaning materials. Identify which of these substances are corrosive and noncorrosive and compare the emergency procedures listed on the containers. Label noncorrosives (NC) and corrosives (C).

BATHROOM	KITCHEN	STORAGE AREA
_____	_____	_____
_____	_____	_____
_____	_____	_____
_____	_____	_____

Treatments for corrosives: _____

Treatments for noncorrosives: _____

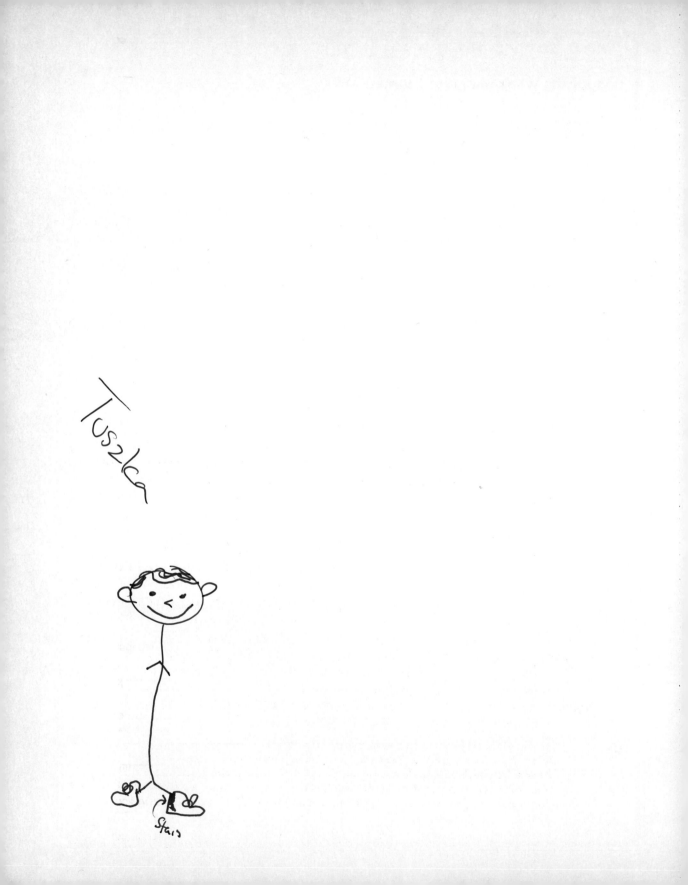

Tuszka

Stan

5 ◆ Fire Safety

Developing effective ways to prevent and reduce fire losses requires a continuing examination of the magnitude and characteristics of the fire problem—where fires occur, what causes them, and who the victims are.

U.S. Fire Administration: Fire in the United States

Fire! Whether you live in a house, mobile home, or apartment or whether you work in a 40-floor office building or a one-story industrial plant, you're not immune—it could happen to you. There are nearly 3 million fires in the United States each year, causing an estimated $7.3 billion in damages and resulting in more than 6000 fire deaths. More than 200,000 Americans require medical attention for burns and other injuries received in these fires. Although the risk of death from fire has steadily decreased in North America during the past 20 years, the United States and Canada still have the highest fire death rates in the industrialized world.

Failure to minimize the risk of death, injury, and property loss caused by fire is not the result of inadequate technology, because many sophisticated methods of fire control have been developed in this country; rather, it is caused by: (1) failure to perceive the danger of fire as a personal threat—"It will never happen to me!" (2) failure to take preventive measures to reduce fire risks, and (3) failure to prepare a plan of action in case of fire. As one investigator for the United States Fire Administration noted, "Most people are so completely unprepared for a fire, they almost never do any of those things they've been told to do. Because fire safety equipment and procedures are not used on a regular basis, people tend to forget them in an emergency situation."[1]

An example that illustrates these human failures was a fire that claimed three lives in an off-campus house at an East Coast university. In a postfire analysis, investigators determined that a grease fire had started around 2:30 in the morning in a stovetop skillet that had been left unattended. The fire quickly spread to the curtains and a paper towel dispenser near the stove. As one of the roommates attempted to extinguish the blaze, another tried to warn the six other occupants of the home. Fifteen minutes after the start of the fire a neighbor noticed heavy smoke and flame coming from the structure and alerted the fire department. Because of the rapid and heavy smoke involvement, three of the roommates who had been sleeping became disoriented, were unable to escape, and died of smoke inhalation.

The fatal errors included the following: (1) Food cooking on the stove should never be left unattended; (2) no one in the house attempted to notify the fire department; (3) a kitchen door was left open, allowing toxic smoke to travel up a stairway to the bedrooms; (4) batteries were missing from both the downstairs and upstairs smoke detectors; and (5) there were no fire extinguishers in the house.

Another example of inadequate preparation to handle a fire emergency involved seven members of a Kentucky family who perished in an early morning house fire. A visiting relative fell asleep while smoking a cigarette; hot ashes ignited the basement couch upon which she was sleeping. The parents were awakened by the smoke and attempted to rescue their five children. The father was able to locate two of his sons and get them outside. While he went to a neighbor's house to phone the fire department, the young boys went back inside the structure for the family dog. The rescue personnel later found the bodies of the mother, the five children, and an elderly aunt who was visiting for Christmas.

A fire marshal's report on the incident indicated that all of the victims died of smoke inhalation and that they probably could have been saved if the home had had some type of smoke detection system. Also, had the two boys been trained to stay outside the burning structure once they had escaped, they would have survived with their father. A few simple precautions could have prevented these deaths.

As you read Chapter 5, continue to think of the four factors of safety. One needs to understand fire hazards to minimize the risk of death, injury, and property damage from fire. Escape techniques and fire-fighting skills must be learned. In terms of the state of the performer, factors such as age and alcohol consumption should be considered. Finally, environmental factors such as the characteristics of combustion, including smoke and hazardous vapors, must be understood. In this chapter we will address how and where fires start, hazards that increase the likelihood of fire, preventive measures that can be taken to reduce these hazards, and actions that should be taken in case of fire.

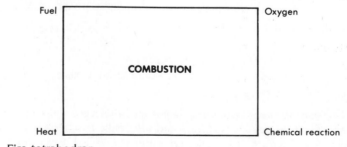

FIG. 5-1   Fire tetrahedron.

PRINCIPLES OF COMBUSTION

Certain elements and conditions are needed before a fire can occur: fuel, heat, oxygen, and an uninhibited chain reaction of molecules. They make up what is commonly known as the "fire tetrahedron" (Fig. 5-1). The combination of these elements under certain conditions results in a chemical reaction between fuel and oxygen known as "combustion." **Combustion** is a continuous, self-sustaining process in which fuel and oxygen molecules combine to yield heat, gas, smoke, and flame.

For fuel and oxygen to react, a heat source is needed to activate the fuel molecules. The minimum temperature to which fuel must be heated before it reacts with oxygen and starts to burn is its **ignition temperature** or **kindling point.**

Every fuel has a specific ignition temperature. The kindling points of some of the more common fuels are: wood (390° F), paper (450° F), cotton fiber (752° F), nylon (797° F), gasoline (536° F), alcohol (689° F), kerosene (410° F), and natural gas (900° F). By contrast, the temperature produced by a match or spark is around 2000° F; that of a cigarette may exceed 1000° F.

Combustion occurs only when fuel is in a gas or vapor phase. Although it has a higher ignition temperature, natural gas can be easily ignited with a small amount of heat from a spark or match because its molecules are in an active gaseous state.

For liquids and solids, sufficient heat must be applied to convert a part of the fuel to vapor before ignition can take place. The chemical decomposition of matter through the action of heat is called **pyrolysis.** As the fuel vaporizes, continued heating will cause it to react with available oxygen molecules, resulting in combustion. The form or structure of a fuel plays a significant role in the process of combustion. The more densely packed it is, the harder it will be to ignite. As an example, let's take a look at a fuel such as wood. A thick block of wood, like a log, does not burn easily; it takes an extremely large quantity of heat to cause vaporization and have the log ignite. Wood shavings or small twigs are less dense in form and can be ignited with the quantity of heat produced by a lighter or match. Wood dust, which is the least dense of the wood products, will ignite explosively from the heat produced by a spark. This is known as the surface-to-mass ratio of a fuel—i.e., the less the mass and the greater the surface area, the more easily a product will ignite.

Unlike solid fuels that vaporize at temperatures very near their kindling points, flammable liquids can produce hazardous vapors at much lower temperatures known as **flash points.** Although these vapors will not burn until their ignition temperatures have been reached, it takes a much smaller amount of heat to start them burning; for example, the ignition temperature of gasoline is 536° F, yet its flash point (the temperature at which easily ignitable vapors are formed) is only −45° F. Even in relatively cold weather, one must take care in filling a gas tank. The vapors that you see around the opening of the tank are highly flammable and can be ignited by a spark, the flame from a match, or ashes from a lighted cigarette.

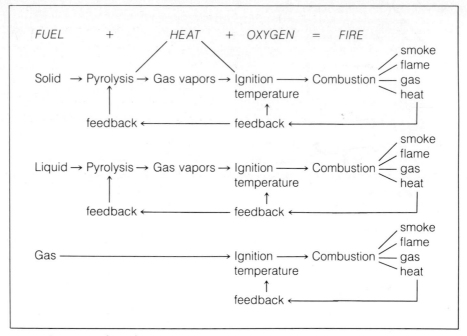

FIG. 5-2 Process of combustion.

Once the combustion process starts, it produces enough heat to continuously activate more fuel molecules, causing the fire to spread. The process that uses heat generated from a fire to prepare adjacent fuel for burning is called **feedback.** Fig. 5-2 illustrates the process of combustion.

HOW AND WHERE FIRES START

The major fire problem in the United States is residential. Home fires occur with much greater frequency than public building fires. Nearly 80% of all fire deaths and 65% of fire injuries occur in residences.[19]

Annually, cigarette ignition is the leading cause of residential fire deaths—accounting for 30% of the total. Other causes listed in order of occurrence are heating (14%), incendiary/suspicious (12%), children playing (9%), cooking (8%), electrical distribution (7%), and all other causes (20%).[13] Table 5-1 defines each of these fire causes.

In terms of property damage, fires caused by heating equipment account for the biggest monetary losses, nearly $700 million annually. As homeowners have gone to a number of alternative heat sources such as wood stoves and portable electric or kerosene heaters, an increasing number of fires are occurring each year because these devices are installed incorrectly, poorly maintained, or misused. Incendiary fires, or those of suspicious origin, also cause significant dollar losses. Many people are surprised to learn that arson is as much a problem in the residential area as it is in business and industry.

Though fire-related deaths in the residential setting are most often associated with smoking, fire-related injuries occur more readily in the kitchen as a result of contact with cooking equipment (23%). Smoking accounts for 17% of the injuries, and 13% of the injuries are associated with heating equipment.[13]

In a study of 7700 fatal home fires, researchers for the National Fire Protection Association reported that almost 70% started in either a living room or bedroom. In the majority of cases, upholstery or bedding was ignited by discarded smoking ma-

Table 5-1 Definitions of cause categories for structural fires*

Cause category†	Definition
Exposure	Caused by heat spreading from another hostile fire.
Incendiary or suspicious	Fire deliberately set or suspicious circumstances.
Children playing	Includes all fires caused by children playing with any items listed in the categories below.
Smoking	Cigarettes, cigars, pipes as accidental heat of ignition.
Natural	Caused by sun's heat, spontaneous ignition, chemical, lightning, or static discharge.
Heating	Includes central heating, fixed and portable local heating units, fireplaces and chimneys, and water heaters as sources of heat.
Cooking	Includes stoves, ovens, fixed and portable warming units, deep-fat fryers, an open-fired grills as sources of heat.
Electrical distribution	Includes wiring, transformers, meter boxes, power switching gear, outlets, cords, plugs, and lighting fixtures as sources of heat.
Appliances, tools, A/C	Includes televisions, radios, phonographs, dryers, washing machines, vacuum cleaners, hand tools, electric blankets, irons, electric razors, can openers, air conditioning and refrigeration units, dehumidifiers, and water cooling devices as heat sources.
Other equipment (also referred to as process or service equipment)	Includes special equipment (radar, x-ray, computer, telephone, transmitters, vending machine, office machine, pumps, printing press); processing equipment (furnace, kiln, other industrial machines); service, maintenance equipment (incinerator, elevator); separate motor or generator vehicle in a structure.
Open flame, heat	Includes torches, candles, matches, lighters, open fire, ember, ash, and rekindled fire.
Other flame, heat	Includes fireworks and explosives,‡ heat or spark from friction, heat from molten or hot material, and other heat from spark or hot objects.
Unknown	Cause of fire undetermined or not reported.

* From the U.S. Fire Administration. This list is a hierarchy for use in assigning fires to the appropriate cause category. Each fire is tested to see if it fits into the first category, then the second, etc.
† "Cause" used here as a shorthand notation for what is sometimes a complex chain of events leading to a fire.
‡ In actual sorting, fireworks and explosives are given a higher priority, after "children playing," but are included in this category for presentation.

Table 5-2   Where fatal home fires start

What ignites first in fatal home fires (%)		Where fatal home fires start (%)	
Furniture	27	Living room	39
Bedding	18	Bedroom	28
Combustible liquid or gas	14	Kitchen	16
Interior finish	9	Storage areas	4
Part of the structure	7	Furnace area	2
Clothing being worn	5	Structural areas	2
Waste, rubbish	5	Elsewhere	9
Electrical insulation	2	Total	100
Other	13		
Total	100		

From the National Fire Protection Association.

terials or nearby heating units, such as fireplaces, wood stoves, or portable kerosene or electric devices.

An additional 16% of fire-related fatalities resulted from fires that started in the kitchen. Heat generated by appliances, especially the burners on stoves, often ignites cooking liquids, clothing of persons working at or near the stove, and combustible paper or textile products placed near burners. Table 5-2 lists areas of the home where fatal fires are likely to start and what ignites first in these fires.

Fire Prevention in the Home

As evidenced by the figures listed in Table 5-2, the three most hazardous rooms in the home (with regard to fire) are the living room, bedroom, and kitchen. Over 80% of fatal home fires originate in one of these three rooms. Other locations that must be considered for their fire potential are basements, storage areas, and garages. Following is a discussion of some of the major fire hazards that are most likely to occur in these areas of the home and preventive measures for reducing their fire potential.

Living room. With cushioned and fabric-covered chairs and sofas, the living room is a prime target for the dozing smoker. Burning ash from a cigarette, cigar, or pipe may reach temperatures in excess of 1000° F and can easily ignite most conventional chairs and sofas. Flammability studies have shown that large pieces of furniture may be completely consumed in less than 10 minutes.[23]

If anyone in your house smokes, be sure to provide a number of large, sturdy ashtrays throughout the house. Ashtrays of improper design may allow a partially consumed cigarette to fall or roll off the tray. Preferably, ashtrays should have center grooves to hold burning cigarettes, or sides steep enough for smokers to have to place cigarettes entirely within the tray, rather than around the edges.

If you have been entertaining friends who smoke, you may want to check chair and sofa cushions for smoldering cigarettes before you retire for the night. If you do not have a metal container in which you can place cigarette butts, ashes, and other smoking materials, leave them in the ashtrays overnight to ensure they will be extinguished and safe for disposal the next day. Never risk putting freshly extinguished smoking material in paper sacks, plastic wastebaskets, or on top of other trash.

Other precautions that need to be considered in this area of the home include the storage of items on or around the television. Heat emanating from the back of a television set over a period of time may ignite accumulations of dust on the back cover of the set or newspapers stored on or near the television. Be sure to dust the back of the set regularly and do not use the top of the TV for storing mail or newspapers.

Malfunctioning extension cords and overloaded electrical outlets are responsible for nearly 20% of the electrical fires that occur each year.[13] Overloaded outlets cause an excessive build-up of heat in the wiring that supplies them with electrical current. After a period of time, the insulation on this wiring, which is located within a building's walls, may deteriorate and ignite. Blown fuses or circuit breakers may be an indication that outlets are overloaded. To remedy this situation, the number of appliances using current from these outlets should be reduced.

Extension cords are used in homes to connect electrical appliances. If the insulation on a cord is damaged, it may lead to **arcing** (the discharge of electricity across a gap in an electrical circuit) and the ignition of nearby combustible materials. If you notice that an electrical cord is starting to wear, replace it immediately. To prevent rapid wear or damage to cords, never place them under rugs, through doorjambs, or across paths where people are continually walking.

Wood stoves and fireplaces. With the ever-increasing cost of fuels, such as oil, gas, and electricity, more people are turning to wood-burning appliances like Franklin stoves or fireplaces to heat their homes. Since 1978, the use of wood-burning stoves and fireplaces has doubled; today these fires are more common than those associated with any other heating fuel (Fig. 5-3). Because the fuel in some of these devices can go from glowing embers to 1000° F within minutes, it is important that these units be properly installed and maintained.

Two of the more common fire hazards associated with wood-burning appliances are hot coals or ashes that may be expelled into a room and the extremely high temperatures to which a stove can be heated. The use of a spark screen in a fireplace or wood stove will keep coals and ashes inside the fire chamber. Removal of ashes is an additional hazard. Never place ashes in a paper sack or plastic bag. Even ashes from a fire several days earlier can contain warm embers. If ashes are placed in a sack or plastic bag, they may ignite combustible trash or the bag itself. The confusing part of all this is how those seemingly cool ashes can remain dormant for 2 or 3 days in the sack, slowly generating heat, until an ignition temperature is reached.

Mr. Achmad Fuquad of Burke, Virginia, had recently purchased his "dream home" for $280,000. His favorite part of the house was the family room, which had a wall-length fireplace. He religiously removed the ashes from the fireplace every Saturday morning, storing them in a plastic bag in the attached garage until Monday when the trash was collected. Last Monday, at 3:30 A.M., he was awakened by the sound of the first-floor smoke alarm. By the time Achmad, his wife, and three children were out of the house, the *garage—which contained a BMW 325i convertible and a Mercedes 190—was totally involved, and flames were spreading to the kitchen and family room. Part of the home was saved; however, Mr. Fuquad's losses were set at over $500,000, including the cars and other personal belongings. Investigators stated that fire had spread from the trash bag to a workbench and then to the rest of the structure.*

Do not store ashes and coals in anything but a metal container with a tight-sealing lid. Be sure to keep the container outside, away from combustible material.

Because wood stoves can become red hot during a fire, they should never be installed near combustible building materials. They should be placed on a fire resistant floor and 3 feet from walls. A stove placed too close to an unprotected wall or in direct contact with the floor creates a fire hazard. To minimize these dangers, have a wood stove installed by a qualified professional. And be sure to get the necessary building permits and inspections from your local governmental agency.

With wood-burning heating units, problems frequently arise when equipment is not properly maintained. Failing to replace loose bricks or mortar in a firebox or fireplace pit allows intense heat to travel to adjacent walls and wood structures in the

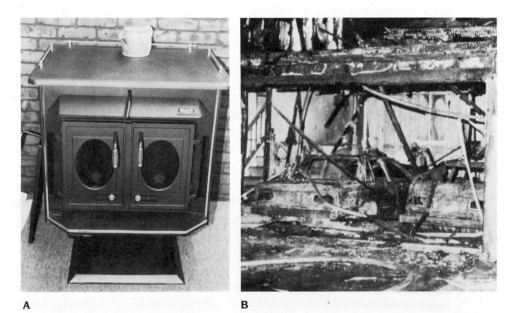

A   **B**

FIG. 5-3   A, Note the brick wall and the noncombustible flooring on which this new wood stove is being installed. Before this stove is in operation, the clay teapot will have to go! **B,** This $400,000 fire was caused by fireplace ashes that had been inappropriately stored in this garage.

A, Courtesy MBC Aquatics and Hot spot, Inc., Fairfax, VA.
B, Courtesy of Paul Torpey Photos.

home. A wood stove's fire clay adapters, which surround the stovepipe as it enters a home's existing chimney, may split or crack, transferring heat from the pipe to the nearby wood framing.

Creosote buildup is another problem that can result from inadequate maintenance. When wood burns, this flammable substance is deposited inside stoves, pipes, and chimneys. Over a period of time, a rather thick residue of creosote will build up. If these deposits are not removed periodically, a chimney fire may result. Sparks and flames will erupt from the chimney and imperil the roof. If there are cracks or chinks in the chimney, the flames may ignite wood beams or rafters. To reduce creosote buildup and the risk of a chimney fire, use only seasoned hardwood in your fireplace or wood stove.

New homeowners need to be especially aware of both chimney installation and maintenance. Instead of masonry chimneys, most new structures have metal chimneys. These chimneys are constructed with two or three concentric metal layers (a tube within a tube). Insulating material is used between the layers of double-wall chimneys, while air acts as an insulator between the layers of triple-wall chimneys. Heat from improperly installed metal chimneys can ignite wood joists, ceiling materials, and other combustibles. To prevent these occurrences, a yearly inspection and cleaning of chimneys, stovepipes, fireplaces, and stoves should be completed by personnel from a reputable heating equipment company.

Misuse of wood-burning heating equipment presents other problems. People like to move their stuffed chairs near the fireplace to feel its warmth, then forget to move the chair back when they leave. Newspapers and magazines are often placed in racks that are too close to wood-burning stoves.

Always make sure there is adequate clearance between your fireplace or wood stove and combustible materials, at least 3 feet. When you're finished sitting near the fire, move your chair back to its original position. Always keep newspapers and magazines away from the heating unit. Finally, never let a fire burn unattended.

Electric and kerosene heaters. Many people are turning to portable electric and kerosene room heaters as economical, alternative sources of heat. Depending on their size, these appliances can heat one or two large rooms easily, thus reducing the need to operate a home's central heating system.

Unlike wood-burning stoves and fireplaces, these units are unvented and do not require major installation costs. The heaters can be moved from room to room and are relatively inexpensive to operate.

In spite of all the benefits, these heating units do present some serious hazards. With its glowing coils (similar to those of a toaster), an electric heater can be quite attractive to a young child. Spaces between the protective bars on the front of older electric heaters allow little hands to touch red hot coils, resulting in severe burns. Even in newer models, the protective screen covering the heating coils may reach temperatures near 500° F.[21] Consequently, if these heaters are placed near combustibles such as drapes, bedspreads, or magazine racks, a significant fire hazard is

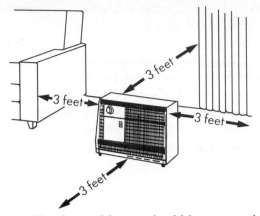

FIG. 5-4   This portable electrical heater should be operated at least 3 feet away from upholstered furniture, drapes, bedding, and other combustible materials.
Courtesy of the U. S. Consumer Product Safety Commission.

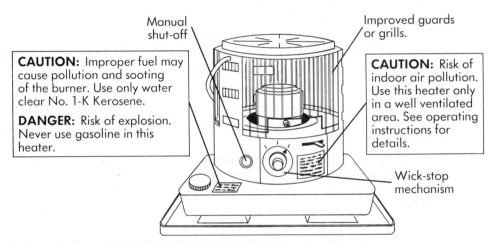

Manual shut-off

Improved guards or grills.

CAUTION: Improper fuel may cause pollution and sooting of the burner. Use only water clear No. 1-K Kerosene.

DANGER: Risk of explosion. Never use gasoline in this heater.

CAUTION: Risk of indoor air pollution. Use this heater only in a well ventilated area. See operating instructions for details.

Wick-stop mechanism

FIG. 5-5   One of the new generation of portable kerosene heaters.
Courtesy of the U. S. Consumer Product Safety Commission

created. If you have children or pets around, buy one of the new electric heaters that shuts off when it is tipped over (Fig. 5-4).

As electricity costs have risen, making the electric space heater less of a bargain, a popular alternative has been the reintroduction of the kerosene heater (Fig. 5-5). In the early 1900s, portable kerosene heaters were used widely as a supplemental heat source in American homes. However, because of the extreme fire hazards they presented, many states had banned the use of such heaters in homes by the 1950s.

In the late 1970s a number of major changes in the design of kerosene heaters again made them a marketable heating alternative. These models had a low center of gravity and were hard to overturn. They had automatic flame cutoffs that were activated when the heater was jarred or upset. Their fuel tanks were designed to be leakproof if the heater tipped over.

Even with these positive changes, kerosene heaters still present some major concerns for safety personnel. Tests have shown that regardless of their safety design a number of kerosene heaters leak fuel when tipped over, and some of the automatic flame cutoffs are not dependable.[10,24] Add to this the misuse of the heaters by consumers, and one can begin to see the difficulties that may arise.

In-depth investigations by the U.S. Consumer Product Safety Commission (CPSC) indicate that ''flare-up'' (an uncontrolled eruption of flames outside the heater casing) is the most frequent fire hazard involving kerosene heaters.[11,12] Although the causes of flare-up are still not well understood, there are a number of possibilities, including the use of gasoline instead of kerosene as fuel, fuel-tank leaks, overfilling of fuel tanks, and incorrect wick adjustment.

In an attempt to correct some of these problems, the CPSC and the kerosene-heater manufacturers have developed additional safety features that now appear on the newer heaters. Manual shutoff devices, located on the front of new heaters, allow for rapid action in emergency situations, such as high flaming in the wick or burner area. Also, heaters are equipped with positive wick-stop mechanisms that prevent the wick from being retracted to a hazardously low setting causing high internal heater temperatures. Warning labels have been added to the units specifying the use of *only* water-clear 1-K kerosene and cautioning that gasoline should *never* be used in these devices.

If you are going to use a kerosene heater in your home, there are some important points to remember[2,5,24]:

1. The heater should be placed out of heavy traffic areas to avoid overturning.
2. Never refuel a heater while it's in operation or still hot. Some exterior parts of the device may reach 500° F, a temperature that exceeds the kindling point of kerosene.
3. Never fill a fuel tank to the top with cold kerosene because it will expand as it warms, causing fuel to spill over the heater.
4. Use only high-quality, low-sulfur kerosene in your heater; poor quality kerosene will gum up the heater's wick, causing a heavy smoke discharge into the room.
5. Never, never use gasoline to fuel the heater. There have been a number of cases where this has been attempted. The results have been tragic, because the highly volatile gasoline vapors explode when ignited.
6. Be sure to keep children and combustible materials at least 3 feet away from heaters.
7. Never leave a kerosene heater unattended, and do not go to bed while it is in operation.
8. If a flare-up does occur, do not attempt to move or carry the heater; activate the manual shut-off switch. If this fails to extinguish the flames, leave the room immediately and call the fire department.

Because they are not vented to the outside, kerosene heaters allow pollutants to be emitted into the indoor atmosphere. Three gases that are of particular concern are carbon monoxide, nitrogen dioxide, and sulfur dioxide. Carbon monoxide is the result of incomplete combustion of a fuel. This gas replaces oxygen in the red blood cells and can cause death by starving tissue of O_2.

Nitrogen dioxide forms when fuels are burned at high temperatures. This gas is especially irritating to the moist tissues in the throat and lungs. Chronic exposure may result in serious lung damage, especially in children.

Another waste product generated by a kerosene heater is sulfur dioxide. Sulfur dioxide constricts respiratory passages, making breathing difficult, especially for those who have respiratory illnesses such as asthma or bronchitis.[5]

The problem of pollutant emission is magnified in the newer, better insulated homes that allow for minimal air exchange in rooms. Wisconsin now prohibits the use of kerosene heaters in homes built after June 1, 1980, because they do not provide adequate ventilation for the use of such devices.[2] If you use a kerosene heater in your home, be sure to have a window opened an inch or so to allow for an adequate air exchange. Before you purchase a kerosene heater, make sure that local building and fire codes permit their use in your community.

Bedroom. The likelihood of a fire occurring in the bedroom is greatly increased if there are smokers in residence. Sheets, mattresses, and sleepwear can be ignited by ashes from a cigarette. The elderly are exceptionally vulnerable to this hazard. Fire death rates for older persons (65 and older) are approximately five times higher than those for the general population.[22] When smoking, older persons may be inattentive and fail to recognize the danger involved. Also, reaction time is generally slower, and an elderly person may be unable to move quickly enough to prevent or control a fire situation. Alcohol and drug consumption by a smoker may also present a hazard. If the smoker is impaired by drugs or alcohol, coordination, reaction time, and level of consciousness are all affected to some degree, thus increasing the likelihood that a lighted cigarette might be dropped, misplaced, or forgotten and left burning. It is conservatively estimated that at least 10% of the victims of fatal fires were impaired by drugs or alcohol.[23] If you have smokers in your home, do your best to prevent them from smoking in bed, especially if they have been drinking or have taken medication.

All smoking materials, including matches and lighters, should be kept out of reach of children. Too often these materials are left around the home for the convenience of the smoker and, consequently, are also a temptation for little ones. A disturbing trend over the past 5 years has been a continued increase in child-play fire deaths related to both matches and cigarette lighters.[13] Children like to imitate adults (smoking, using matches and lighters); however, children are not always able to foresee the consequences of their actions. Like the elderly, young children (under 5 years old) have a significantly higher death rate than other age groups.[13] Young children often do not have the necessary skills to perform certain tasks, nor have they been trained to react to the dangers of fire.

Three other possible fire hazards in bedrooms are overloaded electrical circuits, portable heaters, and nightlights in children's rooms. Be sure that your residence has sufficient electrical outlets in each room to handle the demand from appliances. Use a minimum number of extension cords and do not plug too many appliances into any one outlet.

Electric heaters that are used in the bedroom as a secondary heat source should never be placed near combustible materials, especially bedspreads, drapes, and clothing. They should be placed a minimum of three feet away from these items.

A nightlight should be placed in an area where there is little chance that a child will come in contact with it. Also, the light should be installed away from curtains, bedding, toys, and other combustibles, as bulb temperatures may exceed 450° F.[26]

Kitchen. In the kitchen, the stove top, oven, and small appliances such as broilers and toasters are major heat sources. When using any of these devices, be aware of the location of combustible materials such as curtains, wall-hangings, and paper towels. If the stove is near a kitchen window, a quick gust of wind on a warm spring or summer day may bring curtains in contact with heat from one of the burners. Likewise, if the toaster is stored on the counter top in close proximity to the paper towel dispenser, there is an excellent chance for combustion to occur.

A fatal mistake that many people have made while cooking is to wear loose-fitting or flowing garments. As they reached above or across the stove, portions of their garments were ignited by heating coils or open flames. When cooking, wear either short sleeves or tight-fitting long sleeves.

Another preventive measure that should be taken when preparing a meal is to be sure that handles of pots, pans, and skillets are turned inward on the stove. This serves two purposes: (1) Small children will not be tempted to reach up and grab the handle of a pan, and (2) adults will be less likely to run into the handle of the pan and knock the hot contents from the stove.

The stove is not the only place associated with burns from hot liquids. Hot tap water from faucets injures nearly 3000 persons annually (the majority of whom are children under 5 and the elderly). Many of these injuries are severe; approximately 40 deaths are attributed to tap water scalds each year.[13]

To reduce this burn hazard in your home, lower the temperature setting on your hot water heater so that water coming from the tap does not exceed 120° F.[18] If your water heater doesn't have a specific water temperature setting, adjust the control mechanism to "low" and then check the water temperature at the faucet with a candy or meat thermometer.

Storage areas. Each person in the household can help to reduce the risk of fire in storage areas (for example, basement, garage, or attic) by keeping accumulations of combustible materials to a minimum. Discard old papers, clothing, boxes, and nearly empty containers of flammable liquids. If it is necessary to store these materials, be sure to locate them away from any heat source, such as a furnace, water heater, or space heater.

Storage of materials such as clothing, rags, and paper presents a special hazard. Under certain conditions these materials start to burn even without any external source of heat to stimulate them. This process is known as **spontaneous combustion.** Almost all organic matter (substances that contain carbon), including rags and papers, mixes with oxygen in the atmosphere and goes through a heat-producing process called oxidation. Generally the process is so slow that the heat produced is rapidly transferred into the atmosphere and there is no increase in the temperature of the material being oxidized. However, if the heat is not allowed to escape, the temperature of the material may increase to its kindling point and ignite. This is often the case with loosely packed bundles of oily rags. As the oil starts to oxidize, the loose rags act to insulate or hold in the heat, thus allowing the ignition temperature to be reached. If you must store rags or clothes, be sure they are cleaned first and then bundle them tightly. This will reduce the risk of spontaneous heating because the oxygen supply to the inner layers of fabric will be reduced.

Flammable liquids also present special hazards when stored in the home. Besides being easy to ignite, flammable-liquid vapors, such as those from petroleum products, are invisible and can easily travel the length of a basement or garage floor before dissipating. Because they are heavier than air, the vapors travel at ground level—a perfect condition for ignition by a furnace or water-heater pilot light. Flammable liquids should never be stored in an area that contains a heating unit. Preferably, they should be stored in a shed or garage that is detached from the house.

Planning for Fire Emergencies

A plan of emergency escape can give a family a significant measure of protection against the toxic smoke and flames of a residential fire. This is especially important when there are small children at home. However, an escape plan will not be very effective unless it has been practiced by family members on a regular basis. A well-known program established by the National Fire Protection Association is called Project **EDITH: exit drills in the home.** It consists of a number of basic steps that can be applied, not only in the home, but in the workplace as well.

Following is a list of important points to follow when planning and practicing exit drills:

1. Install smoke detectors in key areas of the home. Tell children what the alarms are for and how they work.
2. Draw a floor plan of your residence marking all exits and escape routes. Have at least two methods of exit from each room in the house where possible (Fig. 5-6). For upper story escape, have a portable ladder available in each occupied bedroom.
3. When a fire is discovered, immediately alert everyone in the house; you may want to use a special signal, such as a whistle.
4. When attempting to escape, stay low (preferably on hands and knees) to avoid breathing in smoke or heated air.
5. Before opening a door, check to see if it is hot with the back of your hand; if it is, use an alternate escape route. If the door is cool, brace yourself against it and open it slowly. Be ready to shut it quickly if smoke or heat start to enter the room.
6. If smoke is entering your room through spaces around the door, stuff rugs, blankets, or clothes in them to slow the smoke entry and attempt an alternate escape.
7. Have a prearranged meeting place well away from the structure so that you can account for everyone.

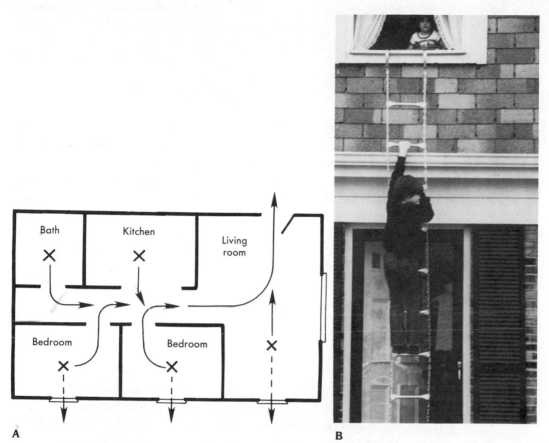

FIG. 5-6 **A,** Fire escape plan for a two-bedroom apartment.
B, Children in this family are learning to use a portable escape ladder.
Courtesy of Fairfax County Fire and Rescue Department

8. Never allow anyone to go back into the house for valuables, pets, and so on, once they have escaped.

9. Once you're outside the structure, immediately notify the fire department from a neighbor's house.

Although Project EDITH is relatively simple to implement, it will not be effective unless people take the time to familiarize themselves with each procedure. Family members should practice escaping from different locations in the home using a variety of planned escape routes. After initial training, in which fire drills are announced, it is advisable to have unannounced sessions from time to time. Since the majority of fatal fires occur between the hours of 11 P.M. and 6 A.M., fire drills held late at night or early in the morning will add a realistic touch.[20] Fire drills should be held several times a month in the home and at least once a month in hotels, schools, and office buildings.

Another fire emergency plan that is used by hospital and office personnel as well as students in university dormitories is called **RCA: rescue, confine, alarm.** It is a three-step procedure that is used when anyone discovers a fire, sees smoke, or smells unusual fumes. The RCA method can be used to train a large number of people about the basics of fire escape in a short period of time. The three steps of RCA are:

1. Rescue: Warn or rescue those in immediate smoke or fire danger.
2. Confine: Close doors to prevent the spread of the fire or smoke.
3. Alarm: Operate the nearest fire alarm or call the fire department.

Hotel and Motel Fire Safety

The principles of planning for fire emergencies can also be used when you are traveling. If you are staying in a hotel or motel, ask the desk clerk about the building's smoke detection, fire alarm, and sprinkler systems. Notice where fire alarms and extinguishers are located on the way to your room.

Once you drop the luggage in the room, go back into the hallway and locate the nearest stairwells and exits. Count the number of doors you pass on the way to the exit and notice on which side of the hallway it is located. A fire can produce heavy smoke that can completely obscure your vision; if you don't know the number of doors to the exit, you may miss it, thus delaying or preventing escape.

When you return to the room, check the window and make sure you can open it. Look for ledges outside the window and note how high you are from the ground. Take a few minutes to visualize the escape routes you could use in a fire emergency. Be sure to keep your room key within easy reach and take it with you anytime you leave the room.

If a fire occurs in your hotel or motel, here are some key procedures to follow[15,20]:

1. If you hear a smoke alarm or wake up to find smoke in your room, grab your key (which should always be kept by the bed), roll off the bed, and head for the door on your hands and knees.
2. Feel the door with the back of your hand. If it is hot or even warm, do not open it. If it is cool, crack it open slowly. Remember, you may have to slam it shut quickly if there is heavy smoke or fire in the hallway.
3. Make your way (on hands and knees or stomach) to the exit. Remember to stay against the wall on the same side as the exit, counting the doors as you go.
4. When you reach the exit door, close it behind you and walk down the stairs (be sure to hold onto the handrail). You don't want people who may be in a panic knocking you down the stairs. When you reach the outside exit, cross the street and wait until it is clear to return.
5. If you encounter heavy smoke on your way down the exit stairwell, turn around and go up to the roof. In taller buildings, smoke that has entered a stairwell may not rise very high before it cools and becomes thick and heavy. This phenomenon is known as ''stacking.'' When you reach the roof, leave the door open so that any rising smoke will vent itself. Find the side of the building away from the smoke and wait for the firefighters.
6. If you cannot leave your room safely, fill the bathtub with water, soak towels, and place them under the door and between the cracks to reduce smoke entry. With an ice bucket bail water onto the door and walls to keep them cool.

7. If smoke continues to seep into your room, place a wet handkerchief or washcloth over your nose and mouth to make breathing easier and stay close to the floor. If possible, open your window to ventilate the room, but do not break it, because you may have to close it again if smoke starts coming into the room from outside.

8. If your room is higher than the third floor, chances are you will not survive a jump. You will be better off fighting whatever fire and smoke has entered your room.

If you are visiting the home of friends or relatives, ask if they have a smoke alarm or fire extinguisher; if so, where is it located? As a final precaution, familiarize yourself with the floor plan of the home and the routes of escape you could use in a fire emergency.

Fire Detection Devices

In recent years, researchers have developed two types of devices to warn of fire: heat and smoke detectors.

Heat detectors sound an alarm when their sensing devices are activated at a specific temperature or rate of rise in temperature. They are widely used in industries that handle or produce flammable materials, but they are not recommended for use in residences. A major problem with using heat detectors in the home is that a fire may be too far away to activate the heat sensors, but it still may be producing large amounts of toxic fumes and smoke.

Poisonous gases and smoke rising ahead of a fire often overcome victims before they have a chance to realize what is occurring. Statistics from the U.S. Fire Administration indicate that smoke inhalation causes 75% of all fire deaths.[23]

Smoke detectors work by sensing the first traces of smoke produced by a fire. The alarm is activated long before toxic concentrations of smoke and gas develop. There are two basic designs for smoke detectors: the photoelectric apparatus and the ionization chamber (Fig. 5-7).

The **photoelectric smoke detector** consists of a thin beam of light and a photocell. When smoke particles disturb the beam of light, they reflect part of the light onto a photocell that activates the alarm.

The **ionization chamber smoke detector** contains a small amount of radioactive material that produces a beam of electrically charged air particles. When smoke

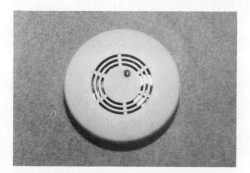

FIG. 5-7   Standard model smoke detector.

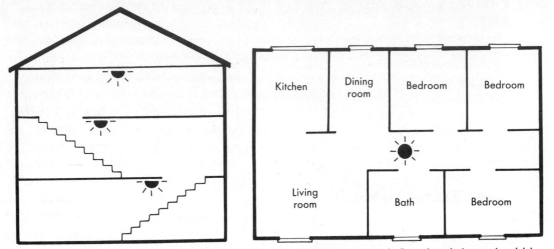

FIG. 5-8   Location of smoke detectors in the home. At each floor level there should be at least one smoke detector.

particles enter the beam, they interrupt the flow of electrical current and activate the alarm.

Photoelectric detectors are more sensitive to the large smoke particles produced by smoldering fires, while ionization chamber detectors respond more quickly to the smaller smoke particles produced by flaming fires. Because most fires produce both large and small smoke particles, studies by the National Institute of Standards and Technology have shown that ionization chamber and photoelectric smoke detectors are equally effective in detecting most fires.

Both of these smoke detectors have battery-powered models as well as models powered by household current. Battery-operated models are easy to install and will operate during a power failure; however, many homeowners fail to replace worn out batteries. Although more expensive to install, electrically powered smoke detectors are more reliable in the long run because power failures caused either by utility company problems or the early stages of a home fire are very rare. Smoke detectors that use household current can be installed with backup battery-powered systems that will activate if there is a power outage.

It is advisable to purchase at least one smoke detector for each level of your home. If this is not financially feasible, one detector can be purchased and placed near the bedrooms (Fig. 5-8).

Because smoke rises during a fire, smoke detectors should be placed on the ceiling or on a side wall between 6 and 12 inches from the ceiling.[26] Never put a smoke detector in the upper corner of the room where the ceiling and wall meet. Smoke is prevented from circulating to this area by an invisible layer of air. The smoke detector should also be placed at least 3 feet from registers and air vents so that drafts will not affect its proper functioning (Fig. 5-9).

How effective are smoke detectors? Increasingly, evidence indicates that detectors do save lives and property. Data from the Federal Emergency Management Agency (FEMA) show that when a fire occurs, the risk of dying in a home where detectors are not installed is twice that in homes where detectors are installed. In addition, the National Institute of Standards and Technology's Center for Fire Research estimates that between 40% and 55% of fire deaths could be prevented by the installation of smoke detectors.[26] In 1985 this could have meant saving as many as 3000 lives if every residence in the United States had had an operable smoke detector.

With the advent of cable television and reasonably priced electronic components, fire detection has taken a step into the future with remote alarm systems for homes. Known as the "automatic remote residential alarm system" (ARRAS), this program is designed so that alarm signals from smoke detectors in a home can be sent via a cable television link or phone lines to a central facility. Operators at the central facility then notify the fire department. Even if no one is home or if family members are asleep or incapacitated, the system will notify the fire department early in the fire's development.

As we have seen, the combination of planning for fire emergencies and the use of fire detection devices can significantly reduce our fire losses each year. In the following sections we will identify the different classes of fires and discuss methods that can be used to control them.

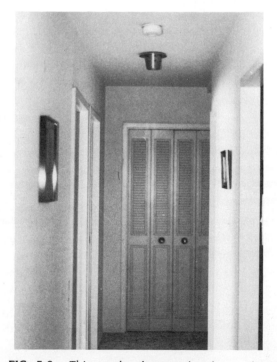

FIG. 5-9 This smoke detector has been placed on the hallway ceiling, away from air vents and registers.

CLASSIFICATION OF FIRES

Identification of the class of fire in which one is involved is very important because this will determine the type of extinguishing agent that should be used to control it. There are basically four classes of fires, and they are identified by the type of fuel being burned.

Probably the most common type of fire is the **class A fire,** which consists of burning wood, paper, or textile material.

Class B fires are often called flammable-liquid fires because they result from the ignition of products such as oil, gasoline, grease, paint, and alcohol. When heated, these materials break down, forming vapors that are easily ignited.

Class C fires involve the use of electrical equipment, including wiring, appliances, and machinery. When the power source is shut off and this equipment no longer has electricity running through it, then it becomes a class A or B fire.

The least common fire is the **class D fire,** which consists of combustible metals such as magnesium, zirconium, titanium, sodium, and potassium. Usually occurring in the industrial setting, class D fires result when metal chips, shavings, and turnings are ignited.

Fire extinguishing agents and their uses

When attempting to extinguish a fire, one or more of the following principles may be used: (1) cooling the fuel below its kindling point or ignition temperature, (2) excluding the oxygen supply, (3) separating the fuel from the oxygen or heat sources, and (4) interrupting the chemical reaction between fuel and oxygen molecules.

Cooling the fuel below its ignition temperature stops the release of combustible vapors, thus preventing the chemical reaction between fuel and oxygen molecules.

When the oxygen supply to the fuel is removed or reduced, one of the primary elements in the combustion process has been eliminated. Many flammable liquids will not burn when the oxygen level is lowered below 15%.

Separation of fuel from oxygen or heat may be accomplished by physically excluding the fuel from the fire (for example, draining diesel fuel from storage tanks). A modified form of fuel removal occurs when certain extinguishing agents are used to cover fuel vapors, thus preventing them from combining with oxygen.

Interruption of the chemical reaction in the fire process is only partially understood. Combustion involves the active combination of hydrogen and oxygen atoms and hydroxyl radicals. When certain liquefied gases, known as halogens (bromine, chlorine, and fluorine), are added to the fire, they attach to the hydrogen and oxygen ions and stop combustion almost immediately.

In each of the above situations, one or more elements of the combustion process have been affected. Using these principles, fire research personnel have developed a number of different fire-extinguishing agents for use on the four classes of fire.

Class A fires (wood, paper, textiles). Two agents are generally used on class A fires: water or a multipurpose dry chemical (for example, ammonium phosphate). Water-based extinguishers lower the temperature of a fire below its kindling point, whereas the dry chemical extinguisher has a smothering effect by covering the burning surface and separating the fuel from both oxygen and heat sources.

Water-based extinguishers are commonly found in schools, apartment buildings, and dormitories. These extinguishers are usually very effective on class A fires and are relatively easy to refill. However, there are some disadvantages to these devices. When filled they may weigh as much as 30 pounds, and if they are to be stored outside, an antifreeze mixture should be added. Probably the greatest disadvantage with water-based extinguishers is that they cannot be used to fight class B or C fires. Water can splash and spread burning liquid, causing a worse flare-up. Because water is an electrical conductor, it can carry an electrical current from the fire source directly back to the extinguisher.

For home use, the dry chemical extinguisher is, by far, the wisest selection. It is very effective in fighting class A fires and is light enough for most members of the family to handle. Before you purchase a dry chemical extinguisher, be sure it is triple-rated; that is, it can be used on class A, B, and C fires. Several types of dry chemical extinguishers are only effective on class B and C fires because of the type of extinguishing agent used in them.

Class B fires (flammable liquids). Three common extinguishing agents may be used with class B or flammable liquid fires; dry chemical, carbon dioxide (CO_2), and foam. Carbon dioxide extinguishers emit a cloud of heavy gas that excludes the oxygen supply from the fire, whereas the dry chemical and foam cover the flaming liquid surface, giving a blanketing or flame-interrupting effect.

Carbon dioxide and foam extinguishers are found in industrial or commercial settings, especially around equipment, where large amounts of oil or flammable fluids may be present. Although these extinguishers are effective in fighting class B fires, they have several drawbacks that make them inappropriate for home use.

The carbon dioxide extinguisher has a rather limited range so that a person must stand close to the fire for adequate coverage. It is also necessary to discharge this apparatus for a longer period of time over a fire to prevent flashback (the quick return of flames). This extinguisher should be used only on small fires in a confined space, since the carbon dioxide can be dissipated quickly.

When operating a foam extinguisher, you must take special precautions not to splash the burning liquids. Consequently, a certain amount of training is needed to use foam successfully. This extinguisher is heavy and cumbersome to manipulate.

For home use, a number of lightweight and highly effective dry chemical agents are the best choice. Besides the multipurpose ABC (triple-rated) extinguisher (for example, ammonium phosphate), manufacturers have developed several other dry chemical extinguishers that are intended specifically for class B and C fires. Two of these are the "regular dry chemical" (sodium bicarbonate) and the purple "K" dry chemical (potassium bicarbonate) extinguishers.

A somewhat expensive, but highly effective, agent in controlling class B and C fires is a liquefied gas called "halon." When discharged, this chemical rapidly turns to a gas and inhibits the chemical reaction between the fuel and oxygen molecules.

The major advantages of this extinguishing agent are that it leaves no residue on electrical contacts, involves little or no clean-up, and has minimal toxicity for humans. Halon is the agent of choice for those industries using highly sensitive and sophisticated electrical equipment.

Class C fires (electrical equipment). When live electrical equipment is involved in a fire, it is of utmost importance that only a nonconducting extinguishing agent be used. Of those discussed so far, only the CO_2, dry chemical, and halon extinguishers meet this requirement.

Water-based and foam extinguishers should never be used on a class C fire, since both agents conduct an electrical current. However, if electrical power to the burning equipment is shut off, these extinguishers may be used to extinguish the fire.

For the homeowner or apartment tenant, the most practical fire extinguishers for controlling class C fires are the ABC and BC multipurpose dry chemical units. They are relatively inexpensive, easy to use, and highly effective.

Class D fires (combustible metals). A laboratory or industrial setting is generally where combustible-metal fires occur. There are specific types of extinguishing agents for the various metals. Dry graphite, soda ash, powdered sodium chloride, and magnesium carbonate are some of the more common extinguishing agents. They are applied to the fire with scoops or hand shovels to create a smothering blanket or coating for the burning metal. Apply only the specified extinguishing agent to these fires, because other agents may intensify or spread the flames.

Fire Extinguisher Operation and Maintenance

Standing in front of a couch that is on fire is not the time to be reading the instructions for using your extinguisher. A delay of less than 1 minute can be the difference between survival and death. Unless it is a small fire, the major function of an extinguisher is to "knock down" or slow the fire's spread, thus allowing you and others to escape safely. Since the total discharge time of most fire extinguishers is 30 seconds or less, it is of extreme importance that people know how to use them correctly.

Though extinguishers vary in size, shape, and contents, principles for their operation and use are very similar (Fig. 5-10). Following is the standard procedure for using most fire extinguishers:

1. Before you approach the fire, break the seal and pull the pin on the extinguisher handle. Then briefly squeeze the handle to make sure the extinguisher works.
2. As you approach the fire, stay in a low, crouching position to avoid inhaling heat or smoke. Never get closer than 6 to 10 feet from the fire, and always leave yourself an escape route.
3. Staying low and holding the extinguisher firmly in an upright position, aim the discharge at the base of the flames, using a sweeping motion to cover the burning area. (If a wall is on fire, start at the bottom and sweep side to side in an upward direction.)

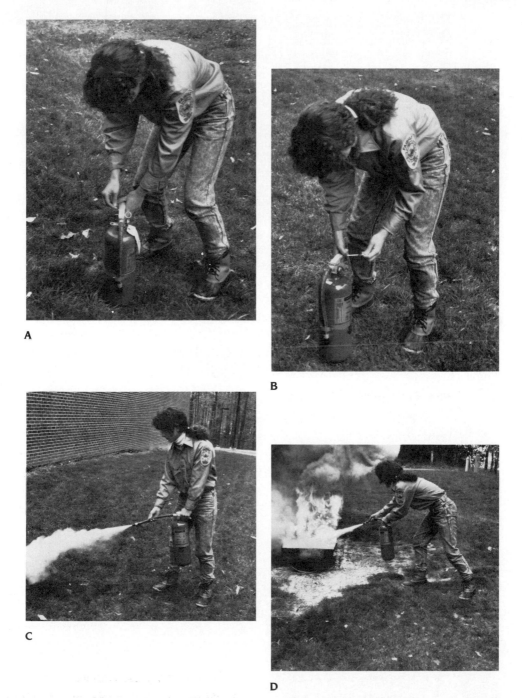

FIG. 5-10   Procedures for fire extinguisher use. **A,** Break the plastic safety seal. **B,** Pull the pin. **C,** Test the extinguisher. **D,** Aim the discharge at the base of the fire, using a sweeping motion.

4. When the extinguisher has been expended, quickly back away from the area. Never turn your back to the fire.

An important point to remember is that most extinguishers will not function properly unless they are held in an upright position.

To ensure that your extinguisher will be functioning properly when you need it, several items should be checked regularly:[19]

1. If the extinguisher has a pressure gauge, check to see that the needle registers in the green, operable area. If it does not have a gauge, weigh it to check for proper charging. A plate on the extinguisher should specify the proper weight. If either of these tests are negative, have your extinguisher recharged immediately.

2. Check the hose or nozzle on the apparatus to make sure no one has placed an obstruction in the opening. An extinguisher is useless if its contents cannot be discharged.

3. Check the plastic wire or lockseal holding the pin in place. If it has been broken, check to see whether someone has discharged the extinguisher.

Purchasing an Extinguisher

Before you purchase a fire extinguisher for your home, apartment, or car, there are several important points to consider. Of primary concern is the type of extinguisher you purchase. Unless there are special hazards in your home, the best choice would be a multipurpose dry chemical unit (Fig. 5-11).

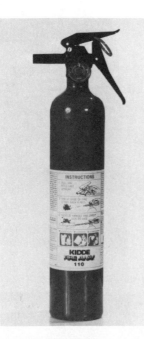

FIG. 5-11 A multipurpose dry chemical extinguisher is the best choice for the home since it can be used with class A, B, and C fires.

Another consideration is the classification of the extinguisher. This refers to the number of square feet the extinguisher can effectively handle for a particular class of fire. This figure will be found on all approved fire extinguishers. An example of this would be "classification: 4A, 60 BC." This figure tells you that the extinguisher can control 4 square feet of a class A fire or 60 square feet of a class B or C fire. A smaller extinguisher may actually be able to cover more surface area than a larger one, so be sure to compare classification ratings before choosing a particular model.

A final check is to make sure that your extinguisher carries the Underwriters Laboratories (UL) or Factory Mutual (FM) seal of approval. Either of these seals ensures that the extinguisher meets rigid standards of construction and performance.

Residential Sprinkler Systems

Sprinklers were primarily developed for property protection. In recent years their importance in protecting human life has been illustrated in a rather tragic manner by the MGM Grand Hotel fire in Las Vegas (1981) and the Dupont Plaza Hotel fire in San Juan, Puerto Rico (1986). In each incident nearly 100 lives were lost when fires (that could have been controlled quickly by sprinkler systems) raced through these structures. Consequently, building codes for most larger commercial structures now require the extensive use of sprinkler systems.

Although great attention has been paid to the issue of commercial-structure fires, the heart of the problem lies in the residential setting. Each year 80% of the fire deaths and 65% of the fire-related injuries occur in residences.[19] In the past few years, sprinkler systems designed for homes have become a reality. Used in conjunction with smoke detectors, residential sprinklers have the potential to make a significant impact on U.S. fire deaths.

In the past, the major reason that residential systems were never considered practical was cost. However, improved plastics technology has provided a number of low-cost, high performance materials that can be easily installed in a structure. In addition, sprinkler manufacturers have developed quick-response sprinkler heads that react as much as five times faster than older models.

Plastic piping placed above ceiling panels provides a readily available water supply throughout the house. Sprinkler heads are then located in the ceilings of each room. If there is a fire, rising heat along the ceiling will melt a composition metal pellet that normally blocks water flow from the sprinkler head. The temperature of the composition metal must reach 160° F to 165° F before it melts away; consequently, there is little chance for the system to go off unless there is an actual fire. As the water drops down from the opening in the sprinkler head, it hits a deflector sending it in a widespread pattern to cover the room and douse the flames. An additional benefit provided by sprinkling of a fire-involved room is that concentrations of toxic gases such as carbon monoxide will be reduced significantly, allowing for a better chance of escape. In the 1990s a number of states have begun to require the installation of sprinkler systems in all newly constructed apartments, condominiums, and multifamily dwellings. Though legislation requiring sprinkler systems in single-family dwellings and duplexes is not likely to be enacted in the near future, consumer demand from an educated public could significantly influence builders to add this technology to new home construction.

ARSON: FASTEST GROWING CRIME IN AMERICA

Statistics presented at a recent conference sponsored by the United States Fire Administration indicate that almost 30% of all fires are the result of arson.[3] An arson fire is a fire that has been deliberately or intentionally set. Property losses totaling an estimated $1.4 billion annually are attributed to fires of suspicious origin.[8] It is also estimated that close to 1000 fire deaths occur each year in "set fires."

With figures like these, it is easy to see why arson has been labeled "the fastest growing crime in America." Fire investigators have long been aware of the problem; however, they have developed few strategies to combat this crime. There is no particular profile for an arsonist. The arsonist may be a local factory owner who has been hurt financially by competition from foreign imports, or it may be a homeowner who is having trouble making mortgage payments. Arson has become such a profitable business that a number of people have become professional fire setters. For a fee, these people, known as "torches," will create a fire in a building and do it in such a way that a large fire loss is sure to occur. Although arson for profit has received the most attention, vandalism and revenge have been, by far, the most frequent motives for arson (Fig. 5-12).

Some of the more effective approaches used to combat the arson problem have consisted of three phases: (1) an arson task force, (2) an early warning analysis system, and (3) a public education program.

Arson task forces consist of fire and police investigators who have been specially trained in determining fire causes. In many cases their investigations may require elaborate testing procedures.

Analysis of insurance data about fire code violations and the fire histories of buildings and their owners can be used to identify patterns associated with suspicious fires. In a number of major cities, computerized profiles have been developed to target commercial businesses that are at risk for arson. Factors included in these arson-prediction models are any previous fires in the structure, vacant apartments in the building, fewer than 3 years at the location, food-related business, history of suspicious fires at other locations, and financial difficulties. The sharing of such information by insurance companies has proved helpful in determining why a particular fire was likely to have been arson rather than accidental in nature. Additionally, these computer profiles have helped to reduce the number of commercial arson fires. Using the prediction scores, fire marshals and insurance companies are able to broadcast subtle warnings to targeted businesses that there will be a swift and thorough investigation if their companies are suspected of having had an arson-related fire.

Public education includes efforts to make the community aware of the magnitude of the arson problem and efforts to seek citizen cooperation in providing investigative leads for specific arson cases. If a fire is termed arson, rewards are offered for

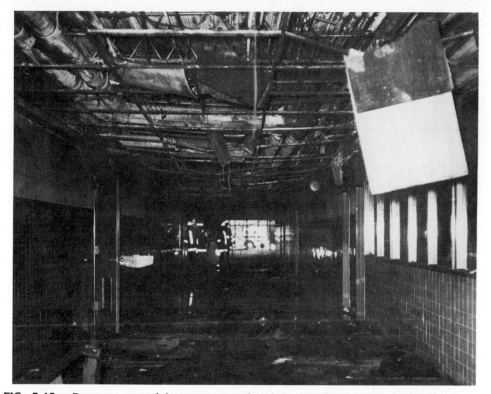

FIG. 5-12   Damage caused by an arson-related fire in this Virginia high school was estimated to be in excess of $4 million.

information leading to the arrest and conviction of the persons responsible. Although it will take some time to develop a network of local arson programs throughout the United States, this seems to be the most viable alternative for solving such a malicious crime.

HIGH-RISE SAFETY

On Wednesday, May 4, 1988, a blaze in the 62-story First Interstate Bank building in Los Angeles killed 1 person, injured 40 others, and caused damage estimated at more than $200 million. Built before a 1974 city ordinance requiring sprinklers in all new high-rise construction, the building was in the process of being retrofitted with a sprinkler system.

The fire, caused by an electrical malfunction, completely gutted the twelfth to the seventeenth floors of the structure. Because of the open-air design of the building, the fire was able to spread rapidly from floor to floor. More than 300 fire fighters worked throughout the night to bring the blaze under control.

Luckily, the fire occurred late in the evening when the only occupants were 50 maintenance personnel. Had it started during working hours, nearly 7000 people

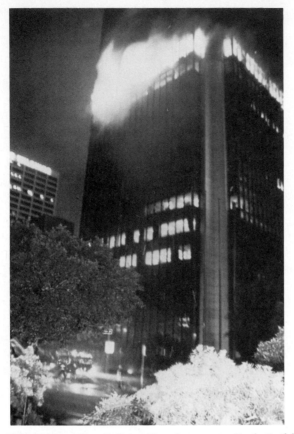

FIG. 5-13   The 62-floor First Interstate Bank Building in downtown Los Angeles was severely damaged on the evening of May 4, 1988.

Courtesy Los Angeles City Fire Department, Los Angeles, Calif.

would have been in the building; a significantly higher death and injury toll would have occurred (Fig. 5-13).

As the population density of cities increased and the cost of property continued to escalate, the advent of the high-rise structure was a practical alternative for housing large numbers of people in a rather small area. However, as with other technological breakthroughs, some new problems were created while alleviating old ones. Although some research has attempted to determine the best ways to control fires in high-rise dwellings, researchers and fire personnel have drawn few definite conclusions.

If you are planning to move into a high-rise or are currently working in such a structure, you may want to direct the following questions to the building maintenance personnel:

1. Since total evacuation of a high-rise is usually not feasible, are there designated ''safe areas'' within the building for occupants?

2. Is there complete coverage of the building with sprinklers?

3. Is the building adequately compartmentalized with fire resistant materials to limit the spread of fire?

4. Is there a building emergency-control center and an occupant-training plan? If so, how often is it tested?

5. Does the building have a fire detection system, including smoke and heat detectors?

WHAT DOES THE FUTURE HOLD?

In terms of fire-fighting technology, the United States continues to be a leader; yet sadly, we continue to have the most fire deaths as well. A nationwide effort is needed in fire prevention to turn this around, and it must come from two directions: public education and legislation.

To be effective, fire safety education needs to be an ongoing process. The annual presentations given to students by local fire departments during National Fire Prevention Week (the first week in October) may heighten awareness momentarily, but they do little to develop positive behaviors. Fire safety should be an integral part of the health curriculum, not only at the elementary level, but at junior and senior high schools as well. It is critical that students receive hands-on instruction in fire safety. It is not enough to discuss the use of fire escape techniques or fire extinguishers; students must have practical experiences. Instruction can be developed on a more sophisticated and technical level for older students. A key to the success of such a program is to use fire fighters as fire safety resource persons to work in conjunction with school health educators (Fig. 5-14).

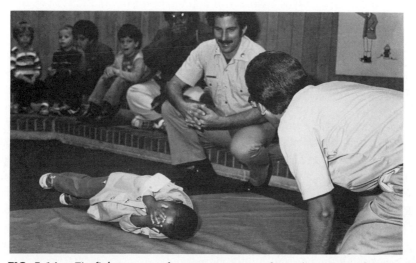

FIG. 5-14   Firefighters can play an important role in the community education process. Courtesy Fairfax County Fire and Rescue Department.

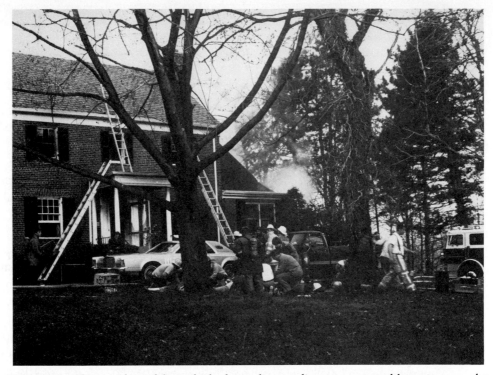

FIG. 5-15   This residential fire, which claimed seven lives, was started by someone who fell asleep on a couch while smoking a cigarette. The home had no smoke detectors.
Courtesy Fairfax County Fire and Rescue Department.

Adult education involves a variety of approaches. Presentations to church groups, civic clubs, and community organizations can do much to increase public awareness. Other fire department programs include free inspections to identify fire hazards in the home and media promotions about such topics as changes in local and state fire safety codes, the development of new fire safety equipment, and the discovery of fire hazards in new consumer products.

Because public awareness and education programs are voluntary for the most part, many people ignore fire safety practices unless they are required to follow them as a result of legislation. Looking to the 1990s, we will probably see an increased emphasis on fire safety legislation. Many jurisdictions around the country have strengthened fire safety codes by requiring that new homes and all multiple family dwellings have smoke detectors. Many state building codes now require the installation of sprinkler systems in new offices, hotels, nursing homes, apartment complexes, and other multiple occupancy structures. As sprinkler system technology continues to improve, there will be legislation to provide quick response sprinkler systems for all newly constructed homes and mobile homes.

On a national level the Consumer Product Safety Commission is currently considering the development of federal standards for fire-resistant upholstered chairs and sofas. This is a result of U.S. Fire Administration estimates that as many as 1500 deaths per year can be attributed to fires that start in upholstered furniture (Fig. 5-15).[23]

With the increasing use of wood stoves and kerosene heaters as alternative sources of heat, it would not be surprising to see the introduction of national legislation that more closely regulates the manufacture, installation, and operation of such devices in the home.

In recent years, smoking—the leading cause of fire deaths in the United States—has come under close scrutiny by a number of national organizations, including the International Association of Fire Chiefs, the Burn Council, the International Association of Fire Fighters, the National Fire Protection Association, and the Citizens' Committee for Fire Protection. Cigarettes have been involved in over 85% of smoking-related fatalities.[9] Unlike cigar and pipe tobacco, cigarette tobacco contains added chemicals that keep it burning—even when the cigarette is not being smoked. A freshly lighted cigarette will burn for approximately 20 to 45 minutes when placed on a flat surface. Without the added chemicals, cigarettes would go out within minutes of the last puff, as do cigars and pipes.

The most likely legislation concerning the cigarette hazard would be a national performance standard requiring manufacturers to develop a cigarette that would self-extinguish when not being actively smoked. Studies indicate that development of such a cigarette is within the realm of present manufacturing technology. With the Fire Safe Cigarette Act of 1990, Congress has taken the first step. It has authorized the National Institute for Standards and Technology's Center for Fire Research to begin the development of a prototype cigarette that will have a reduced propensity to ignite upholstered furniture and mattresses.

Unless greater effort is placed on fire safety education and legislation, we will not likely see a significant decrease in fire deaths, injuries, and property loss in the 1990s.

SUMMARY

Although the fire death rate has been decreasing in recent years, the United States still has a serious problem in terms of lives lost, people injured, and property damaged as a result of fire. The problem is not one of technological inadequacy but of human failure—failure to perceive the dangers of fire and failure to prepare for handling those dangers.

To perceive the dangers of fire, one must have an understanding of the process of combustion and the roles played by fuel, heat, and oxygen. A person must also realize that the major fire problem is in the home or residential setting, where almost 80% of all fatal fires occur.

Each area of the home presents its own distinct set of hazards. Nearly 70% of fatal home fires start in either the living room or a bedroom, discarded smoking materials being the primary cause. Cooking appliances are major heat sources in the kitchen and are capable of igniting paper towels, wall hangings, and clothing. Garages and basements deserve special attention if they are used to store flammable liquids or materials such as rags or paper. Because flammable liquids are capable of producing hazardous vapors well below their ignition temperatures, it is important to keep them away from heat sources such as furnaces and water heaters. Under certain conditions, rags and papers that are stored in loose bundles may go through a heat-producing process (spontaneous combustion) and start to burn, even though there has been no external source of heat to stimulate them. To prevent this from happening, accumulations of combustibles must be kept to a minimum.

Regardless of the precautions taken to reduce the risk of fire, there is always a chance that one may occur. Prefire planning involves: (1) fire emergency escape routes, (2) fire detection devices, and (3) fire extinguishing agents.

A well-known plan for developing escape routes is Project EDITH (exit drills in the home). Although most plans of exit from a dwelling are usually simple, they will not prove effective unless people familiarize themselves with the program and actually go through the escape drills.

Based on the fact that 75% of all fire deaths are caused by smoke inhalation, it is likely that a significant number of fire deaths could be prevented by the installation of smoke detectors. These devices are activated by the first traces of smoke from a fire long before toxic concentrations of smoke develop.

Before you attempt to control a fire, it is important to know what type of fuel is being burned so that you can use the correct extinguishing agent. For home use the triple-rated ABC dry chemical extinguisher is the best choice; it is effective on a wide range of fires, easy to handle, and relatively inexpensive. An important fact to remember about all extinguishers is that they are designed to *slow* a fire's progress, not to put it out. It is important that people familiarize themselves with the techniques for handling different fire extinguishers. If you have not practiced the skills, chances are you will not be able to use them in a fire emergency.

Labeled the "fastest growing crime in America," arson accounts for nearly 30% of all fires. The $1.4 billion cost of these "set fires" is paid through increased insurance premiums for all of us. To combat this situation, many cities are developing a three-phase program consisting of arson task forces, early warning analysis systems, and public education.

As the population increases and property prices escalate, the high-rise structure will remain a practical alternative for housing large numbers of people. If you are planning to move into a high-rise, it would be wise to become familiar with the types of fire protection offered by such a facility.

A nationwide effort in fire protection must concentrate on public education and legislation. A key to the success of public education is the use of fire fighters as fire safety educators. Legislative efforts must address issues such as stricter fire safety codes and nationwide performance standards for consumer products that may present fire hazards.

Key Terms

Arcing   The discharge of electricity across a gap in an electrical circuit.

Arson fire   A fire that has been deliberately or intentionally set.

Class A fire   Consists of burning wood, paper, or textile material.

Class B fire   Flammable liquid fires.

Class C fire   Involves the use of electrical equipment, including wiring, appliances, and machinery.

Class D fire   Consists of combustible metals.

Combustion   A continuous, self-sustaining process in which fuel and oxygen molecules combine to yield heat, gas, smoke, and flame.

Exit drills in the home (EDITH)   This educational program assists families in developing fire exit plans for their homes.

Feedback   The process that uses heat generated from a fire to prepare adjacent fuel for burning.

Flash point   The temperature at which a flammable liquid becomes an easily ignitable vapor.

Halogens   Certain liquified gases that stop combustion almost immediately.

Heat detector   Sounds an alarm when it is activated at a specific temperature or rate of rise in temperature.

Ignition temperature or **kindling point**   The minimum temperature to which a fuel must be heated before it reacts with oxygen and starts to burn.

Ionization chamber smoke detector   Contains a small amount of radioactive material that produces a beam of electrically charged particles. Smoke particles interrupt the flow of electrical current and thereby activate the alarm.

Photoelectric smoke detector   Smoke particles disturb a beam of light to activate the alarm.

Pyrolysis   A chemical decomposition of matter through the action of heat.

Rescue, confine, and alarm (RCA)   A three-step procedure that can be used by anyone who discovers a fire, sees smoke, or smells unusual fumes.

Spontaneous combustion   Under certain conditions, materials begin to burn even though there has been no external source of heat to stimulate them.

References

1. Bryson, W., Jr.: Fire! Tips that can save your life, Parade Magazine, Feb. 10, 1980, p. 4.
2. Burke, B.: Some things you should know about kerosene heaters, Family Safety, Fall 1982, p. 12.
3. Callahan, J.: Elusive goal: proving fraudulent claim, Fire Chief 30(7):44, 1986.
4. Coleman, R.: Residential sprinkler ordinances: successes and failures, Fire Chief 30(7):31, 1986.
5. Consumer Reports: Are kerosene heaters safe? Oct. 1982, p. 499.
6. Consumer Reports: Fire extinguishers, Feb. 1988, pp. 101-104.
7. Fire, F.: Plastics and fire investigations, Fire Engineering 138(1):46, 1985.
8. Hammett, T.: Pulling together against arson, Firehouse, Aug. 1986, p. 44.
9. Howard, B.: Feasibility study of cigarette-ignited fires, Washington, D.C., May 1987, U.S. Consumer Product Safety Commission.
10. Harwood, B.: Flare-up fires involving kerosene heaters, Washington, D.C., March 1987, U.S. Consumer Product Safety Commission.
11. Harwood, B., and Kelly, S.: Fire hazards involving kerosene heaters, Washington, D.C., 1985, U.S. Consumer Product Safety Commission.
12. Harwood, B., Kale, D., and Kelly, S.: Hazards involving kerosene heaters, Washington, D.C., 1983, U.S. Consumer Product Safety Commission.
13. Hoebel, J. F.: National estimates: 1988 fire losses, Washington, D.C., July 1990, U.S. Consumer Product Safety Commission.
14. Kale, D.: Fires in woodburning appliances, Washington, D.C., Dec. 1982, U.S. Consumer Product Safety Commission.

15. Kauffman, R. H.: Warning: hotels could be hazardous to your health, Aide, Spring 1981, p. 20.
16. Laughlin, J. W., ed.: Firefighter occupational safety, Stillwater, Okla., 1979, Fire Protection Publications.
17. Mulrine, J.: Residential sprinklers: plastic pipe dreams? Firehouse, Sept. 1982, p. 116.
18. National Fire Protection Association: Automatic sprinklers: save lives, save property, Batterymarch Park, Quincy, MA, 1988.
19. National Fire Protection Association: Facts about fire, Boston, 1979, Pamphlet No. 500M-FP-470-FPW-4.
20. Naughton, T.: Can your family escape a fire? Family Safety and Health 42(3):4, 1983.
21. Smith, L., and Kramer, J.: Hazard analysis: fires associated with portable electric heaters, Washington, D.C., April 1986, U.S. Consumer Product Safety Commission.
22. Tinsworth, D. K., and Kelly, S.: Hazard analysis: fires in mattresses and bedding, Washington, D.C., July 1984, U.S. Consumer Product Safety Commission.
23. U.S. Consumer Product Safety Commission: Upholstered furniture fire loss estimates, Washington, D.C., 1986.
24. U.S. Consumer Product Safety Commission: What you should know about kerosene heaters, Washington, D.C., Aug. 1987.
25. U.S. Consumer Product Safety Commission: Special analysis: kerosene heaters, June 1982.
26. U.S. Consumer Product Safety Commission: Your home fire safety checklist, Washington, D.C., Sept. 1987.

Resource Organizations

American Insurance Association
85 John Street
New York, NY 10038

Factory Mutual System
1151 Boston-Providence Turnpike
Norwood, MA 02062

Fire Equipment Manufacturers Association
c/o Thomas Associates, Inc.
1230 Keith Building
Cleveland, OH 44115

Fire Marshals Association of North America
1110 Vermont Avenue, NW, Suite 1210
Washington, DC 20005

International Association of Fire Chiefs
1329 18th Street, NW
Washington, DC 20036

International Association of Fire Fighters
1750 New York Ave., N. W.
Washinton, DC 2006

National Association of Fire Equipment
Distributors
c/o Smith, Bucklin and Associates, Mgrs.
111 East Wacker Drive
Chicago, IL 60601

National Institute of Standards and Technology
Center for Fire Research
Commerce Department
Washington, DC 20234

National Burglar and Fire Alarm Association
1120 19th, NW, Suite LL-20
Washington, DC 20036

National Fire Protection Association
Batterymarch Park
Quincy, MA 02269

Society of Fire Protection Engineers
60 Batterymarch Street
Boston, MA 02110

CHAPTER 5

Applying What You Have Learned

1. In the space provided draw up an emergency escape plan for your home, apartment, fraternity/sorority house, or the dormitory floor on which you live.

[blank box]

2. Examine the fire extinguishers and smoke detectors in your home, apartment, fraternity/sorority house, or the dormitory floor on which you live.

SMOKE DETECTORS

a) How many do you have? _____

b) Where are they located? Ceiling _____ Side wall _____

Are they at least 3 feet from registers or air ducts? _____

Are the side wall detectors at least 6 to 12 inches from the ceiling? _____

SMOKE DETECTORS

c) What is the power source? Battery _____ Household current _____

d) Were they (was it) in working order? _____

FIRE EXTINGUISHERS

a) How many do you have? _____

b) Where are they located? _____

c) What are their classifications? 1A10BC _____ 10BC _____

   5BC _____ 4A60BC _____ Other _____

3. Go to a local retail store that sells smoke detectors and fire extinguishers and compare prices of the following items:

SMOKE DETECTORS		FIRE EXTINGUISHERS	
Battery operated	$_____	1A10BC	$_____
Household current	$_____	10BC	$_____
Combination battery/current	$_____	5BC	$_____
		Halon	$_____
		Other	$_____

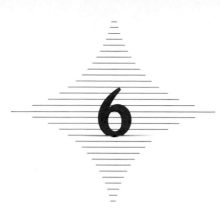

Personal Protection and Firearm Safety

Clearly, crime remains a serious problem for our society. The evidence is that we are making progress, but much remains to be done.

Bureau of Justice Statistics: Criminal victimization in the United States

"Burglaries Jump 36%," "Rise in Child Shootings," "High School Student Shot at School Assembly," "Rapes Here Twice U.S. Average," "Boy, 11, Shot Fatally by Friend, 10," "District Crime on the Rise," "Firm Offers Mugging Insurance." These headlines appear every day in newspapers across the country. Crime victimization is one of the most common negative life events confronting families in the United States. Victims of violent crime are about as common as victims of motor vehicle accidents (Fig. 6-1).[21] Although we saw a slight decrease in the crime rate in the early 1980s, there has been a steady increase over the last 5 years and into the 1990s. The most recent data from the Federal Bureau of Investigation, known as the *Uniform Crime Reports,* indicate more than 14 million crimes being reported annually; an increase of 15% from the mid-1980s.[27]

It is important to stress that in many cases victims do not report crimes to the police. This is especially true for crimes in which no one is injured or the criminal attempt fails. The Bureau of Justice Statistics of the U.S. Department of Justice has developed a program, known as the National Crime Survey, to measure the crimes that go unreported. Last year the National Crime Survey estimated that there were more than 35 million attempted or completed crimes in the United States.[28] Do you realize what that statistic indicates? It means that as many as one out of seven Americans became a crime victim during the year.

Before we proceed, we must answer an important question: Why is a chapter on criminal activity included in a safety text? Looking at the definition of safety, the answer is simple: Safety includes actions that minimize our risks while maximizing our quality of life; thus threats to our well-being or property are a safety concern. Whether a person was injured in a motorcycle accident or during a robbery, his or her

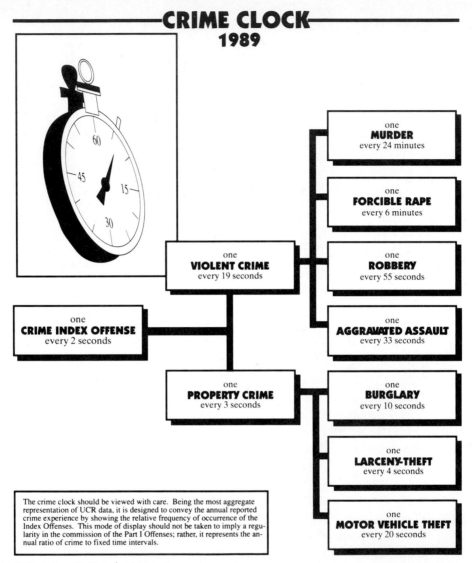

FIG. 6-1   National crime rate.

Source: Federal Bureau of Investigation: Uniform crime reports.

well-being has been affected. We must develop strategies to protect people and their property from a wide variety of threatening situations including deliberate and non-deliberate acts of personal violence or property damage.

The four factors of safety (understanding the difficulty of the activity, the ability level and immediate state of the performer, and condition of the environment) certainly come into play when addressing the issues of crime and violence. It is essential to understand how people may be victimized and what is their potential for becoming victims. Protection from the criminal element requires us to develop certain skills that comprise both preventive measures and techniques of self-defense. Depending on the circumstances, the state of the performer (both mental and physical) may be the factor that determines whether he or she will become a victim. An environment such as a home with deadbolt locks and a security system may reduce our chances of victimization, while another environment, such as a poorly lighted underground parking garage, may increase our potential for victimization.

Among the similarities in a wide range of crimes are: (1) The victims failed to take the necessary preventive measures and precautions, believing that such a thing could not or would not happen to them, or (2) they were unable to react appropriately when accosted. This chapter attempts to make you ''street-wise'' to the criminal elements threatening you and your property. Criminal victimization is not limited to a particular ethnic group, socioeconomic level, age, or sex. Everyone must take an active role in dealing with crime, because no one is immune to the danger.

In this chapter we will investigate both violent and nonviolent crimes, stressing prevention and self-protection. Since the use of weapons, particularly handguns, has received a great deal of publicity in relation to criminal activity and self-protection, we will also address the issue of firearm safety.

VIOLENT CRIMES

Violence may be defined as the use of physical force or the threat of force to inflict injury on or cause damage to persons or property. The *Uniform Crime Report* (an FBI publication) defines **violent crimes** as those offenses including murder, forcible rape, aggravated assault, and robbery. Following a pattern set in recent years, violent crime rates have continued to increase. Recent studies have indicated that a growing number of Americans (as many as 75%) fear becoming victims of violent crimes.[5] The crimes of rape, robbery, and assault have been designated ''crimes of high concern'' by the U.S. Department of Justice, because so many people consider them the most threatening.[21] This fear is evident in the increased sales of handguns, tear gas sprays, guard dogs, security systems, and many other protective devices.

The introduction of these gadgets and devices has not curbed the increasing crime rate. A guard dog at your apartment will not protect you as you are walking home from work. A loaded pistol in the dresser drawer won't be of any use as you are riding the subway home late at night. A can of mace or tear gas will not be an effective deterrent to a mugger if you don't know how to operate it. What most Americans need is a knowledge and awareness of the characteristics of violent crime, not a loaded .357 magnum.

Some questions need to be answered before we can effectively protect ourselves against crime. Who are the victims? Who are the assailants? Under what circumstances do these crimes occur? Awareness will help you to determine how to protect yourself realistically.

Patterns of Violence

In this section we will examine some of the characteristics of persons who become victims and persons who are the assailants. This information will provide a framework for our discussion of violent crimes.

Relative to their number in the population, persons under 25 years of age are the most frequent victims of criminal attacks.[12] These victims are twice as likely to be males, and nearly 88% of them were alone at the time they were victimized. We might find credence in the adage: "There is safety in numbers."

As a group, urban residents are the most vulnerable to crime; people living in central areas of major cities are twice as likely to be victimized as residents of nonmetropolitan areas. Rural residents are the least likely to be victims of violent crimes.

Most violent crimes occur during the evening (between 6 P.M. and midnight). Specifically, the most violent time span is the 2-hour period between 10 P.M. and 12 A.M. In terms of location, victims are more apt to be on the street, in a parking lot, or in a wooded area when they are accosted. Almost 60% of robberies and 50% of assaults and rapes occur in these settings.[30]

In most violent crimes, the characteristics of the assailants are very similar to those of the victims. Most violent crimes (90%) are committed by men, nearly 70% of whom are under 30 years of age.[27] They generally victimize those of their own race; that is, whites victimize whites, blacks victimize blacks, Hispanics victimize Hispanics and so on. A long-standing myth that needs to be dispelled is that most crimes are **interracial.** According to the U.S. Department of Justice, more than 80% of all violent crimes are **intraracial.**

In the past 15 years, weapons used in violent crimes have become increasingly deadly; a relatively large number of assailants and criminals now carry handguns. It is not surprising to find that injuries resulting from these crimes tend to be more serious.

In addition, alcohol is an important factor in crimes of violence. A study of violent offenders in California indicated that more than 60% of the assailants had ingested alcohol, either alone or with other drugs, before their assaults. A positive correlation was also established between the use of alcohol and the subsequent use of firearms.[22, 26] Additionally, the National Institute of Justice estimates that 50% of male and female arrestees test positive for drug use. A composite picture of the typical violent criminal yields important information that will be used later in this chapter to develop strategies for self-protection.

The violent criminal is a young male, generally of the same race as his victim. He is likely to be carrying a weapon and to have been drinking before his violent act.

In the next sections we will take a look at some specific acts of violence and investigate the safety procedures that could be used to reduce the chances of victimization.

Robbery

Robbery is defined as "the taking or attempting to take anything of value from the care, custody, or control of a person or persons by force or threat of force or violence and/or by putting the victim in fear."[27] A robbery may involve the use of a weapon, or it may involve the use of force with hands and feet. The former is called "armed robbery"; the latter is termed "mugging."

The impact of robbery cannot be measured in terms of monetary loss alone. While the object of a robbery is to obtain money or property, the crime involves force or the threat of force. Many victims suffer serious personal injury; approximately one third of all robbery victims sustain some sort of physical injury.[28] The use of weapons in robberies has increased significantly in recent years. In 1976, 48% of all robberies involved the use of a weapon; in 1989, this figure rose to nearly 60%.[27]

Predisposition to attack. Research has indicated that certain conditions, situations, and actions may contribute to a person's chances of becoming a robbery victim.[28] The following conditions tend to increase the chances of victimization:

1. After dark: The cover of darkness gives the robber an increased advantage by making it harder to be identified by potential victims or witnesses.
2. Elderly and handicapped: These persons are extremely vulnerable because they are less likely to have the ability to forcefully resist an attacker.
3. Impediments: Carrying items such as luggage or groceries inhibits the ability either to flee or fight.
4. Well-attired individuals: Why attempt to hold up someone wearing blue jeans when it is just as easy to rob a businessman wearing a three-piece suit and carrying a leather briefcase?
5. Being alone: A lone individual is much easier to control. This is especially true in robbery, since nearly half of these cases involve two or more assailants.
6. Neighborhoods with mixed social classes: This is a classic case of the "haves" versus the "have nots." Areas of urban redevelopment commonly have higher robbery and burglary rates. Sometimes known as "urban pioneers," upper- and upper-middle-class professional people will buy older structures in poorer downtown areas and refurbish them so that they are closer to their work. Since they are usually in the minority in terms of socioeconomic level, they become likely candidates for victimization.

Even a person's body language can increase his or her chances of being victimized. In a recent study of convicted armed robbers at Rahway State Penitentiary in New Jersey, researchers identified a number of characteristics that were frequently seen in robbery victims.[13] Among them were:

1. Exaggerated stride when walking (either too long or too short)
2. Putting the entire foot down when walking instead of using the more normal heel to toe foot movement
3. Staring down at their feet while walking
4. Having little or no awareness of their surroundings

Described as "easy hits" by the convicts, the robbery victims consistently exhibited a less than confident and awkward style of walking. To support the hypothesis that robbery victims give signals of their vulnerability, many of them had been robbed or assaulted on several previous occasions.

Rape: The Most Underreported Crime

Called "the most underreported crime in America," forcible rape has increased more than any other offense during the past 10 years. Most states define it legally as sexual intercourse, achieved or attempted without the victim's consent and with the use or threat of force. The definition of **forcible rape** comprises three elements: (1) the use of force (it doesn't have to be physical; it can be strictly verbal), (2) an absence of consent by the victim, and (3) penile-vaginal penetration. Since 1971 reported rapes have increased from 42,260 to 100,433 in 1990. However, this may only be the tip of the iceberg. Victimization studies completed by the Law Enforcement Assistance Administration of the U.S. Department of Justice estimate that 54% of rapes go unreported.[28] Using 1990 statistics, that means that as many as 218,333 women may have been victims of rape or attempted rape.

Victims' fear of their assailants and their embarrassment about the incidents are two factors that may stop them from contacting law enforcement personnel. After a sexual assault many victims have no idea of what to do or where to turn for help. Rape victims often fear being blamed for not fighting hard enough or for being somewhere they shouldn't have been. Many victims choose not to tell their families, friends, or co-workers about their assaults.

In this section we will attempt to investigate the nature of rape. Who are the victims? Who are the offenders? How can a woman protect herself? What can be done after a rape occurs?

Victims and offenders. Some people think that a man rapes because of sexual desire. It is not uncommon to hear statements like: "She asked for it," "She was dressed too seductively," or "All women want to be raped." Rape is *not* a sexually motivated crime. It is primarily a crime of power, a hostile attack intended to injure and humiliate the victim.

Generally unemployed or unskilled,[4,30] the rapist has little self-esteem and feels that he has little control over his life. Having suffered many frustrations as a result of competing in society and enjoying little personal recognition, he is able to regain some of that self-esteem by controlling and dominating someone else. Sex is the weapon in this violent crime.

Rape can happen to anyone—children, mothers, grandmothers, working women, students, housewives, the rich, the poor. Ages of reported rape victims have ranged from as young as 9 months to 97 years.[15,28] Nearly 70% of the victims are under 25, single, and live alone. The majority of them are employed (65%) or attend school (20%). The victims do not have a particular occupation, but women who are waitresses, students, sales persons, and nurses are more likely to be coming home late at night and are at greater risk. Almost half of all rapes and rape attempts take place outside: on a street, park, field, playground, school ground, or parking lot. Walking and jogging paths through wooded areas are prime locations for rapists. Another 32% of sexual assaults take place in or near the victim's home; women living in ground-floor or first-floor apartments tend to have an increased risk.

The pattern of rape is somewhat cyclical or time-oriented. The greatest number of rapes occur during the months of July and August, after which the volume drops continuously through the end of the year. Another time factor is that most rapes occur on weekends between the hours of 8 P.M. and 2 A.M.

In the past, rape has been considered mainly a problem of cities. Women living in metropolitan areas were twice as likely to be raped as their counterparts in smaller communities. However, as populations have shifted to suburban and rural settings, so has the incidence of rape. Although women living in large cities are still at greater risk, rapes in suburban and rural areas have increased significantly in recent years.

Like their victims, most rapists are under the age of 25. They also tend to be unmarried. As with other violent offenders, rapists generally assault persons of their own race.

Two major differences in the demographic characteristics of rapists and their victims are employment and educational level. Nearly three quarters of rapists are unemployed or work as unskilled laborers, whereas their victims are usually employed and come from a broad range of socioeconomic backgrounds.[4,30] While most rape victims have some college education, many rapists have not graduated from high school.

Although the majority of reported rapes (60%) involve strangers, they are not impulsive or chance confrontations. In most cases the rapist plans his attack; he is familiar with the area where he attacks his victims, or he may have even observed them for a period of time. In cases where the victim knows her assailant (for example, "date rape"), the assailant has an even greater advantage because the victim does not expect a person she knows to force her to have intercourse. Victims of acquaintance rape often feel that they will have a credibility problem if they try to tell anyone about their experience; consequently, most authorities feel that victimization surveys significantly underestimate the proportion of rapes committed by "nonstrangers."

Victims versus avoiders: what are the differences? The Department of Justice estimates that for every rape there are at least two rape attempts. What makes one person a victim and another an avoider? Two studies comparing women who have been raped with those who avoided rape have uncovered a number of interesting findings.[4,21]

The major finding from both studies was that women who used physical resistance immediately at the beginning of an attack were twice as likely to escape rape as women who did not resist.[4,16] Although a woman's physical resistance is associated with a somewhat higher possibility of minor injuries (cuts, abrasions, contusions), she will have a substantially higher probability of avoiding the rape.

The studies also found that serious injury was generally not a consequence of victim resistance. Of the 414 women interviewed in these studies only 26 (6%) received injuries serious enough to require hospitalization. Only half of the women who required hospitalization had attempted to physically resist. Since the aggression and hostility of an attacker tend to escalate as the encounter progresses, women who made no attempt to physically resist were as likely to be seriously injured as women who did.[4] In fact, a recent report by the U.S. Department of Justice indicates that victims of rape were twice as likely to be injured as women who avoided rape.[30]

Physical resistance isn't limited to fighting with the rapist; it includes attempts to flee or run, screaming, and verbal aggression. The more of these strategies that can be used, the greater a woman's chances of avoiding rape.

In her study of victims and avoiders, P. B. Bart found that women who possessed skills that enabled them to be independent and self-sufficient were more likely to be rape avoiders, whereas women who were reared in a more traditional, dependent role were more often victims.[4] Rape avoiders were likely to have had major household responsibilities as children; they were more likely to have participated in contact sports; and their parents tended not to intervene in their fights and tended to counsel them to fight back. Rape victims, on the other hand, had few childhood responsibilities, were not involved in sports, and had parents who intervened in their fights or punished them for using violence.

As adults there was a continuation of these patterns of independence for rape avoiders and dependence for rape victims. For example, avoiders were twice as likely to have had training in safety and first aid. And they were more likely to have participated in some type of athletic activity on a regular basis. It seems that an action-oriented lifestyle, which develops a self-confident attitude, is a key factor in the ability to handle the stress of a rape attack.

What about some of the more traditional, passive strategies for dealing with a rapist, such as reasoning with him, trying to gain his confidence, pleading with the assailant, or going along with the rapist? Although some of these techniques are effective to a degree, they force the victim to play along with the rapist and generally suffer a certain amount of humiliation. Let's be realistic, in certain cases there may be no other choice. Submitting to a rape out of fear for your safety or your family's does not mean that you consented. It is still a rape and still a crime. Victims who do not resist should never feel guilty; it is the rapist who committed the crime.

So what should you do if you're attacked? The answer is: *It depends*. It depends on you. It depends on the attacker. It depends on the situation. Without knowing the situation, no one can say what you can or should do. The following discussion gives you some things to consider.

Active resistance. Active resistance consists of four basic strategies: fleeing, fighting, screaming, and verbal aggression. The key to these strategies is that they must be used at the beginning of an attack. Although the rapist will generally have the element of surprise, a rapid and forceful response by the intended victim will not allow him to gain immediate control. The use of verbal aggression in combination with one of the more physical strategies is an added benefit. The use of violent epithets, swearing, and commanding language will put the attacker on the defensive psychologically, while the victim's fighting will keep him occupied physically.

An example of this technique was used by Carol, a waitress who was attacked late one night in the parking lot of the supper club where she worked. As she was unlocking her car door, the attacker grabbed her by the hair and tried to force her into the car. Her first move was to turn toward the man, and as she pushed away she screamed, "Keep your goddamn hands off me!—Now!" His startled reaction was to release his grip from her hair, thus allowing her to run back to the restaurant.

At this point a word of caution is needed. Carol was successful for several reasons. She reacted immediately and used at least three methods of active resistance: fighting, verbal aggression, and fleeing. She was in an open area when the attack occurred. The attacker had no weapon. Also, at 5 feet 9 inches, Carol is taller than the average woman.

Let's look at some of the situational factors that favor the use of physical resistance by the victim: being outside, absence of a weapon, only one assailant, and training of the victim.

In her study of 320 rape victims and avoiders, J. J. McIntyre found that any enclosed area is potentially more dangerous than an open space, although a person usually doesn't have a choice of where an attack occurs.[16] However, when women entered cars, either voluntarily or by force, their chances of being raped were significantly increased because their mobility was greatly reduced. This is why there is such risk in accepting rides from strangers.

The introduction of a weapon in a sexual assault does not occur as frequently as you might think. Weapons are used in less than 25% of reported rapes; the most common weapon is a knife rather than a gun.[15,30] What about physical resistance in this case? There is no easy answer. Although the victim's resistance does not seem to be related to whether or not she will receive serious injuries, weapons were more often used in attacks where serious victim injuries occurred.

Related to the weapon issue is the number of assailants in an attack. Multiple offenders are involved in roughly 23% of sexual assaults, and they possess weapons more often than single assailants.[15,30] Women who have escaped multiple assailants have usually been attacked outside, where they could more easily attract someone's attention. When weapons or multiple attackers are involved, passive resistance may be the only viable alternative. When there is a greater potential for danger in a given situation than in another, it is unrealistic to ignore that danger.

Although a woman does not need to be a self-defense expert to use some type of active resistance, it is important that she develop both physical and psychological skills to deal with a sexual assault. While men are often accustomed to physical struggle because of their lifelong involvement in contact sports, women are generally not combat oriented.

To use the skills to resist an attacker, a woman must practice regularly. Too often women will take a 6-week self-defense course at the local YWCA and then never practice what they have learned once the course is over. To maintain proficiency a person should practice several times per week. Do you have that kind of perseverance?

The development of psychological skills is probably the most difficult thing to do. How does a woman change 18 to 20 years of social conditioning in which she has been told to act like a lady? Be polite, be gentle, and above all don't fight! To deny control to an assailant, a woman needs mental toughness to go along with her physical skills. Perhaps the answer is to add some type of assertiveness training to current self-defense programs, thus giving a woman the confidence to take more control in her life—including situations where she must defend herself.

Passive resistance. Someone has a gun to your head and says, ''Take off your clothes.'' Scary, isn't it? But what would you do? This is probably not the time to use violent physical resistance. This may be a time to use one of the methods of **passive resistance:** verbal persuasion, pleading, or submission. Author Frederick Storaska offers five closely interwoven principles to use in such a situation. They are as follows:[24]

1. Retain your emotional stability.
2. Treat the rapist as a human being.
3. Gain his confidence. (Assure him that you are not a threat.)
4. Go along until you can safely react. (This may involve some sexual contact on your part.)
5. Use your imagination and good judgment.

Storaska suggests that women are better prepared to use subtle negotiation techniques in a sexual assault. By going along with the rapist, the potential victim may have the opportunity to talk her way out of the situation, or at least have the time to set him up so that she can escape. Some of the tactics that women have used to escape include asking the rapist to let her go to the bathroom to remove a tampon, asking the rapist to get a couple of beers from the refrigerator before they had sex, and pretending to be a deaf-mute. However, as research has shown, this passive method of resistance is not as effective as the more violent methods, and it does not seem to reduce the likelihood of victim injury.[4,16]

A passive method that is even less likely to work is that of pleading with the rapist. This action tends to acknowledge to the rapist his ability to dominate; consequently the victim's pleas go unheeded and the attacker continues with the rape.

If all else fails, submitting to penetration must be considered a viable alternative in terms of reacting safely. At this point your goal should be survival, because that's the only way you can ensure that you will have an opportunity to see that he pays for his crime. Try to remain calm, pay attention, and gather evidence that will help police find the assailant.

As you can see, there are many variables that must be considered in an attack situation. Whether you decide to actively or passively resist is up to you.

Help for the rape victim. If you have been sexually assaulted, seek help as soon as possible. Your first call should be to the police. They can take you to the hospital, put you in touch with community services, and collect information from you that will help them apprehend the rapist. Many police forces now have officers who are specially trained in rape investigation; often they are female officers.

If you prefer not to call the police right away, get help from a friend or call your community rape crisis center. These programs generally have a 24-hour hotline number. Rape crisis counselors will explain your choices, contact the police for you, and even escort you to the hospital. These centers can also provide invaluable support for the victim in the days after the rape.

The most important thing to remember after an attack is that you should not touch anything, change your clothes, douche, or shower until you have been to the hospital for an examination. A woman's body and her clothing provide most of the evidence in a rape case.[32]

Recent reforms in state sexual assault laws are starting to favor the victim instead of the criminal. These laws have broadened the definition of rape to include such things as forced oral-genital or anal contact. Some states now have varying degrees of sexual assault defined by law. Although the attacker may not be convicted of rape, he will, at least, receive a certain amount of punishment for his crime. In 1991 both the Senate and House of Representatives introduced legislation to combat violence and crimes against women on the streets and in the home. Known as the Violence Against Women Act of 1991, this bill will provide funds to encourage women to prosecute their attackers, create new penalties for sex crimes, strengthen rape prevention and security programs on college campuses, and protect women from abuse by spouses.

Although there is still a long way to go, society is beginning to realize that sexual assault is no different than any other violent crime and must be treated as such.

Campus rape: what's the story? Traditionally university campuses have been thought of as safe havens in a relatively violent U.S. Society. As more than a few students have said it: "What the hell, the university's not the real world; I can do whatever I want and nothing will happen."

Well, it's time to wake up; what happens in the community happens in the university. Violence and sexual assault occur on every campus. Probably the greatest difference between these crimes on campus versus those off campus is that victims know, or are at least acquainted with, their assailants. Because of this factor it is estimated that as many as 90% of the women who are sexually assaulted at universities never report the incidents.[3] A victim will blame herself for not resisting forcefully enough, using poor judgment, or contributing in some way to the assault. Additionally, the woman who is raped by her date is likely to feel that no one will believe her. Often victims of acquaintance/date rape are left with feelings of helplessness, rage, and humiliation—emotional trauma that is not easily healed.

How can such a situation occur on university campuses in the 1990s? Much of the problem can be associated with the traditional sex-role stereotypes that exist on college campuses just as they do in the rest of society, i.e., men should dominate and women should be submissive. In the decade of the 90s institutions of higher learning should take the lead in dispelling these myths and educating men and women about mutual respect and sexual equity. In the meantime pay attention to these basic rules of sexual behavior and communication:

Women

1. Early on, clearly communicate your expectations about sexual activity and what you want in the relationship.
2. Don't send mixed messages; if you mean *no,* say it forcefully.
3. When dating someone for the first time, a group situation is a better way of getting acquainted.

4. Be wary of a companion who attempts to control or dominate your behavior.

5. If you drink, drink responsibly and remain in control!

Men

1. Clearly communicate your attitudes and expectations about sexual behavior.

2. When a sex partner says that's as far as we go, that's as far as you go.

3. If you sense that your sex partner is uncomfortable with the situation (i.e., obviously not enjoying it), stop and communicate your concern.

4. Sex with a partner who does not consent is sexual assault.

5. Sex with a partner who is unconscious or incapacitated by alcohol or drugs is nonconsensual sex/sexual assault.

Aggravated Assault

Aggravated assault is defined as an unlawful attack by one person upon another for the purpose of inflicting severe bodily injury.[27] It is a violent crime in which men are 2.5 times as likely to be victimized as women. This type of assault is usually accompanied by the use of a weapon or by means likely to produce death or great bodily harm. However, it is not necessary for an injury to result when a gun, knife, or other deadly weapon is used; the threat of its use is considered aggravated assault.

An important point for college or university students to remember is that a conviction for aggravated assault at a fraternity or sorority party or local bar can drastically affect your career as well as your financial situation. If you knock out a person's teeth, break his nose, or require him to have hospital emergency-room treatment, many jurisdictions will consider this an aggravated assault—especially if you started the incident. With an aggravated assault conviction, you are now open to civil litigation for damages to your victim. You may regret your actions, especially when you see what an attorney will charge for defending you. So, unless you are in imminent danger of bodily harm, avoid these confrontations.

Unlike the violent crimes of rape and robbery, where offenders are generally strangers, in aggravated assault the assailants are usually known to their victims. Nowhere is this brought out more clearly than in the case of domestic violence against women. In a recent 4-year study, the U.S. Justice Department reported that an estimated 2.1 million women were assaulted by spouses, ex-spouses, boyfriends or ex-boyfriends.[11]

Only 50% of the victims of domestic violence ever call the police. As in the case of rape, many of the women consider the crime a private or personal matter that cannot be resolved by police intervention. However, researchers have found that just the opposite holds true. An estimated 41% of women who did not call police were subsequently assaulted again by the same man; for women who did call police, only 15% were reassaulted.[23] Whether you're a man or woman, married or unmarried, no one has the right to assault you. If you are ever assaulted, contact the authorities immediately; outside intervention is the only way to ensure that this will not be repeated.

SELF-PROTECTION VERSUS SELF-DEFENSE

Self-Protection

Traditionally Americans have taken pride in being independent; *liberty, freedom,* and *individual rights* are words frequently used to describe this sentiment. We can go where we want, when we want! The idea of restricting one's behavior goes against the principles on which this nation was founded; however, it is unrealistic to ignore danger.

In our discussions of violent crimes such as rape and robbery, it was found that certain conditions or situations can increase the chances of victimization. In this section we will discuss measures that can be taken to reduce the chances of victimization. A number of these strategies of self-protection may restrict our behavior somewhat, but if we are to deal with the situation realistically, that's what must be done. Ultimately, you have to weigh the benefits of an activity against the risks involved.

In your home or apartment

1. Keep doors and windows locked, even when you are at home. An unlocked door is an invitation for an intruder, and you will not hear him if you are vacuuming upstairs or are in the shower. Apartment dwellers are often guilty of leaving doors unlocked when they go down the hall to the laundry room.
2. When answering a knock at the door, make sure the caller is legitimate. If you are expecting a repairman, insist on proper identification. If the person wants to use your phone, tell him or her you will make the call for him or her, but do not let the person inside. Installation of a peephole viewer will help to alleviate this problem.
3. Train your children not to open doors to strangers.
4. If you are a woman living alone, do not advertise the fact by putting your full name on mail boxes and in telephone directories; instead, use only initials.
5. If possible, have your locks changed or rekeyed when you move into a new home or apartment.
6. If you live in an apartment, avoid being in the laundry room or garage by yourself, especially late at night.

Outside

1. The most important point to be stressed here is to be alert to your surroundings and the people around you.
2. Know the area in which you are traveling. In most cities there are areas or neighborhoods that have consistently high crime rates; these areas should be avoided.
3. There is safety in numbers. It is a rare occurrence when three or more people are attacked.
4. When you are in an unfamiliar area, always act and walk in a confident manner. An attacker will be looking for someone who seems vulnerable.
5. Walk on the side of the street facing traffic, and walk close to the curb. This will reduce your chances of harrassment from people in cars as well as protect you from persons hiding in doorways, alleys, and bushes.

6. Do not burden yourself with too many packages or pieces of luggage. Try to keep one arm free.

7. The best way to carry a purse is to hold it in place firmly under your arm with the carrying strap over your shoulder. If a man is going to carry a wallet in his hip pocket, he should transfer most of his money and major credit cards to his front pocket.

8. When you're in a bar or other public facility, do not display large amounts of cash.

9. Avoid walking through secluded areas.

10. Rely on your instincts. If you think you are being followed, walk quickly to areas where there are lights and people. If you feel that you're in immediate danger, don't be reluctant to scream and run. A robber or attacker does not want commotion.

11. The elderly and handicapped have a special vulnerability because of their condition. Community services which provide able-bodied individuals to escort them to stores, clubs, and theaters have been successful in reducing criminal assaults on the elderly and handicapped.

12. If you are a jogger, try to run with a partner, vary your route and the time you run, and if you run at night, be sure the area is well lighted.

Your motor vehicle and self-protection

1. Keep the doors of your car locked at all times, even when you're in it.

2. Park your car on a well-lighted, busy street or in a well-illuminated parking lot. Avoid underground or enclosed parking garages at night, since there are usually no security personnel available.

3. Even if you're only going to be gone 5 minutes, lock the car. And when you return, check the back seat before you enter.

4. When walking to your car at night in a large parking lot, have a security guard escort you. If one is not available, walk to your car with a friend and then take the friend to her car.

5. If you get lost, drive to a well-lighted service station to ask directions.

6. If your car breaks down on the road, raise the hood or attach a white cloth to the car's antenna and then wait inside the vehicle. If a stranger approaches to assist, roll the window down slightly and ask him to call road service or the police department. Do not get out of your car.

7. Never pick up hitchhikers and never be a hitchhiker yourself.

If You Are Attacked

So far in this section we have dealt with measures of self-protection (actions that help to eliminate risks as well as to recognize and avoid danger). But what happens if these measures don't protect you or you have failed to take the necessary precautions? Ultimately you may find yourself encountering a robber or rapist. Although your options are relatively few, there are still choices to be made. These choices concern your self-defense. There are basically three actions that can be taken: (1) You can submit to the attacker's demands, (2) you can flee from the attacker, and (3) you can fight the attacker. At a given time any of these actions can and should be considered viable alternatives under the definition of *self-defense* (the act of preventing aggression or attack). Let's examine each of these alternatives.

Why should a person submit to an attacker's demands? Have you ever heard the statement: "Discretion is the better part of valor?" Well, it is, especially when a person is pointing a .357 magnum at you from a distance of only a few feet and is requesting your wallet. Most police authorities agree that an armed-robbery victim is less likely to be injured if he or she cooperates with the attacker. Often the armed robber may feel as threatened as his victim; consequently, aggressive or hostile acts by the victim may scare him into shooting. Submitting to an attacker's demands makes the criminal no less guilty of his crime, but it may give you the opportunity to remember details that can be used to apprehend and convict him. Although handing over your possessions to a criminal is a frustrating and maddening experience, those valuables can be replaced—your life cannot.

Fleeing an attacker is also a legitimate way to protect yourself. If you return home and find your door ajar, do not enter and attempt to challenge the intruder; use a neighbor's phone to call the police. *They* get paid to take those risks.

If you think you are being followed, either on foot or in a car, don't hesitate to go quickly to the nearest well-lighted residence or business and call the police to report your suspicions. In a case where you are being followed on foot, if that person has made threatening gestures toward you, scream loudly to draw attention to your situation. The last thing a potential assailant wants is attention and possible recognition.

The last alternative is to physically attack your assailant. An attack may consist of using weapons, such as guns, knives, and tear gas sprays, or it may mean using personal weapons such as hands, feet, and knees.

Violent force in self-defense. When should you use violent force against an assailant? There are no hard and fast rules; a general guideline is that violent force can be used if a person feels that he or she, family members, or friends are in imminent danger of bodily injury. No one can make that decision for you; it must be made when the situation arises.

Regardless of the type of violent force with which you decide to defend yourself, the key factor is that of preparedness. It does absolutely no good to buy a weapon if you don't know how to use it properly. The same holds true for personal defense techniques. If you don't practice these skills on a regular basis, they will be of no use in an attack.

Currently two of the most common weapons used for self-defense are handguns and tear gas sprays. Both weapons present a number of problems of which many people are not aware; for instance, in most states, persons over 18 years of age and without a criminal record can buy handguns, but few of them will be able to get licenses to legally carry the weapon. For all practical purposes, handguns are not an option for self-defense outside the home. Furthermore, if we look at handgun potential for home defense, the likelihood of confronting an intruder is at best rare. Only 4% of burglaries involve victim-intruder confrontations.[18]

Another pertinent question is, "How easy is it to shoot an assailant with a handgun?" Most experts agree that if an assailant is more than 2 or 3 feet away and moving, the chances that an inexperienced marksman will shoot him are very slim. Is having a gun in the home worth the added danger? Nearly 2000 people die annually in gun-related accidents; most of these deaths are caused by handguns.[18] We will address the issue of firearm safety in a later section.

Although there are not as many problems with tear gas sprays as there are with guns, they do not seem to be as effective as manufacturers would have us believe. Studies in California, Maryland, and Virginia have indicated that while the sprays do irritate the eyes and cause some respiratory discomfort, they neither work instantly nor do they completely incapacitate an attacker. Another finding was that these sprays had no effect on assailants who were intoxicated or highly agitated because of drug ingestion, anxiety, or nervousness.

Other difficulties that have been reported by various law enforcement agencies involve the handling of the spray apparatus by its users. Common problems were not being able to get to the spray can, incorrect operation of the device, and conditions that reduced its effectiveness, such as strong winds and the wearing of glasses by the attacker.

With as many as 6 million people purchasing these devices each year, it is important to emphasize that while these sprays can briefly distract an attacker, they will not paralyze or stop him. Also, to properly operate this equipment, training is a necessity.

The most viable form of violent force in self-defense is the use of personal weapons such as hands and feet. Wherever you go, these weapons are available. However, as is the case with the use of any weapon, preparation and continual training are essential.

Most self-defense experts agree that mental preparedness is an important part of any program involving techniques of personal protection. An individual involved in such training must develop a certain amount of assertiveness; it is not enough to hurt an assailant, he or she must be immobilized.

Another important aspect of psychological preparation is the ability to imagine an actual attack and to feel the anxiety it would trigger. By making attack training as realistic as possible, students are able to develop greater confidence in their skills and, at the same time, reduce the likelihood of panic in a dangerous situation.

The other essential element is skill development, including repetition of each skill until a technique is mastered. Once these defensive techniques are developed, they must be maintained with regular training sessions.

In our discussion of personal defense techniques we can only scratch the surface. If you are interested in pursuing instruction in self-defense contact your local police department, YWCA, or YMCA for information on classes in your area. (See the box on pp. 180-181.)

PROPERTY CRIMES

Burglary and Larceny-Theft

Burglary. The crimes of burglary and larceny-theft are referred to as **property crimes.** The FBI's *Uniform Crime Report* defines **burglary** as the unlawful entry of a structure to commit a felony or theft.[28] Typically burglary is associated with the theft of property from a residence; however, in a situation such as a rape where the attacker entered unlawfully, two specific crimes would have been committed: rape and burglary.

The estimated 3.2 million burglaries in the United States in 1989 accounted for nearly 23% of the reported crimes. This is a decrease of over 16% since 1985. The decrease results in large part from a variety of community-oriented crime prevention programs across the country. Nonetheless, with the increasing number of women in the workforce, it is not surprising to find that daytime residential burglaries remain a problem.

Burglary represents a substantial financial loss. In 1989, burglary victims suffered losses estimated at $3.4 billion; the average dollar loss per burglary was $1060. In 10 years this figure has more than doubled; the average dollar loss in 1979 was $505.[27] Who pays for these losses? The answer is that we all do, through higher insurance premiums. Contributing to this loss figure is the fact that only 14% of all burglaries are cleared by arrest. Victims contribute to this situation by not marking and identifying their property. If a suspect is arrested with 50 stereo receivers, 12 portable televisions, assorted cameras, guns, or silverware, how can the rightful owners be found? Without having some way of identifying their property (serial numbers or special marking), most burglary victims cannot reclaim it even if it is found; thus their particular burglaries technically go unsolved.

Who are the burglars and who are the victims? Residential properties (homes, condominiums, and apartments) account for 67% of all burglaries, while businesses account for most of the remainder.[27] Major metropolitan areas have the highest burglary rates; however, there have been substantial increases in suburban areas in recent years. The burglar goes where the money is and today that is in the suburbs.

Studies by the Law Enforcement Assistance Administration indicate that more than 75% of burglaries require forcing a door or window to gain entry; yet most houses and apartments are protected by simple and ineffective door and window locks.[19] Law enforcement personnel feel that a significant decrease in burglaries would occur if people used more effective window and door locks. As we will see in the next section, it is relatively easy to make forced entry difficult.

Larceny-theft. The other property crime that will be addressed is **larceny-theft.** This is the unlawful taking, carrying, leading, or riding away from the possession of another.[27] It includes crimes such as shoplifting, pocket picking, purse snatching, bicycle theft, and thefts of equipment and parts from motor vehicles. Although the actual theft of motor vehicles is considered in a separate crime-reporting category by the FBI, we will include it in our discussion at this time.

Self-defense hints

Before you can use violent force on an assailant, you must know what personal weapons are available and on what areas of the attacker's body they will be most effective. Your key defensive weapons include your hands, feet, fingers, thumbs, knees, and voice.

Surprisingly, the voice is a strong psychological weapon; loud, animal-like screams as you attack will not only affect an assailant's concentration, but it may alert others to your plight. Remember, you're not yelling for help; it is an act of aggression against your attacker, and the screams must be loud and violent. You may find it helpful to practice this skill, since it is not something most people can easily do.

Vulnerable areas include the eyes, groin, nose, neck, and knees. The two most sensitive areas are the eyes and groin. A problem that occurs with both men and women students is that they are somewhat reluctant to practice the skills that involve damaging an assailant's eyes (Fig. 6-2, A and Fig. 6-2, B). Nevertheless, you must remember that in a real attack, your life is in danger—it's either you or the attacker, you have no other choice.

Women are also hesitant to attack the genital area, as there are certain sociocultural overtones involved with this action (Fig. 6-2, C). It is important to remind students that an assailant is not worried about inflicting severe injury on *them*.

Improvisation is another important part of self-defense training. Many household articles can be used as weapons in an emergency. Textbooks, purses, magazines, keys, umbrellas, and brooms are just a few of the common articles that can be used against an assailant.

A textbook or a purse held in both hands can be jabbed into the nose or throat of an attacker; a rolled up magazine will work in the same manner (Fig. 6-2, D). An umbrella or broom makes a very efficient spearing device. Held with both hands spread approximately 18 inches apart along the length of the broom or umbrella, these objects can be thrust forcefully and quickly toward the face or groin of an approaching attacker (Fig. 6-2, E). Never swing these items at a assailant; he or she can easily block the blows and even if they land, they will do little damage. Remember, the most effective action is to jab or spear.

Keys can be used in several ways. The most commonly mentioned method is to place keys between your fingers with the sharp ends protruding from the knuckles before walking to your car or home from class. If you are attacked, hold the keys firmly in place and punch into the attacker's eyes (Fig. 6-2, F).

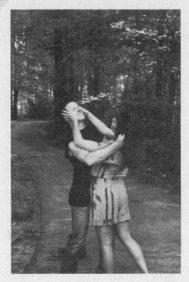

FIG. 6-2   A, Gouging an attacker's eyes.

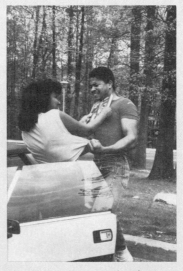

FIG. 6-2   D, A textbook is a common article that can be jabbed into the attacker's throat or nose.

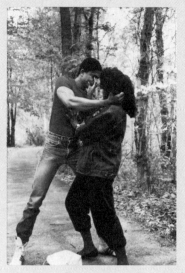

FIG. 6-2   B, Attacking the assailant's eyes.

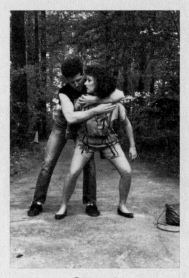

FIG. 6-2   C, Attacking the assailant's genital area.

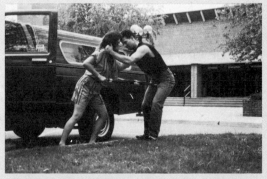

FIG. 6-2   E, Jabbing forcefully at the oncoming attacker.

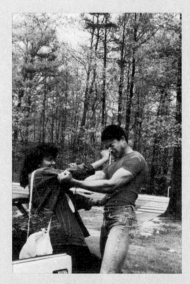

FIG. 6-2   F, Using keys, another common article, to jab the attacker's eyes.

In 1989, there were an estimated 7,872,442 larceny-theft offenses in the United States.[27] As is the case with burglary, larceny-theft has two peak seasons, the midsummer months of July through August (when people are vacationing) and December (when people, including thieves, are doing their Christmas shopping). The loss to victims nationally is estimated at $3.6 billion. While some of the goods stolen are recovered, the frequent absence of owner identification on recovered property indicates the overall loss caused by this criminal activity is not substantially reduced. In addition, other studies have indicated that many thefts, particularly when the value of the stolen goods is small, never come to police attention. Have you ever had something ripped off, but never reported it?

Thefts from motor vehicles and buildings, and shoplifting account for nearly 65% of these crimes. Car stereos, tape decks, and CD players are popular targets; what makes it even easier is the number of people who do not lock their cars.

A serious problem in shopping malls and their surrounding parking lots are "boosters," professional shoplifters and those who specialize in stealing from automobiles. During the Christmas shopping season, "boosters" have a field day with shoppers who leave packages in their cars. They will usually steal only what they can see; if your valuables are out of sight, the boosters are more likely to pass you by.

Thefts are generally based on supply and demand; what is currently popular is more likely to be stolen; that is, the increased popularity of bicycles in the 1970s led to an increase in the rate of bicycle thefts. Shoplifting shows a similar pattern. (Go into a store and see which products are locked in cabinets or are attached to some type of security device.) With the increased popularity of VCRs, video tapes, and computer equipment, more stores are putting these items in locked glass cases. More often than not, you will also find leather goods secured.

The advent of highrises and multistoried office buildings has also made it easier for thieves. A large number of people and their many possessions are concentrated in a rather small area. A condominium complex or high-rise dormitory with its rows of bicycle racks increases the thief's chances of finding an unlocked bike and decreases his or her chances of being caught. An office building with 30 or 40 different firms renting space gives the thief who steals computers, word processors, and other office equipment the advantage of anonymity.

As is the case with burglary, everyone becomes a victim when people steal. We all pay higher prices in stores to offset the losses from shoplifting. It will take a concerted effort by all Americans to change the situation. People can no longer worry only about themselves; we have to look out for our neighbors as well. In the following sections we will investigate a number of preventive strategies that could significantly reduce both violent and property crimes.

Preventive Measures for the Home

Doors and windows. Most authorities agree that delaying a burglar for 4 minutes is usually sufficient to prevent entry into a house or apartment.[19] Delaying a burglar increases his or her chances of being observed and possibly captured.

Since doors and windows are the burglar's usual means of entrance, these are appropriate places to start with preventive measures. All outside entrance doors should be solid wood or metal-covered if they have a hollow core. Security screening or grills should cover glass panels in or around the entrance door, or one of the newer extra-strength laminated glass products such as Saflex should be used. This will reduce the possibility of someone's gaining entrance by breaking a glass panel and reaching in to unlock the door.

Every entrance door should have a deadbolt lock. When this device is operated, a 1-inch throw or bolt moves into the door frame. To gain entrance when the deadbolt is being used would mean tearing away part of the door frame, the kind of commotion a burglar doesn't want to make. The most frequently used lock for entrance doors is the key-in-the-knob latch lock. These locks can be forced by breaking off the knob, or they can be opened by prying or slipping a piece of plastic between the door jamb and the latch. Do you know anyone who has used a credit card to get into his apartment when he locked himself out? Key-in-the-knob locks can be supplemented effectively by the addition of a deadbolt. (See Fig. 6-3, A, B.)

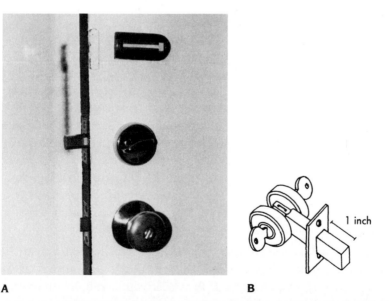

A   **B**

FIG. 6-3   A, This door has three locking devices. At the bottom is the standard key-in-the-knob lock; in the middle is a single cylinder or thumb-turn deadbolt; and at the top is a chain lock. **B,** This illustration is an example of a double-cylinder deadbolt lock. To operate this device from the inside a key is also needed. If a burglar is able to break a glass panel near the door to reach inside, he will be unable to unlock the door without a key for the deadbolt. A note of caution: When you use this type of deadbolt, remember where you put the key at night. In an emergency you will need that key to unlock the door.

Source: U.S. Department of Justice, Office of Justice Assistance, Research, and Statistics.

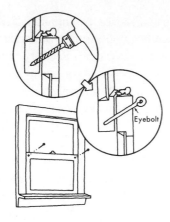

FIG. 6-4   Eyebolts securing these windowframes can be removed quickly in an emergency to allow the window to be opened.

Source: U.S. Department of Justice.

Sliding glass doors present a major security problem if they do not have the proper locks and if steps are not taken to prevent removal of the door. The best lock for a sliding glass door is a modified deadbolt mechanism. An additional method of securing sliding glass doors is the use of removable locking drop bars that fit into the track on which the door slides.

Many people do not realize that even when a sliding glass door is locked, it can be lifted from the track and removed. To prevent this, metal screws should be inserted in the top of the door frame at both ends and in the middle. The screws should be adjusted so that the door barely clears them when it slides along the track.

Two types of windows that are found most often in homes and apartments are the double-hung sash window, which operates in an up-and-down motion, and the sliding window, which is moved in a horizontal motion in the same way as a sliding door. The most effective protection for double-hung windows is a key-locking security sash lock. Unlike the simple sash lock, which is on most double-hung windows, this device cannot be "jimmied" loose. Another method for securing double-hung windows is to drill holes through the overlapping frames, then insert a nail or eyebolt so the windows can't be opened (Fig. 6-4). Security measures for sliding windows are the same as those taken for sliding doors.

Landscaping and lighting. When planting trees, bushes, and flowers, remember to keep doorways, windows, and porches clear. Privacy for you may give a burglar a place to hide. Also, if you have large trees near your home, lower limbs should be removed, since they may provide second-story access.

Exterior lighting is extremely important in residential security. Each exterior doorway, including the garage door, should be illuminated to prevent a burglar from concealing his activities. Yard lights or flood lights mounted under the eaves of your house will provide extra protection. A good habit to develop is to leave a light on outside every night. Yard and entrance lights can be equipped with sensors that will turn them on at dusk and off at dawn. When you do this, people are unable to tell whether or not you're at home. A second advantage of dusk-to-dawn lighting is that your chances of being burglarized while you sleep and when you're away from home are greatly reduced. Outside lights can also be equipped with motion detectors. They come on with any movement nearby, then turn off several minutes after the movement ceases.

When you're away from home. Whether it's a night on the town or a 3-week vacation, a residence that has a ''lived-in'' appearance is a deterrent to burglars. By practicing the following preventive measures, your chances of becoming a burglary victim will be reduced. When you're going out at night:

1. Leave one or more interior lights on and perhaps have a radio playing.
2. Leave exterior lights on so that the area around your home is well illuminated.
3. Never leave notes that can inform a burglar that your house is unoccupied.
4. Do not hide door keys outside your home.
5. Make certain all windows and doors are secured before departing. An empty garage advertises your absence too, so close and secure the garage door.

When planning a vacation or prolonged absence:

1. Do not publicize your plans. Some burglars specialize in reading newspaper accounts of people's vacation activities.
2. Discontinue all deliveries ahead of time; for example, newspapers and laundry.
3. Notify the post office to forward your mail or hold it until you return.
4. Arrange for lawn and landscaping care.
5. Set a radio and various indoor and outdoor lights on automatic timers.
6. Inform neighbors of your absence so they can be alert for suspicious persons.
7. Leave a key with one of your relatives or a neighbor so that your residence can be periodically inspected. Ask them to vary shade and blind positions.

Burglar alarms. A specialized form of home protection is the burglar alarm system. When an intruder activates a sensing device, an alarm is sounded both inside and outside the home. It may be a loud bell, buzzer, siren, or horn. The system can also be programmed to turn on household lights when the alarm sounds. More sophisticated systems may include silent alarms that alert an off-premises monitoring source. Burglar alarms have been around for quite a while; however, in the past, most were too expensive for home installation. With the advent of more sophisticated electronic technology the cost of alarm systems has become more reasonable, especially when compared to the cost of replacing stolen items such as silverware, jewelry, and antiques.

There are basically two types of burglar alarms: a perimeter system and an interior system. Probably the best alarm is the **perimeter system,** which uses sensing devices attached to all doors and windows leading into the home. The most widely used sensing devices are called contacts. These are electromechanical devices composed of a simple switching mechanism that operates in the same manner as a hidden light switch on a refrigerator door. When an intruder opens a door or window the electric circuit is disturbed and an alarm sounds.

Two other perimeter systems involve the use of metal foil and vibration detectors. The metal foil is attached to various surfaces including glass, door panels, and walls.

The foil is designed to break when an attempt is made to gain entry by means of the surface to which it is attached. Vibration detectors react to vibrations similar to those that result when an attempt is made to gain entry. Because they are more sensitive, the foil and vibration detectors may be activated more easily. Family pets and children can easily tear the ribbonlike metallic foil and activate the system, and if the vibration device is not properly set, a large clap of thunder or a sonic boom can set off this system.

The second type of burglar alarm is the **interior system,** which consists of pressure mats, photoelectric beams, and motion detectors. Pressure mats are basically sensing devices that react to the weight of a person's footsteps. They are commonly placed in doorways, under windows, and at the bottom of staircases. Photoelectric burglar alarms work in the same way as a photoelectric smoke alarms. They cast a beam of light across rooms, hallways, and stairwells. When the beam is interrupted, an alarm is sounded. A relatively new device is the motion detector. This device emits high-intensity sound waves (microwaves) throughout a room in a specific pattern. When a moving object enters the room, the pattern is changed and an alarm sounds.

Although they work well, interior systems have two distinct disadvantages: (1) They allow an intruder to enter the home before an alarm is sounded, and (2) they cannot be used without limiting activity in the home, such as that of children and pets moving around in the middle of the night. Consequently, from a practical standpoint the perimeter system offers the greatest degree of protection.

Neighborhood Watch Program

Developed in 1972, the National Neighborhood Watch program focuses on the prevention of residential crime, especially burglary. It has three major components: (1) community vehicle and foot patrols, (2) home security checks, and (3) identification of valuables.

The police cannot be everywhere; therefore, success against crime depends on citizen cooperation and involvement. Community patrols consist of volunteers who travel through their neighborhoods on foot or in vehicles to report crimes or suspicious situations to the police. Patrol members do not possess police powers and are instructed *not* to pursue or challenge anyone. However, just by their presence on the streets these highly visible citizen observers (who wear identification) can be an effective deterrent to crime. Another component of this program is known as ''Block Watch.'' Neighbors on each block are encouraged to report to police any suspicious persons or events they may observe (Fig. 6-5). A recent inmate interview project in Colorado involving convicted burglars revealed that a neighborhood watch program is one of the most effective deterrents against burglary. The majority of the inmates stated that merely being noticed by a neighbor was enough to deter them.[6]

Home security checks consist of surveys or questionnaires that help the home-owner locate weak points that may be advantageous to a burglar. These checklists systematically cover the common areas of weakness in residential security, including

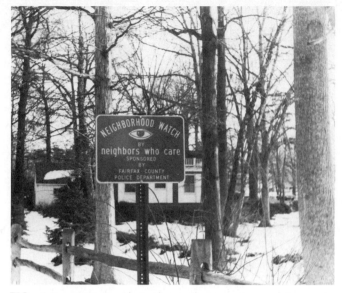

FIG. 6-5 Citizens throughout the country are becoming actively involved in the protection of their neighborhoods. Does your community have a neighborhood watch program?

doors, windows, lighting, and landscaping. The box on pp. 188-189 is an example of a home security checklist. In many communities a person can arrange for a free home security inspection by calling the local police department. They will send an officer who will inspect your home and make recommendations for improving security.

The third component of the Neighborhood Watch program is known as ''Project Identification.'' It consists of marking all of your valuables with a specific identification number and making a record of these items.

The preferred method for marking your valuables is to use an electric engraving pen. These devices can be used on metal, plastic, or wood. It is recommended that your social security number be used as the identifying mark because of the speed with which the property owner's name and address can be obtained through police computer systems. When marking the valuable, be sure to engrave the identification number directly on the object rather than on an easily removed part, such as a back panel, or metal nameplate.

Your owner's inventory record should list all valuables that you have engraved. Pertinent information should include a description of each item, brand name, model and serial numbers, as well as the location of your identification number (box on p. 190).

Another important measure that can be taken is the photographing or videotaping of valuables. In this way you not only have a written record of these possessions, you

Burglary Prevention Checklist for Homes

Survey your home with this checklist. Every "no" check mark shows a weak point that may help a burglar. As you eliminate the "no" checks, you improve your protection. Go through this list carefully and systematically. You may want to look over this situation in daytime, when most house burglars work, as well as in the night. Remember, this checklist only points out your weak points—you are not protected until they are corrected. Complying with these suggestions will not, of course, make your property burglar proof, but it will certainly improve your protection.

Doors

1. Are the locks on your most used outside doors of the cylinder type? Yes ☐ No ☐

2. Are they of either the deadlocking or jimmyproof type? Yes ☐ No ☐

3. Can any of your door locks be opened by breaking out glass or a panel of light wood? Yes ☐ No ☐

4. Do you use chain locks or other auxiliary locks on your most used doors? Yes ☐ No ☐

5. Do the doors without cylinder locks have a heavy bolt or some similar secure device that can be operated only from the inside? Yes ☐ No ☐

6. Can all of your doors (basement, porch, french, balcony) be securely locked? Yes ☐ No ☐

7. Do your basement doors have locks that allow you to isolate that part of your house? Yes ☐ No ☐

8. Are your locks all in good repair? Yes ☐ No ☐

9. Do you know everyone who has a key to your house? (Or are there some still in the possession of previous owners and their servants and friends?) Yes ☐ No ☐

Windows

10. Are your window locks properly and securely mounted? Yes ☐ No ☐

11. Do you keep your windows locked when they are shut? Yes ☐ No ☐

12. Do you use locks that allow you to lock a window that is partly open? Yes ☐ No ☐

13. In high-hazard locations do you use bars or ornamental grille? Yes ☐ No ☐

14. Are you as careful of basement and second-floor widows as you are of those on the first floor? Yes ☐ No ☐

15. Have you made it more difficult for the burglar by locking up your ladder, avoiding trellises that can be used as a ladder or similar aids to climbing? Yes ☐ No ☐

Garage

16. Do you lock your garage door at night? Yes ☐ No ☐

17. Do you lock your garage when you are away from home? Yes ☐ No ☐

18. Do you have good, secure locks on the garage doors and windows? Yes ☐ No ☐

19. Do you lock your car and take the keys out even when it is parked in your garage? Yes ☐ No ☐

Source: The National Sheriff's Association and The Law Enforcement Assistance Administration, U.S. Department of Justice.

Burglary Prevention Checklist for Homes—cont'd

When You Go on a Trip

20. Do you stop all deliveries or arrange for neighbors to pick up papers, milk, mail, packages? Yes ☐ No ☐

21. Do you notify a neighbor? Yes ☐ No ☐

22. Do you notify your sheriff? They provide extra protection for vacant homes. Yes ☐ No ☐

23. Do you leave some shades up so the house doesn't look deserted? Yes ☐ No ☐

24. Do you arrange to keep your lawn and garden in shape? Yes ☐ No ☐

Safe Practices

25. Do you plan so that you do not need to "hide" a key under the door mat? Yes ☐ No ☐

26. Do you keep as much cash as possible and other valuables in a bank? Yes ☐ No ☐

27. Do you keep a list of all valuable property? Yes ☐ No ☐

28. Do you have a list of the serial numbers of your watches, cameras, typewriters, and similar items? Yes ☐ No ☐

29. Do you have a description of other valuable property that does not have a number? Yes ☐ No ☐

30. Do you avoid unnecessary display or publicity of your valuables? Yes ☐ No ☐

31. Have you told your family what to do if they discover a burglar breaking in or already in the house? Yes ☐ No ☐

32. Have you told your family to leave the house undisturbed and call the sheriff or police if they discover a burglary has been committed? Yes ☐ No ☐

This checklist was designed to help you go through your home and make a check to see that you are not inviting a burglary by having an "open house." The checklist covers the common areas of weakness in residential security.

If you would like professional advice and assistance in a thorough home security inspection, call your local law enforcement agency.

To keep your guard, take a critical look at your home security every 3 to 4 months. Don't become lax—crime prevention is a continuous process.

Owner's Inventory

Household and Personal Items

ITEM	BRAND NAME	MODEL #	SERIAL NUMBER	$ VALUE
Television				
Television				
Stereo/phono				
Tape recorder				
Radio				
Radio				
CB radio				
Countertop oven				
Vacuum cleaner				
Sewing machine				
Clock				
Watch				
Watch				
Camera				
Camera				
Lawn Mower				

Automobiles, Motorcycles, RVs, and Bicycles

MAKE	YEAR	MODEL	SERIAL NUMBER	LICENSE NUMBER	$ VALUE

Appliances, Tools, Power Equipment, and Miscellaneous

ITEM	BRAND NAME	MODEL #	SERIAL NUMBER	$ VALUE

also have a visual record that can be used to identify valuables. As a precaution, file one copy of the inventory and photos in a safe place at home and keep a duplicate set of these materials in a bank safe-deposit box or with another family member.

IF A CRIME OCCURS

Successful efforts to combat crime require the cooperative involvement of police and citizens. Whenever you observe suspicious events, call the police. People often fail to call because they are unsure what constitutes suspicious activity, and the police lose valuable response time. Here are some examples of suspicious activities: strangers entering the home of a vacationing neighbor, people carrying televisions or stereos late at night, anyone attempting to use a device other than a key to get into a car, individuals fighting or screaming, and noises such as breaking glass, gunshots, or explosions. If you are in doubt, call the police anyway; investigation is their responsibility.

Following is a list of some information you need to include when reporting a crime to the police:[6, 7]

1. What happened?
2. When?
3. Where?
4. Is anyone hurt?
5. License numbers
6. Vehicle descriptions
7. Direction of travel
8. Description of suspects
9. Were weapons involved?

Additional information that you should provide is your name, address, and phone number in case further police contact is necessary. All of this information will be kept in confidence by the police department.

If a crime is in progress, police will respond quickly; however, if it has already occurred and there are no injuries, there may be some delay. The first priority for police are situations, whether accidental or criminal, that involve risk of injury to the public.

While waiting for the police to arrive, it may be helpful to write down as much descriptive information as you can while it is still fresh in your mind. Facts gathered in the early stages of an investigation generally contribute most to the subsequent arrest of an offender. It is not easy to identify and arrest a suspect, especially when the person has not been seen by anyone and has not left any usable fingerprints or other identifying traces.

If an arrest is made as a result of a police investigation, you may be required to attend one or more court hearings to testify about the offense. Questions that you may have about these hearings should be directed to the district attorney's office of the city or county in which you reside. From time to time hearings may be postponed; such court delays can be very discouraging. Nevertheless, remember that without your testimony the case may be dismissed and the offender will not be held accountable for his wrongdoing.

FIREARM SAFETY

Washington, D.C.: A man died from gunshot wounds inflicted during an argument that developed after a minor dispute. The fatal assault occurred as the two drivers argued over a parking space at a shopping mall. When one of the drivers refused to back his car away from the empty slot, the other driver returned to his vehicle, pulled out a pistol, and shot the other driver four times.

Chicago, Ill.: Two men were shot in an argument with a third man over tickets to an M. C. Hammer concert. One man died from his wounds; the other suffered serious internal injuries.

Indianapolis, Ind.: In a heated argument during a card game with his uncle and cousin, a local man shot and killed both relatives with a handgun he had recently purchased to protect his home from burglars.

Miami, Fla.: Irritated by the blaring sounds of a stereo in the house next door, a Miami man shot and killed his neighbor in an argument over noise.

Arlington, Va.: While playing in his parents' bedroom, a 12-year-old boy accidentally shot and killed his 10-year-old playmate. The loaded handgun was kept in the bedroom so that the young man's father could protect the family from intruders.

If we look at the statistics for 1989, we can see that 62% of the 21,500 Americans who were murdered, died from wounds inflicted by guns. Of these, 48% were committed with handguns, 8% involved shotguns, and 6% were committed with rifles.[27] Another 2000 people die in gun-related accidents, and at least 30,000 are wounded each year.

A myth that has been promoted over the years is the claim that "guns don't kill people; people kill people." In a technical sense this may be true; however, the simple fact is that Americans now own more than 70 million handguns, with another 2 million being purchased each year. The increased availability of firearms is believed to be related to an increased incidence of not only homicides, but suicides and accidental deaths as well.

Although shotguns and rifles are as effective as handguns for killing people, their lack of concealability and their cumbersome nature make them less likely to be involved in murders, suicides, or accidents. They cannot be pulled quickly from a jacket pocket or used impulsively like handguns.

Handgun design maximizes the ability to cause serious or fatal wounds with a minimum of effort and planning. The intent to discharge a gun need be present only momentarily—if at all—to accomplish the pulling of a trigger. This enhances the probability of an unplanned discharge of a weapon, whether during an argument, a robbery, or while you are cleaning it.[2] Supporting this statement is the fact that over 35% of all murders were preceded by altercations, domestic quarrels, and arguments between acquaintances or relatives.[27,28] In most cases the killer reached for an available handgun and impulsively shot his victim. Few of the killers had considered what they were going to do or what might happen to them after the act. Considering the increased availability of handguns, it is not surprising that the murder rate has doubled in the past 20 years.

A handgun bought for protection is six times more likely to kill you, a member of your family, or a friend than it is to kill an intruder. In fact, more than 90% of burglaries occur in unoccupied houses. In half of the remaining cases, the occupants slept through the burglary.[18]

Circumstances under which accidental shootings occur have also changed in recent years. At one time most shooting-accident victims were men injured with rifles or shotguns while hunting. Today more than half of the accidents occur in the home, and the weapon causing much of that damage is the handgun. With women now purchasing handguns in rapidly growing numbers, it is likely that an increasing percentage of them will be injured in gun-related accidents.

Guns: To Control or Not to Control

The ease with which firearms can be purchased stands in marked contrast to measures taken by states to control the possession and use of firearms. Generally states are relatively lenient with gun sale laws. The basis for these laws is the Federal Gun Control Act of 1968. This law prohibits the sale of firearms to persons under 18 years of age, those convicted of specific crimes (including the use of certain drugs), fugitives, and persons termed mentally defective. The mail-order sale of firearms is also prohibited.[2]

Most states concentrate their efforts on possession laws. Their intent is to prevent the possession of firearms by people who are likely to use them illegally; however, these laws are of limited value, since they are difficult to enforce once an individual has purchased a gun. The standard possession laws apply to those seeking to carry handguns. Special permits must be acquired before you can carry a handgun on your person or keep it in the car. Some states even differentiate between ''concealed'' and ''unconcealed'' handguns. In Virginia it is unlawful to carry a concealed handgun without a permit; however, that same weapon can be carried without a permit, provided it is not hidden from view.

Other state laws involve the use of guns; that is, where and when they can be discharged. Increasingly, states are stiffening penalties for crimes committed with guns, since it is recognized that a victim's chances of being seriously wounded are greatly increased when a felon uses a gun. Recently, Detroit went a step further, passing legislation that mandates a jail sentence of up to 90 days for anyone caught carrying a handgun without a permit. Police estimated that Detroit's 1.1 million residents owned 1.5 million guns. The easy availability of handguns, especially among teenagers, was mentioned as a key factor for Detroit's rising murder rate—the highest in the nation in recent years. Giving additional impetus to this legislation was the fact that 338 children under 17 years of age had been shot, 38 of them fatally.[14]

How do these laws work in curtailing the illegal use of handguns and handgun fatalities? Not very well! The problem with this type of legislation is that it works *after* the fact. The possession and use laws will be applied after a shooting incident has occurred—when it's generally too late for the victim. Gun-control groups have a strong case when they say that current legislation has been ineffective in reducing the murder rate in this country.

If we are to reduce the carnage, certain realistic and perhaps unpopular measures must be taken. The banning of the sale or possession of handguns in the United States is not a realistic proposal, although some small cities such as Morton Grove, Ill., have passed legislation in their communities banning the sale and possession of handguns.

The regulation of the manufacture of firearms (in terms of product design and quantity manufactured) could be a feasible first step in eliminating the gun problem. A design issue that will have to be addressed in the 1990s is the development of the plastic gun. Made of high-strength polymers, these guns cannot be easily detected by current airport security systems because they contain few metal parts.

A computer analysis of handguns used in crimes committed in the 1980s indicated that 8 of the 10 most commonly used weapons had snub-nosed barrels measuring 2.5 inches or less.[1] (Weapon concealability seemed to be of prime importance to the criminal.) Although the well-publicized **Saturday night specials** (small-caliber, short-barreled weapons whose parts are imported and assembled in the United States) led the list of crime guns, the majority of the handguns used in crimes were the more expensive American made, short-barreled models.

Legislation proposed in Congress to stop the importation of cheaply made handgun parts may solve part of the problem, but what about the American-made, short-barreled models? Perhaps that legislation should include a limitation on barrel length for handguns produced in the United States. It would be extremely difficult to conceal a weapon with a 6-inch barrel; however, this design change would not affect the sportsman or the person who wanted protection in the home.

If only the answer were that simple! The handgun issue is a multifaceted problem. Other investigations of handgun crimes have found that as many as 80% of the guns used by criminals had been stolen.[18] This is not a surprising statistic when you discover that more than 200,000 handguns are taken from private homes each year. It is a myth that "if we don't allow citizens to have handguns, only the criminals will have them," because criminals get a significant number of handguns by stealing them from law-abiding Americans.

With gun ownership you take on the responsibility of securing the weapon whenever it is not in use. When not cleaning or firing your gun, you should store it, unloaded, in a locked and secure cabinet (*not* a glass display case or under a pillow).

Nationwide, the development of a handgun registration and licensing act could serve two valuable purposes: (1) When individuals purchased handguns, this act would allow authorities to investigate applicants to determine whether they had previous records of violence; and (2) such a registration act would allow authorities to trace lost or stolen guns more easily. Recently Congress has approved a piece of gun-control legislation known as the "Brady Bill." The Brady Bill, named for President Ronald Reagan's press secretary, James S. Brady, who was disabled in an assassination attempt on Reagan, calls for a national 7 day waiting period to buy handguns.

There has been no mention of prohibiting handguns in any of the suggestions discussed thus far. The intent is to reduce the possibility of handguns being used against innocent victims, not to infringe on the Second Amendment right to bear arms for self-protection, guaranteed in the U.S. Constitution.

While the decreased availability of handguns may result in the increased use of such weapons as knives and clubs in murder attempts, the lower fatality rates associated with them would increase a victim's chances of survival from such an attack. Although the strategies mentioned will not eliminate all gun-related deaths, they could substantially reduce them and the injuries caused by firearms.

Guns: Procedures for Safe Handling

Two factors involved in most firearms accidents are carelessness in handling the weapon and a lack of knowledge about its operation. In the case of gun accidents, victims and the persons who shot them often either had no idea that the guns were loaded or they did not know how to handle them properly (Fig. 6-6). There are a number of safety precautions that apply to the handling of any firearm. We will discuss some of the more basic procedures in this section.

Treat every gun as if it were loaded. Never point a firearm at anyone or anything you do not intend to shoot, nor in a direction where unintentional discharge could cause injury or damage. This also applies to guns you know to be unloaded.

Many people accidently shoot themselves or companions while carrying a firearm. To reduce the possibility of such an occurrence, keep your finger off the trigger until you are ready to fire; stumbling may cause you to unintentionally discharge the weapon. Develop a habit of placing fingers on the outside of the trigger guard when walking. As you are moving with the weapon, the barrel should be pointed downward

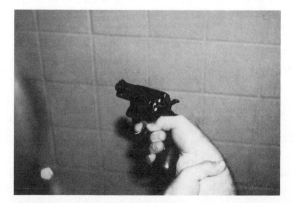

FIG. 6-6 Do you know whether this gun is loaded? What danger do you see in this photograph?

in front of you; an accidental discharge will go into the ground rather than injuring a friend.

When not in use, guns must always be unloaded and stored properly. After shooting a handgun, a simple three-step procedure for unloading the weapon could eliminate many accidents. The procedure is demonstrated in Fig. 6-7 and Fig. 6-8. This practice will assure you that the weapon is unloaded, and it will also prevent you from losing ammunition that might later be found by children.

Unloaded firearms should be stored and locked in a rack, cabinet, closet, or drawer. Ammunition should be stored and locked in a separate facility away from guns. Another precaution is to place trigger locks on weapons when they are not in use. This device locks behind a gun's trigger, thus preventing its rearward movement and discharge of the firearm. Such responsible actions could significantly reduce the likelihood of a weapon's being stolen or used impulsively by its owner.

If there are children in the family, it is especially important that everyone have a clear understanding of both the potential dangers of guns and their proper function and use. An important reason for educating children is to eliminate the mystique about guns. They must learn at an early age that guns are not toys and should never be treated as such. The combination of proper instruction of children and storage of firearms will do much to reduce the hazards of having guns in the home.

Hunting safety. Although nearly two thirds of gun-related accidental deaths occur in the home, another 600 to 800 persons lose their lives each year in hunting accidents. Surprisingly, it is neither the first-time hunter nor the experienced one who has accidents. The most likely candidate is the young hunter (15 to 24 years old) who has at least 3 years of experience and is momentarily careless and fails to follow the rules of hunting safety.

Never assume that people know or follow hunting-safety rules because they claim to have a knowledge of firearms. The priority in any hunting party is to make sure that everyone handles his or her gun in a safe manner.

Before going hunting, you and your companions may want to consider the following points:

1. Be sure to get permission from the landowners on whose property you will be hunting. Ask them what they will allow in terms of game to be hunted and areas on the property in which to hunt. To ensure future hunting opportunities on the land, share your game with landowners or offer to help them with work or clean-up around the property.

2. Never get into a car or truck with loaded weapons. More than a few hunters have blown holes in vehicle roofs in their haste to start hunting. Hunting dogs stepping on loaded guns also have been known to cause discharges in vehicles.

3. Many hunters accidentally shoot themselves or companions when they slip or stumble while carrying a firearm. To reduce the possibility of such an occurrence, keep your finger off the trigger and the gun's safety in the "on" position until you are ready to fire. Develop a habit of placing fingers on the outside of the trigger guard

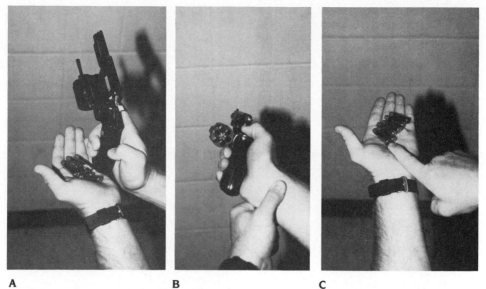

A   B   C

FIG. 6-7   Revolver. **A,** Open the cylinder and eject cartridges into your hand. **B,** Inspect the chambers. Be sure they are empty. **C,** Count the number of rounds in your hand. Verify that none are missing.

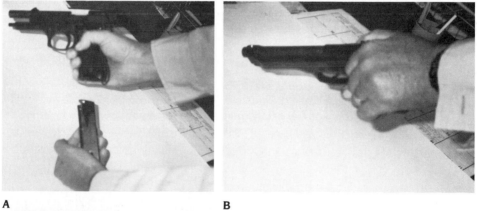

A   B

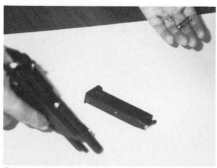

C

FIG. 6-8   Semi-Automatic Pistol. **A,** The first step in unloading a semi-automatic pistol is to remove the magazine. **B,** Next, open the chamber. **C,** Visual inspection of the chamber will show if it is unloaded.

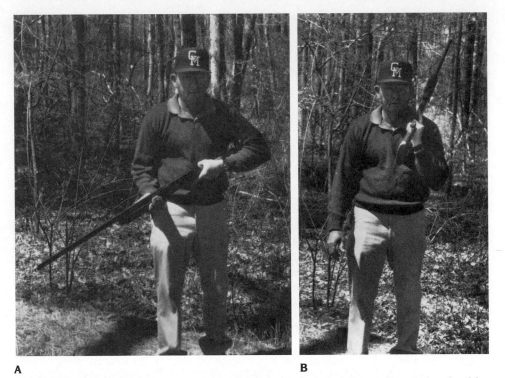

A   **B**

FIG. 6-9 The proper way to carry a gun. **A,** Side-by-side formation. **B,** On the shoulder.

when you are walking, since stumbling may cause you to grip the trigger unintentionally and discharge the weapon.

4. Hunters should also be aware of the proper way to carry a gun. Hunters should preferably be in a side-by-side formation with guns pointed down in front of them. An accidental discharge will go into the ground instead of a friend. A gun may also be carried on the shoulder with the trigger guard facing upward. This position forces the muzzle to point up. If a hunter stumbles, the muzzle will be pointed still higher in the air, reducing the risk of hitting someone (Fig. 6-9).

5. Before attempting to cross a fence, ditch, or stream, a hunter should remove cartridges or shells from the gun, leave the action open, and pass it to the other side. Once you have safely crossed the obstacle, you can then reload. A similar plan of action should be used by hunters who attempt to climb a tree.

6. When hunting with others, ''zones of fire'' must be established so each hunter will not endanger others. After determining zones of fire, each hunter must shoot only within his or her specific zone.

7. *Be sure of your target and what is beyond!* There have been numerous tragedies in which eager hunters, having failed to clearly identify their targets, shot other hunters, children in the woods, or someone's pet. Many hunters also fail to realize how far a bullet can travel; a .22 caliber slug can travel well over a mile.

8. At the end of a day of hunting, before storing your firearm and starting for home, carefully check to ensure that it is unloaded. The same holds true when members of the hunting party gather in camp; weapons should be loaded only when you are in the field.

9. If you are considering purchasing a firearm or you have decided to take up the sport of hunting, contact your local law enforcement agency, county conservation office, or sporting goods store concerning state laws and regulations pertaining to firearms ownership and hunting. Another important person to contact is your local representative of the National Rifle Association. He or she can provide you with information about the numerous programs in firearm and hunting safety offered by the NRA.

A final word of caution: whenever you handle any firearm, always check to see whether it is loaded. Never take anyone's word for it. A gun in your possession is your responsibility.

SUMMARY

In the past 5 years, reported crimes have increased nearly 15%. If you take into account the crimes that go unreported, as many as one out of every seven persons may become a victim this year.

Violent crimes involve either force or the threat of physical force. They include murder, forcible rape, robbery, and assault. Relative to their number in the population persons under 25 years of age are the more frequent victims of violence. The typical victim of violence is young, living in a large metropolitan community, and traveling alone through an isolated area late at night.

In most violent crimes, the characteristics of the assailants are very similar to those of the victims. The violent criminal is usually a young male of the same race as his victim. He is likely to be carrying a weapon and to have been drinking before his assaultive behavior.

With the increased use of weapons in recent years, it is not surprising to find that many victims suffer serious personal injuries during robberies. Before their victimization, persons who are robbed can often be found in a vulnerable situation, such as being alone, carrying packages or groceries, or having some type of physical handicap.

Rape is a violent crime that involves women as the primary victims. Victims of rape are most often young, single, and living alone. They come from a broad range of socioeconomic backgrounds and most of them are employed. The offenders are most often young, single, and unemployed.

Having histories of failure and frustration from competing in society, rapists use sexual violence to gain a feeling of control in their lives. Rape is a crime of power and hostility; it is *not* sexually motivated.

Historically, women have been told not to physically resist an attacker, since this may cause him to react more violently; however, in recent studies researchers have found that women who forcefully resisted were less likely to be raped, with only a slightly increased chance of receiving minor injuries. They also found that serious injuries were as likely to occur to a woman who did not resist as to a woman who did resist.

Self-protection and self-defense involve preventive measures as well as active measures to reduce crimes of violence. The most important point to be stressed is to be alert to your surroundings and the people around you. In this way you can reduce risks and avoid danger.

Although they generally do not involve violence, the property crimes of burglary and larceny-theft account for over $7 billion in losses annually.

Victims of property crimes are as likely to be found in the suburbs as they are in the inner city. Most of these crimes involve the law of supply and demand; what is currently popular is more likely to be stolen. Stereos, TVs, VCRs, gold, silver, and guns are popular items for burglars; whereas ten-speed bicycles, CD players, auto tape decks, clothing, and electronic equipment are the targets of the larcenist-thief.

A wide range of preventive measures can be taken to reduce both violent and property crimes. The use of deadbolt locks, window locks, burglar alarms, and improved lighting are just a few of the measures that can reduce property crime. The Neighborhood Watch Program can be invaluable in tracing stolen items as well as in deterring crime.

Despite the measures that you take, you can still become a victim. If we are to combat crime successfully, the cooperation and involvement of citizens and police are needed. When a crime occurs, call the police immediately; the sooner an investigation can begin, the more likely an arrest will be made. If a suspect is arrested, you are likely to be called to testify. Without your testimony an offender may not be held accountable for his crime.

Whether you have purchased a gun to hunt or to protect yourself, remember that there are certain procedures that apply to the handling of any firearm. A gun in *your* possession is *your* responsibility.

Key Terms

Active resistance   Fleeing, fighting, screaming, and verbal aggression.

Aggravated assault   Unlawful attack of one person by another for the purpose of inflicting severe bodily injury.

Burglary   Unlawful entry of a structure to commit a felony or theft.

Forcible rape   Sexual intercourse achieved or attempted without the victim's consent and through the use or threat of force.

Interior system burglar alarm   Consists of pressure mats, photoelectric beams, and motion detectors inside the home.

Interracial crime   The assailant and victim are of different races.

Intraracial crime   The assailant and victim are of the same race.

Larceny-theft   The unlawful taking, carrying, leading, or riding away the possession of another.

Passive resistance   Verbal persuasion, pleading, and submission.

Perimeter system burglar alarm   Uses sensing devices attached to all doors and windows leading into the home.

Property crimes   Offenses such as burglary and larceny-theft.

Robbery   Taking or attempting to take anything of value from a person by force or threat of force.

Saturday night specials   Inexpensive, small-caliber, short-barreled handguns often used in violent crimes.

Violent crimes   Offenses such as murder, rape, aggravated assault, and robbery.

References

1. Albright, J.: Ban snubbies and solve the great handgun debate, The Washington Post, Nov. 1981.
2. Baker, S. P., Teret, S.P., and Deitz, P.E.: Firearms and the public health, Journal of Public Health Policy 1(3):224, 1980.
3. Bane, V., Grant, M., Alexander, B. and others: Silent no more, People Magazine, Dec. 17, 1990, pp. 94 -104.
4. Bart, P.B.: Avoiding rape: a study of victims and avoiders, Rockville, Md., 1980, National Center for the Prevention and Control of Rape.
5. Citizens Crime Commission of New York City: Crossroads on crime: a report, New York, 1980, The Commission.
6. Duncan, J.T.: Citizen crime prevention tactics, U.S. Department of Justice, National Institute of Justice, Washington, D.C., 1980, U.S. Government Printing Office.
7. Fairfax County Police Department: Neighborhood watch: a community crime prevention program, Fairfax, Va., 1986, U.S. Government Printing Office.
8. Harlow, C.W.: Motor vehicle theft, U.S. Department of Justice, Bureau of Justice Statistics, Washington, D.C., March 1988, U.S. Government Printing Office.
9. Isikoff, M.: Record number of rapes reported in U.S. in '90, The Washington Post, March 22, 1991, p. A-3.
10. Koppel, H.: Lifetime likelihood of victimization, U.S. Department of Justice, Bureau of Justice Statistics, Washington, D.C., March 1987, U.S. Government Printing Office.
11. Langan, P., and Innes, C.: Preventing domestic violence against women, U.S. Department of Justice, Bureau of Justice Statistics Special Report, Washington, D.C., Aug. 1986, U.S. Government Printing Office.
12. Langan, P.: The risk of violent crime, U.S. Department of Justice, Bureau of Justice Statistics Special Report, Washington, D.C., May 1985, U.S. Government Printing Office.
13. Mackay, S.: Patterns of violent crime, SASD Bulletin (6):19, 1980.
14. McAllister, B.: Detroit gun measure signed, Washington Post, Dec. 9, 1986, p. A-3.
15. McDermott, M.J.: Rape victimization in 26 American cities, U.S. Department of Justice, Bureau of Justice Statistics, Washington, D.C., 1979, U.S. Government Printing Office.
16. McIntyre, J.J.: Victim response to rape: alternative outcomes, National Center for the Prevention and Control of Rape, Rockville, Md., 1980, U.S. Government Printing Office.
17. Moore, M.H., and Trojanowicz, R.C.: Policing and the fear of crime, NCJ 111459, U.S. Department of Justice, National Institute of Justice, Washington, D.C., June 1988, U.S. Government Printing Office.
18. National Coalition to Ban Handguns: Facts about handguns, Washington, D.C., 1981, The Coalition.
19. National Sheriffs' Association: How to protect your home, Washington, D.C., 1980, The Association.
20. O'Neill, J.A.: The Drug Use Forecasting (DUF) Program reports 1989 results, NIJ Reports, Summer 1990, pp. 10 -11.
21. Rand, M.: Households touched by crime, 1985, U.S. Department of Justice, Bureau of Justice Statistics Bulletin, Washington, D.C., June 1986, U.S. Government Printing Office.
22. Russell, C.: Gun study hits home, Washington Post, June 12, 1986, p. A-3.

23. Sherman, L: Domestic violence, U.S. Department of Justice, National Institute of Justice, Washington, D.C., Jan. 1988, U.S. Government Printing Office.
24. Storaska, F.: How to say no to a rapist and survive, New York, 1975, Random House, Inc.
25. Timrots, A.D., and Rand, M.R.: Violent crime by strangers and nonstrangers, U.S. Department of Justice, Bureau of Justice Statistics, Washington, D.C., Jan. 1987, U.S. Government Printing Office.
26. Tinklenberg, J.R., and Ochberg, F.: Patterns of adolescent violence: a California sample, Montreal, 1979, University of Montreal, International Center for Comparative Criminology.
27. U.S. Department of Justice: Crime in the United States: 1989, Federal Bureau of Investigation, Washington, D.C., July 1990, U.S. Government Printing Office.
28. U.S. Department of Justice: Criminal victimization in the United States: 1989, Bureau of Justice Statistics, Aug. 1990, U.S. Government Printing Office.
29. U.S. Department of Justice, Report to the nation on crime and justice (ed 2) NCJ-105506 Bureau of Justice Statistics, March 1988, U.S. Government Printing Office.
30. U.S. Department of Justice: The Crime of rape, Bureau of Justice Statistics, Washington, D.C., March 1985, U.S. Government Printing Office.
31. U.S. Department of Justice: The seasonality of crime, NCJ-111033 Bureau of Justice Statistics, Washington, D.C., May 1988, U.S. Government Printing Office.
32. Warner, C.G., ed.: Rape and sexual assault: management and intervention, Rockville, Md., 1980, Aspen Systems Corp.
33. Wright, B.A., and Fesenmaier, D.R.: A factor analytic study of attitudinal structure and its impact on rural landowners' access policies, Environmental Management, vol. 14, no. 2, 1990, pp. 269-277.

Resource Organizations

Academy of Criminal Justice Sciences
1313 Farnam–on–the–Mall
University of Nebraska at Omaha
Omaha, NE 68182

American Association of Retired Persons
1909 K Street, N.W.
Washington, DC 20049

Citizens Committee for the Right to
Keep and Bear Arms
Liberty Park
12500 N.E. Tenth Place
Bellevue, WA 98005

Federal Bureau of Investigation
Uniform Crime Reporting
10th Street and Pennsylvania Avenue,
N.W.
Washington, DC 20535

Feminist Alliance Against Rape
P.O. Box 21033
Washington, DC 20009

National Coalition to Ban Handguns
100 Maryland Avenue, N.E.
Washington, DC 20002

National Crime Prevention Institute
School of Police Administration
University of Louisville, Shelby Campus
Louisville, KY 40292

National Criminal Justice Association
444 North Capitol Street, N.W., Suite 608
Washington, DC 20001

National Criminal Justice Reference Service
Box 6000
Rockville, MD 20850

National Institute of Mental Health
5600 Fishers Lane
Rockville, MD 20857

National Law Enforcement Council
1140 Connecticut Avenue, N.W.,
Suite 804
Washington, DC 20036

Gun Owners Incorporated
1025 Front Street, Suite 300
Sacramento, CA 95814

Handgun Control, Inc.
1400 K Street, N.W.
Washington, DC 20005

International Association of Chiefs of Police
13 Firstfield Road
Gaithersburg, MD 20878

National Association for Crime Victims'
Rights
P.O. Box 16161
Portland, OR 97216

National Association of Neighborhoods
1651 Fuller, N.W.
Washington, DC 20009

National Coalition Against Sexual Assault
c/o Volunteers of America
8787 State Street, Suite 202
East St. Louis, IL 62203

National Organization for Victim Assistance
717 D Street, N.W.
Washington, DC 20531

National Rifle Association of America
1600 Rhode Island Avenue, N.W.
Washington, DC 20036

National Sheriffs' Association
1450 Duke Street
Alexandria, VA 22314

National Shooting Sports Foundation
P.O. Box 1075
Riverside, CT 06878

CHAPTER 6

Applying What You Have Learned

1. Utilize the Burglary Prevention Checklist on pp. 188-189 to systematically inspect your dorm, apartment, home, or sorority/fraternity house. After completing the inspection, list those weak points that may make your living quarters somewhat vulnerable.

a.) _____

b.) _____

c.) _____

d.) _____

e.) _____

2. Using the owner's inventory of personal items found in the box on p. 190, record the brand names, model numbers, serial numbers, and estimated values of your own personal property. You might want to add another page for clothes, jewelry, and miscellaneous items. When you're finished, make a copy and send it to your parents for safe keeping.

a.) What was the estimated value of your personal belongings?

_____

_____

_____

b.) Were there any surprises for you as you completed this project?

_____

_____

_____

Motor Vehicle and Pedestrian Safety

Two out of five Americans will be involved in an alcohol-related crash at some point in their lives.

National Highway Traffic Safety Administration: The conference on injury in America

IMPACT OF MOTOR VEHICLE ACCIDENTS

Since the enactment of the Highway Safety Act in 1966, the motor vehicle death rate (number of deaths per 100 million miles driven) has decreased 60%. In 1966, the fatality rate was 5.58 deaths per 100 million vehicle miles of travel; today the rate has dropped to 2.25.[26] In 1966, 53,000 people were killed on U.S. highways; in 1989 the number was 46,900. If the 1966 fatality rate had been experienced in 1989, more than 115,000 persons would have lost their lives in traffic accidents.

A multitude of factors played a role in this risk reduction. Vehicle design changes included improved steering control systems, bumper systems, and occupant restraints. Highway safety research led to improvements in roadway design and construction, the elimination of hazards such as roadside obstacles, and the development of protective devices such as median barriers, impact attenuators, and breakaway light and utility poles. One of the most important changes was the imposition of the 55-mile-per-hour (mph) nationwide speed limit in 1974. It has been estimated that as many as 55,000 lives have been saved in the last 18 years as a result of slower vehicle speeds.

Now for the bad news! Although statistically one's risks are much lower today than they were in 1966, they are not as low as they could be, considering the technologies that have been available to motor vehicle manufacturers.

Rather than a continuing reduction in the number of highway deaths, as one would expect, there has been an increase as we proceed into the 1990s. Factors contributing to this increase in fatalities include the repeal or weakening of laws requiring motorcycle operators and passengers to wear helmets; an increase in the number of light trucks and vans, which are not subject to many of the safety requirements that apply to passenger cars; an increase in accidents involving heavy trucks; lightweight cars added to a traffic mix of heavier vehicles; slow movement by the auto industry in adopting passive restraint systems; and the eroding of driver compliance with the 55-mph speed limit. A preliminary projection indicates that by the year 2000 vehicle fatalities will increase by 10,000 to 15,000 per year as a result of the likely increase in travel by a growing population, if these factors are not appropriately controlled.

As we will find in this chapter, vehicle safety involves a complex set of factors. Although human error is usually the cause of most accidents, extenuating circumstances such as design hazards and environmental conditions can exacerbate the situation.

Death, Injury, Financial Loss

By far the greatest number of yearly accidental deaths occurs on our nation's streets and highways. Motor vehicle deaths account for nearly 50% of all deaths resulting from accidents.[26] Unlike other major health problems, which take their toll among persons over 40 years of age, highway deaths and injuries primarily strike the young. Drivers between the ages of 15 and 24 represent only 16% of licensed drivers, yet they are involved in 28% of the total fatal crashes.[4]

Not only does age seem to make a difference when one considers the likelihood of being involved in a fatal accident, but also figures indicate that male drivers are involved much more frequently in fatal motor vehicle accidents than are female drivers. In 1989 approximately 76% of the drivers involved in fatal accidents were male, whereas 24% were female.[26] Although the amount of time spent by men behind the wheel exceeds that spent by women, it does not account for the excessive number of fatal accidents in which men are involved. Certain sociocultural factors, including the ''hard-drinking, fast-driving macho image'' of the American male driver as portrayed by the media, have contributed to the problem.

Fatal motor vehicle accidents occur almost twice as often in rural settings as they do in urban areas. The higher speeds at which people travel and the prevalence of two-lane roads make rural areas more hazardous for vehicle operators.

Time of the day and day of the week are two other factors that can increase one's likelihood of having a fatal accident. The most dangerous time of the day is from 10 P.M. to 2 A.M. The next most dangerous time is the rush hour period from 6 P.M. to 10 P.M. As expected, the weekend is the worst time for travel; almost 40% of fatal accidents occur on Friday or Saturday, especially later in the evening.

As smaller passenger cars and motorcycles have become more popular, they have added a new dimension of danger for the motor vehicle operator. The amount of protection afforded operators and passengers of these vehicles is much less than that of full-size cars or trucks. Later in this chapter we will take a close look at this issue and what can be done about it.

If we put these factors together, *the prime candidate for a fatal motor vehicle accident is a male, 15 to 24 years of age, driving on a two-lane, rural road between the hours of 10 P.M. and 2 A.M. on a Saturday night*. If he has been drinking and is driving a subcompact car or motorcycle, the likelihood that he and his passengers will have a fatal accident is even more pronounced. One way to minimize your risks would be to avoid this particular set of circumstances. Think about it; have you ever been in this situation?

In any discussion of vehicle safety we also must consider the injuries and economic losses resulting from accidents. Nearly 2 million disabling injuries resulted from motor vehicle accidents in 1989; 140,000 of these injuries involved some type of permanent impairment.

Losses from motor vehicle accidents in terms of deaths, injuries, and dollars are staggering; however, the major impact of these accidents cannot be measured. No dollar value can be placed on the loss of a brother, sister, father, mother, husband, or wife. A leg amputated as the result of a motorcycle accident cannot be replaced. The loss of potential to society when an infant suffers permanent brain damage from hitting the windshield of a car cannot be estimated. In a motor vehicle accident, the victim isn't the only one to suffer. Have you lost a close relative or friend in a motor vehicle accident, or do you know someone who has? Sadly, the answer far too often is yes.

In the following sections we will investigate the major causes of vehicle accidents and the efforts that can and should be taken to reduce the damage on our streets and highways (Fig. 7-1 and Table 7-1).

MOTOR VEHICLE ACCIDENTS: THE HUMAN ELEMENT

Human error accounts for nearly 85% of all accidents, including motor vehicle accidents. The term most often used to describe the causes of these accidents is *improper driving.* This includes such actions as speeding, failure to yield right of way, driving left of center, incorrect passing, and following too closely.

Although an estimated 2000 to 4000 lives had been saved annually in the years since the 55-mph speed limit was introduced, Congress enacted legislation in 1987 that raises the speed limit on rural interstate highways to 65 mph.

Although speed limits will remain 55 mph on noninterstate roadways, the new law affects as much as 75% of the U.S. interstate system.

Two questions about this legislation must be addressed: (1) Will the increased speed limits have an impact on the highway death toll? (2) Will people comply with the 65-mph speed limit? In a recent report to Congress, the National Highway Traffic Safety Administration estimated that the fatality rates on rural interstates in the 38 states that now have 65-mph speed limits has increased by approximately 15%. This has resulted in an additional 500 motor vehicle deaths per year.[26] In those states that have retained a 55-mph rural interstate speed limit, there has been no change in fatality rates. Additionally the states with higher speed limits have had an increase in the percentage of drivers exceeding the speed limit.

With increased vehicle speed a driver must consider three factors: (1) There will

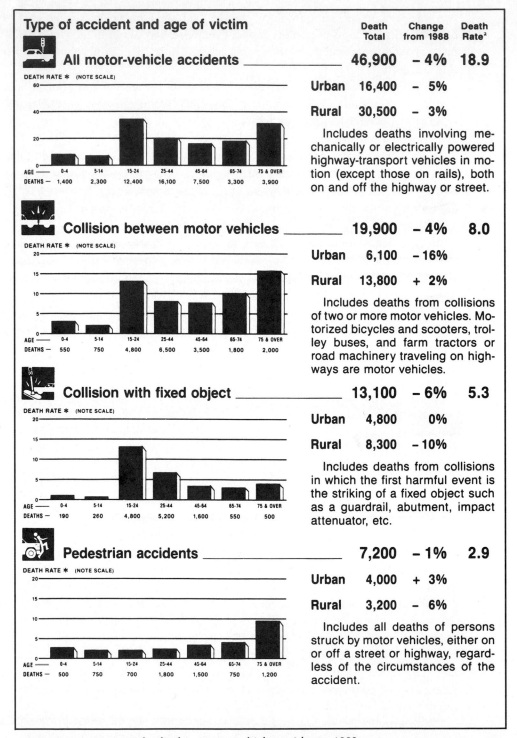

Type of accident and age of victim

	Death Total	Change from 1988	Death Rate[a]

All motor-vehicle accidents —————— 46,900 – 4% 18.9

DEATH RATE * (NOTE SCALE)

AGE	0-4	5-14	15-24	25-44	45-64	65-74	75 & OVER
DEATHS	1,400	2,300	12,400	16,100	7,500	3,300	3,900

Urban 16,400 – 5%

Rural 30,500 – 3%

Includes deaths involving mechanically or electrically powered highway-transport vehicles in motion (except those on rails), both on and off the highway or street.

Collision between motor vehicles ———— 19,900 – 4% 8.0

DEATH RATE * (NOTE SCALE)

AGE	0-4	5-14	15-24	25-44	45-64	65-74	75 & OVER
DEATHS	550	750	4,800	6,500	3,500	1,800	2,000

Urban 6,100 – 16%

Rural 13,800 + 2%

Includes deaths from collisions of two or more motor vehicles. Motorized bicycles and scooters, trolley buses, and farm tractors or road machinery traveling on highways are motor vehicles.

Collision with fixed object —————— 13,100 – 6% 5.3

DEATH RATE * (NOTE SCALE)

AGE	0-4	5-14	15-24	25-44	45-64	65-74	75 & OVER
DEATHS	190	260	4,800	5,200	1,600	550	500

Urban 4,800 0%

Rural 8,300 – 10%

Includes deaths from collisions in which the first harmful event is the striking of a fixed object such as a guardrail, abutment, impact attenuator, etc.

Pedestrian accidents ———————— 7,200 – 1% 2.9

DEATH RATE * (NOTE SCALE)

AGE	0-4	5-14	15-24	25-44	45-64	65-74	75 & OVER
DEATHS	500	750	700	1,800	1,500	750	1,200

Urban 4,000 + 3%

Rural 3,200 – 6%

Includes all deaths of persons struck by motor vehicles, either on or off a street or highway, regardless of the circumstances of the accident.

FIG. 7-1 How people died in motor vehicle accidents, 1989.

From National Safety Council: Accident Facts, Chicago, 1990.

	Death Total	Change from 1988	Death Rate[a]
Noncollision accidents	**4,900**	**– 6%**	**2.0**

DEATH RATE * (NOTE SCALE)

AGE	0-4	5-14	15-24	25-44	45-64	65-74	75 & OVER
DEATHS	130	200	1,700	2,000	650	110	110

Urban	800	0%
Rural	4,100	– 7%

Includes deaths from accidents in which the first injury- or damage-producing event was an overturn, jackknife or other type of noncollision.

	Death Total	Change from 1988	Death Rate
Collision with pedalcycle	**1,000**	**+11%**	**0.4**

DEATH RATE * (NOTE SCALE)

AGE	0-4	5-14	15-24	25-44	45-64	65-74	75 & OVER
DEATHS	20	300	220	280	100	30	50

Urban	500	+ 67%
Rural	500	– 17%

Includes deaths of pedalcyclists and motor-vehicle occupants from collisions between pedalcycles and motor vehicles on streets, highways, private driveways, parking lots, etc.

	Death Total	Change from 1988	Death Rate
Collision with railroad train	**700**	**+17%**	**0.3**

DEATH RATE * (NOTE SCALE)

AGE	0-4	5-14	15-24	25-44	45-64	65-74	75 & OVER
DEATHS	10	30	160	290	130	50	30

Urban	200	0%
Rural	500	+ 25%

Includes deaths from collisions of motor vehicles (moving or stalled) and railroad vehicles at public or private grade crossings. In other types of accidents, classification requires motor vehicle to be in motion.

Other collision _____ **100 0%** (b)

(animal, animal-drawn vehicles, street cars)

Includes deaths from motor-vehicle collisions not specified in other categories above. Most of the deaths arose out of accidents involving animals or animal-drawn vehicles.

Note: Procedures and benchmarks for estimating deaths by type of accident and age were changed in 1990. Estimates for 1987 and later years are not comparable to earlier years. The noncollision and fixed object categories were most affected by the changes.

*Deaths per 100,000 population in each age group.

[a]Deaths per 100,000 population.
[b]Death rate was less than 0.05.

FIG. 7-1, cont'd. How people died in motor vehicle accidents, 1989.

Table 7-1 Current motor vehicle legislation

State	21 Year Drinking Age Since[a]	Happy Hour Ban[b]	Dram Shop Law[c]	Open Container Law[d]	Effective Date	Enforce-ment[e]	Seating Positions	Child Safety Seat Law Date[f]	Effective Date[b]	Applicable Vehicles
		Alcohol Legislation			Mandatory Belt Use Law				65 Speed Limit	
Alabama..........	1985	yes	yes	no	none	...	...	1982	1987	all
Alaska...........	1983	no	yes	yes	none	...	...	7/85	none	...
Arizona..........	(g)	(g)	(g)	(g)	none	...	...	(g)	(g)	(g)
Arkansas.........	1957	no	no	no	none	...	...	8/83	4/87	all
California........	1933	no	no	yes	1/86	2	all	1/83	5/87	some
Colorado.........	1987	no	yes	no	7/87	2	front	7/87	4/87	all
Connecticut......	1985	yes	yes	no	1/86	1	front	1982	none	...
Delaware.........	1983	no	no	yes	none	...	...	6/82	none	...
Dist. of Col.	(g)	(g)	(g)	(g)	12/85	(g)	(g)	(g)	(g)	(g)
Florida	1985	no	yes	yes	7/86	2	front	7/83	4/87	all
Georgia..........	1985	no	no	no	9/88	2	front	7/84	2/88	all
Hawaii...........	1986	no	no	yes	12/85	1	front	1983	none	...
Idaho............	1987	no	yes	yes[h]	7/86	2	front	1/85	5/87	all
Illinois...........	1980	yes	yes	yes	7/85	2	front	7/83	4/87	some
Indiana..........	1934	yes	yes	no	7/87	2	front	1/84	6/87	some
Iowa.............	1986	no	no	yes	7/86	1	front	1/85	5/87	all
Kansas...........	(g)	(g)	(g)	(g)	7/86	(g)	(g)	(g)	(g)	(g)
Kentucky.........	1938	no	no	no	none	...	...	7/82	6/87	all
Louisiana.........	1987	no	no	no	7/86	2	front	1/85	4/87	all
Maine	1985	no	yes	no	none	...	...	9/83	6/87	some
Maryland.........	1982	no	no	no	7/86	2	front[i]	1/84	none	...
Massachusetts	1985	yes	no	no	repealed	...	...	1/82	none	...
Michigan.........	1978	no	yes	yes	7/85	2	front	3/82	12/87	some
Minnesota........	1986	no	yes	yes	8/86	2	front	8/83	6/87	all
Mississippi	1986	no	yes	no	none	...	...	7/83	4/87	all

State									
Missouri	1945	no	yes	9/85	2	front	1/84	4/87	some
Montana	1987	no	no	10/87	2	all	10/83	4/87	all
Nebraska	1985	yes	no	repealed	...	...	8/83	4/87	all
Nevada	1933	no	no	7/87	2	all	7/83	4/87	all
New Hampshire	1985	no	no	none	...	...	(g)	4/87	all
New Jersey	1982	yes	no	3/85	2	front	4/83	none	...
New Mexico	1934	no	yes	1/86	1	front	5/83	4/87	all
New York	1990	no	yes	12/84	1	front	4/82	none	...
North Carolina	1985	(g)	yes	10/85	1	front	1/85	(g)	all
North Dakota	1936	no	yes	none	...	...	1/84	4/87	all
Ohio	1987	no	(g)	5/86	2	front	6/83	7/87	some
Oklahoma	1983	yes	no	2/87	2	front	11/83	4/87	all
Oregon	1935	no	yes	none	...	...	1/84	10/87	some
Pennsylvania	1935	no	no	11/87	2	front	11/83	none	...
Rhode Island	1984	yes	yes	none	...	...	7/87	none	...
South Carolina	1986	no	no	7/89	2	front	(g)	7/87	all
South Dakota	1987	no	no	none	...	...	7/84	4/87	all
Tennessee	1984	no	no	4/86	2	front	1/78	5/87	all
Texas	1985	no	yes	9/85	1	front	1/85	5/87	some
Utah	1935	yes	yes	4/86	2	front	1983	5/87	all
Vermont	1986	yes	yes	none	...	...	7/84	4/87	all
Virginia	1986	yes	no	1/88	2	front	1/83	7/88	some
Washington	1934	no	no	6/86	2	all	1/84	4/87	some
West Virginia	1986	yes	yes	none	...	...	7/81	5/87	all
Wisconsin	1986	no	no	12/87	2	front	4/84	6/87	all
Wyoming	1988	no	no	6/89	2	front	4/85	5/87	all

From Offices of State Governor's Highway Safety Representatives. In Accident Facts, National Safety Council, p. 55, 1990. [a] Year in which original law became effective, not when grandfather clauses expired; [b] includes administrative action as well as legislation; [c] Alcohol server responsibility law; [d] Law prohibiting open liquor containers in motor vehicles; [e] "1" indicates primary enforcement (law can be enforced on its own). "2" indicates secondary enforcement (law enforced only if vehicle stopped for a separate offense); [f] Effective date of original law, not of subsequent revisions; [g] Information not available. [h] Does not include beer; [i] Excluding front center seat.

be a decrease in the time one has to react; (2) there will be an increase in the vehicle's stopping distance; and (3) there will be an increase in the destructive force of the vehicle.

At 30 mph a vehicle will cover 44 feet per second, whereas at 60 mph it will travel 88 feet per second. As you can see, the chances of avoiding a child who darts into the roadway are significantly reduced at higher speeds.

The stopping distances of vehicles are also affected as speed increases. The average braking distance at 30 mph is 80 feet; at 60 mph it is 251 feet, a threefold increase. The stopping distance for a car filled with passengers or traveling on a wet road will be increased even more.

Many people do not realize that even small increases in vehicle speed can significantly increase vehicle destruction in an accident. Tests by the National Highway Traffic Safety Administration (NHSTA) have shown that a crash at 35 mph is 36% more severe than one at 30 mph.[36] Statistics from the National Safety Council indicate that a person's chances of dying in a 55-mph crash are 1 in 50, at 65 mph, 1 in 20, and at 75 mph, 1 in 8 (Fig. 7-2).

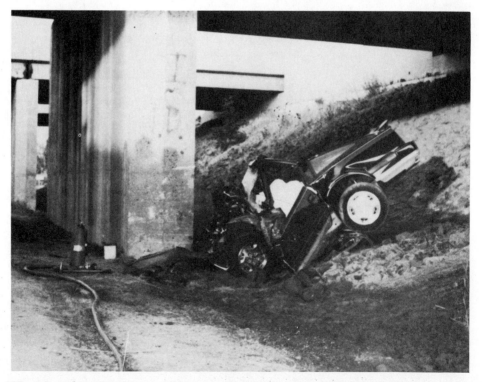

FIG. 7-2 This 1987 Datsun 300-zx was traveling in excess of 100 mph when it hit the overpass support structure.

Courtesy Fairfax County Fire and Rescue Department. Fairfax, Va.

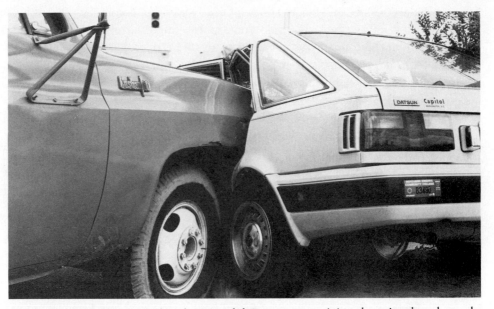

FIG. 7-3 The driver of this late model Datsun was injured seriously when she attempted to beat the changing traffic signal.

Courtesy: Mr. Paul Torpey.

In 1989 speed was considered the major factor in 27% of all fatal motor vehicle accidents. This figure does not necessarily mean that these vehicles were breaking the speed limit. Many of the fatalities resulted from vehicle operators driving too fast for conditions. Wet pavement, traffic congestion, and limited visibility are just a few of the conditions that require reduced driving speeds. The important thing to remember is that no speed limit can be safe under all conditions. The vehicle operator must be able to determine when slower speeds are necessary.

Speeding isn't the only improper driving behavior that leads to motor vehicle accidents. Accidents involving motorists' right of way account for nearly 20% of the annual fatalities. There are basically three types of right-of-way errors: failure to yield, passing a stop sign, and disregarding a signal (Fig. 7-3). Failure to yield accounts for the greatest percentage of these accidents. Too often drivers do not take sufficient time to look for oncoming traffic; instead they stop momentarily, then take a chance and proceed into the path of oncoming vehicles. Another problem associated with failure-to-yield accidents occurs when a driver's vision is obstructed by parked cars, buildings, or trees close to the intersection, or when the driver simply has trouble judging the speed of approaching vehicles.

Disregarding signals and passing stop signs account for approximately 5% of fatal accidents. Have you ever been late for work, and the signal is yellow but you're not at the intersection yet? What did you do—hit the breaks or hit the gas? Chances are you accelerated and made it through the intersection before the other vehicles moved away from the light. What do you suppose might have happened if traffic coming from that side street was already moving and arrived just as the signal turned green for them? The famous T-bone crash into the side of your door!

What can we do about these right-of-way problems? The answer is defensive driving—don't depend on the other person to stop. Anytime you are approaching an intersection or side street, look for vehicles about to enter the flow of traffic. Try to anticipate their movement and be prepared to take evasive action. When you are attempting to get on a main road, wait until there is a wide gap in traffic; then pull out and get up to speed quickly. Also, if there are obstructions in your community or neighborhood that block a person's view of stop signs or oncoming traffic, report these hazards to local or county police so that corrective measures can be taken.

Statistics from the Department of Transportation indicate that over 60% of all motor vehicle fatalities involve a frontal impact.[13, 17] Consequently, it is easy to

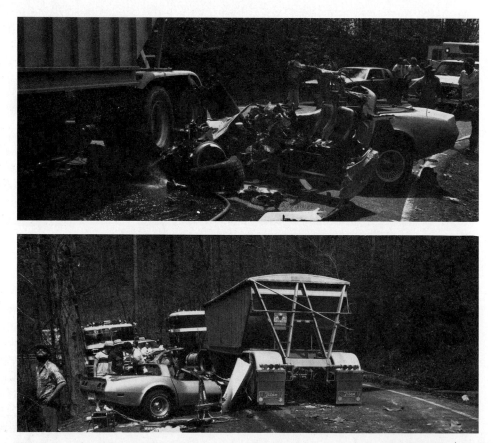

FIG. 7-4   The driver of this Corvette was killed and his passenger was injured critically, when his vehicle drifted into the path of the tractor-trailer as it rounded the curve.
Courtesy Fairfax County Fire and Rescue Department, Fairfax, Va.

understand why driving left of center (with its increased risk of producing a frontal collision) is one of the most deadly errors that a driver can make (Fig. 7-4). This accident most often occurs on rural two-lane roadways; and at higher speeds, a slight error in judgment can quickly put a vehicle into the wrong lane. In 1989 driving left of center accounted for 5% of the fatal motor vehicle accidents.

If you are faced with a driver coming at you in the wrong lane, you have one choice, and that is to get out of the way by going as far to the right as possible. In some cases this may entail driving off the road and into someone's yard or field; at least you will still have some control of the vehicle and an opportunity to avoid a major collision. What about pulling into the left lane to avoid the oncoming car? The answer is *no*—you may hit a second oncoming car or the first driver may suddenly pull back into his lane at the last instant.

An improper driving behavior that may be associated with driving left of center is incorrect passing or overtaking. Whether you are doing the passing or you are being passed by another vehicle, certain rules of the road should be followed. When another vehicle is passing you, take the time to look ahead for oncoming traffic. If it looks like there could be a problem, slow down to ensure that the other driver gets around safely. Many of the newer small-engined vehicles lack the power for quick acceleration, so it is important for these drivers to realize that more time and distance will be needed to pass slower vehicles. Before you attempt to overtake another vehicle, make sure that the passing lane is clear. After signaling, pull into the other lane and accelerate smoothly but quickly. Signal your return to the right lane, but do not pull over until you see the other vehicle in your rear view mirror.

Although it is not often the cause of fatal crashes, tailgating or following too closely is the third most frequent single cause of all vehicle accidents; it accounts for nearly 10% of urban motor vehicle accidents. These accidents usually occur when the lead driver suddenly stops and the driver or drivers following fail to react quickly enough—for example, the rush-hour expressway chain-reaction crash (Fig. 7-5). The

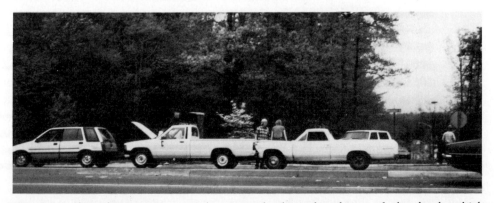

FIG. 7-5 This chain-reaction crash occurred when the driver of the lead vehicle stopped to avoid hitting a dog.
Courtesy Mr. Douglas DeHart.

best way to avoid this type of mishap is to use the "2-second rule." As you are following another vehicle, note when it passes a particular object or landmark on the side of the road and count "one-one thousand, two-one thousand." If you reach the landmark before you finish "two-one thousand," you are following too closely. A nice point about using this rule is that it can be applied to vehicles traveling at any speed. The key is to maintain that 2-second space between vehicles.

Alcohol and Substance Abuse

The persistent hazard of the drunk driver underlies much of the improper driving on our streets and highways. Statistical estimates from the NHTSA indicate that two out of five Americans will be involved in an alcohol-related crash at some point in their lives.[4] Annually 50% of the motor vehicle deaths in this country are alcohol related.

Alcohol is a central-nervous-system depressant; that is, its major effect is on the brain. The greater the amount of alcohol in the body, the more noticeable will be its effects. Unlike other foods, alcohol requires no digestion. It passes quickly from the stomach into the small intestine, where most of it is absorbed into the bloodstream which circulates it to all parts of the body. The liver plays a key role in oxidizing or breaking down alcohol in the bloodstream, and it performs this function at a fairly constant rate. A person of average weight (150 pounds) can metabolize approximately one drink per hour. When the amount of alcohol being absorbed into the bloodstream exceeds the rate at which the liver can oxidize it, this excess alcohol will produce its intoxicating effect on the brain. The quantity of alcohol that is in the blood is known as the **blood alcohol concentration (BAC)** or **blood alcohol level (BAL).** The higher the BAC, the more profound will be the effect on the brain.

Because it can be measured very accurately, blood alcohol concentration has been used to predict the effects of drinking on behavior. For instance, a person with a BAC of 0.01 to 0.03 (%) (one or two drinks) will experience very mild effects from the alcohol. As the BAC increases to a level of 0.05 to 0.07 (three or four drinks), there may be mild sedation with some impairment of fine motor skills (finger movement and hand-eye coordination) and increased reaction time. A number of western European countries, including Finland and Sweden, have set a BAC of 0.05 as the legal limit for intoxication. In the range of 0.08 to 0.10 (four or five drinks), visual and hearing acuity are reduced; there will be a continued decrease in motor skill performance and some problems with balance. Four states, California, Maine, Oregon and Utah, have established a BAC of 0.08 as the legal level for determining intoxication in motor vehicle operators, while 45 states have determined 0.10 to be the BAC at which a person can be charged with driving while intoxicated **(DWI).** Maryland is the only state to specify two separate levels of intoxication. A driver with a blood alcohol level of 0.08 to 0.13 would be charged with driving under the influence **(DUI).** A person with a BAC of 0.14 or higher would be charged with DWI.[1]

At one time many states used 0.15 as the legal level of intoxication. With this level of alcohol in the blood, drivers were found to exhibit major impairment in physical and mental functioning, including difficulty in standing. Although a driver with a BAC of 0.10 was seven times as likely to crash as a driver who had not been drinking, statistics indicated that drivers with a BAC of 0.15 were 25 times as likely to have an accident. This information quickly led legislators to lower the standard to 0.10.

A sad commentary on the drinking and driving problem in the United States is that the blood alcohol levels of drivers involved in accidents frequently exceed 0.15. Studies in California, Maryland, and New Jersey consistently demonstrated that close to 40% of the drivers in fatal injury accidents had BACs of 0.20 or higher.[31] At this level of intoxication, most persons are unable to move or stand without assistance.

Drugs and driving. Only in recent years have researchers begun to investigate the role of drug usage in motor vehicle accidents. During the 1970s a complex array of chemical agents that have the potential to affect driving ability came into use. But unlike alcohol, which can be readily measured in the bloodstream, there is no portable method of testing for the presence of drugs in the system. The **breathalyzer** is a portable instrument that can accurately measure BAC, because there is a constant relationship between the concentration of alcohol in the breath and alcohol in the blood. However, tests for the presence of drugs must be completed in a laboratory.

Laboratory studies have established standard measures of performance in relation to the amount of alcohol in the blood. Whether a person is large or small, at a BAC of 0.15 he is going to exhibit a certain pattern of behavior. In the case of drug ingestion there are no established criteria to determine levels of intoxication. With a particular medication one person may perform normally, whereas another individual will not be able to function.

Although the situation with drugs is not as clear-cut, evidence indicates that they are playing a larger role in motor vehicle accidents than most people thought. A recent California study of male drivers 15 to 34 years of age who were killed in motor vehicle accidents found that 70% of the victims had measurable blood alcohol concentrations. Marijuana was also detected in 37% of the subjects and cocaine in 11%.[39] In most of the cases drugs were used in combination with alcohol.

Currently the National Institute on Drug Abuse and the Department of Transportation are developing instrumentation for the detection and quantification of a wide range of drugs. At the present time chemical analysis alone cannot be used reliably for legal action, because individual variations in tolerance and thresholds for performance decrements vary widely. Other research efforts will concentrate on determining the effects of each drug's use on performance and the role of various factors such as body weight, gender, age, dosage, and time since ingestion.

DWI: enforcement measures and programs. As mentioned earlier in this chapter, alcohol plays a role in almost half of all fatal motor vehicle accidents and one third of serious injury accidents. A question that has no easy answer is: ''What do we do with the drunk driver?'' The primary concern of any alcohol safety program is to get the drunk driver from behind the wheel and off the streets.

The first step in such a program must be the identification of intoxicated drivers. This is generally the responsibility of law enforcement personnel. Detection of the drunk driver on the road is most likely to result from an officer's observation of certain driving behaviors. Stopping without cause in a traffic lane, following too closely, making wide turns, straddling the center of the road or lane markers, and almost striking an object or vehicle are cues that consistently distinguish a drunk driver from a sober driver. A California study that was used to develop a drunk-driver detection guide indicated that as many as 60% of the persons exhibiting the above driving behaviors would have a BAC equal to or greater than 0.10[15] (Fig. 7-6).

If an officer suspects that a vehicle operator is intoxicated, he or she will stop the vehicle and investigate further. A driver exhibiting signs of intoxication such as slurred speech or problems with balance or coordination will be asked to take a blood or breathalyzer test. Most states have "implied consent" laws; if you drive in those states, you are legally obligated to take a chemical test for intoxication when requested by law enforcement personnel. A driver who refuses to take a breath or blood test will be charged with a separate offense in addition to the DWI charge. Some metropolitan police are now videotaping everyone brought into custody under a

1. Turning with wide radius
2. Straddling center of lane marker
3. Appearing to be drunk
4. Almost striking object or vehicle
5. Weaving
6. Driving on other than designated roadway
7. Swerving
8. Speed more than 10 mph below limit
9. Stopping without cause in traffic lane
10. Following too closely
11. Drifting
12. Tires on center or lane marker
13. Braking erratically
14. Driving into opposing or crossing traffic
15. Signaling inconsistent with driving actions
16. Slow response to traffic signals
17. Stopping inappropriately (other than in lane)
18. Turning abruptly or illegally
19. Accelerating or decelerating rapidly
20. Headlights off

FIG. 7-6   Guide for detecting drunk drivers at night.
Source: National Highway Traffic Safety Administration.

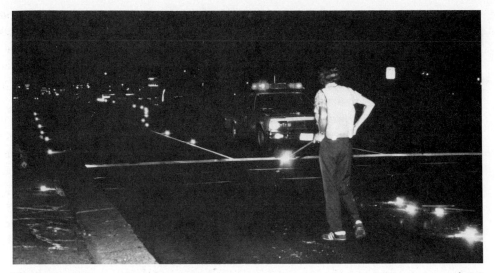

FIG. 7-7 Officers observing vehicle operators for signs of intoxication at a sobriety checkpoint.
Courtesy Fairfax Journal, Fairfax, Va.

charge of driving while intoxicated. If a person refuses the breathalyzer test or has a low BAC, there will be a visual record of the person's inability to function that can be used as evidence in court.

Though sentences vary from state to state, penalties on conviction of driving while intoxicated may include mandatory loss of operator's license for 6 to 12 months, fines from $200 to $1000, and possible jail sentences of up to 12 months. Failure to take a breath or blood test usually carries a mandatory loss of license for 3 to 6 months. Unlike European countries, which regularly jail drunk drivers, the U.S. courts perhaps have been too lenient with their sentences. In fact, fewer than 10% of those who kill someone while driving under the influence of alcohol receive jail terms.

To curb the problem of the drunk driver, two measures must be considered. Stronger efforts by law enforcement agencies must be made to deter drinking and driving, and the courts must become tougher in their sentencing. An innovative measure that was taken in the early 1980s in Montgomery County, Maryland, was the development of a Sobriety Checkpoint Program (Fig. 7-7). It was instituted as the result of a study that indicated that 67% of the DWI arrests and a significant number of fatal and serious-injury accidents occurred on 18 of the county's 1536 streets and roads.

A number of road flares are placed on the shoulder or in the center of the road, and marked police cruisers are parked on the shoulder of the road. No physical barriers are used at the checkpoint. All oncoming traffic is stopped by a uniformed officer, who explains to each driver that this is only a routine stop to check for intoxicated drivers. The entire process takes approximately 20 seconds. If the officer observes signs of intoxication he or she will ask the vehicle operator to pull to the side of the road for further inquiry.

Checkpoints are conducted between 10 P.M. and 4 A.M. for a period as short as half an hour to several hours. Checkpoint locations are selected on the basis of traffic flow, number of vehicle accidents and DWI arrests, as well as the safety with which motorists may be stopped.

Because of the success of such programs in reducing personal-injury accidents involving alcohol consumption, today all 50 states employ sobriety checkpoints as a drunk-driving enforcement tool.

Another countermeasure in dealing with the drunk driver has been the establishment of Alcohol Safety Action Projects (ASAP) throughout the United States. These programs, initially funded by the Department of Transportation, are now self-supporting in most states. Although they address the issue of enforcement, the emphasis of the ASAP programs is on judicial procedures and rehabilitation of the DWI offender.

If your state has an Alcohol Safety Action Project and you are arrested for driving while intoxicated, here is what may happen: If you are eligible for the program (based on prior record and arrest circumstances) and are willing to cooperate with the provisions set by the court, you may be allowed to participate in an alcohol education and/or treatment program that may last from 2 to 6 months. Depending on the program, this may include classroom sessions, group discussions, professional evaluations, and sessions involving other members of your family. During this time you will generally be able to keep your driving privileges, though there may be some restrictions. Each participant must pay a fee for attending the program as well as any additional fines established by the court. At the end of the program you will return to court for a final disposition of your case.

If a person does not request admission to an ASAP program or is found ineligible, the judge may proceed with sentencing. In most states this means a mandatory loss of one's driving license for a minimum of 3 to 6 months and a substantial fine. It is easy to see why most people opt for the ASAP program if they are eligible.

The ASAP programs have been a step in the right direction, but many law enforcement and legal personnel feel that more emphasis must be placed on deterring drinking and driving. An alternative that may be more effective than assigning violators to alcohol education and treatment programs is the prompt suspension or revocation of the driver's licenses of alcohol offenders before court conviction. Known as "administrative per se," these laws require that any driver registering a BAC higher than 0.10 has his or her license automatically suspended for 60 to 90 days, regardless of the subsequent disposition of the case. If the person refuses to take a BAC test, the license is suspended for 180 days. Restricted or hardship permits are not allowed during the period of revocation, since the purpose of these laws is to impress upon people the seriousness of the offense. In the 21 states that have enacted "administrative per se" license suspension laws, alcohol-related fatalities have decreased an average of 30%.[18]

In recent years a number of groups that vocally support and lobby for stronger drunk-driving legislation and the stricter enforcement of existing laws have come into existence throughout the United States. Founded in 1980 by the mother of a young girl who was struck and killed by a chronic alcoholic with three previous arrests for driving while intoxicated, a California-based organization known as Mothers Against Drunk Driving (MADD) has chapters in every state, Puerto Rico, and Canada. Another national organization founded under similar circumstances in New York is known as RID (Remove Intoxicated Drivers). The highly visible campaigns of these groups have had a significant effect on both the courts and state legislatures.

An anti–drunk-driving campaign that has been developed with an emphasis on public awareness of this problem is Students Against Drunk Driving (SADD). Begun as a high school project in Massachusetts, SADD chapters have been developed in high schools throughout the country. During the school year many of these chapters sponsor programs such as "Dial-A-Ride," a service that offers safe, no-questions-asked rides home for intoxicated students. Student-parent volunteer teams provide the service on weekend and holiday nights.

Mandatory drinking-age laws. As changes were being made in the DWI laws, laws concerning the legal drinking age came under close scrutiny by legislators. Evidence from studies in the early 1980s suggested that significant increases in motor vehicle deaths were occurring in those states where the legal drinking age was under 21. In 1984 Public Law 98-363, the Federal Minimum Drinking Age Law went into effect. This legislation encouraged all states to raise the legal drinking age to 21. It also stipulated that if a state had not raised the legal drinking age to 21 by October 1, 1987, it would lose up to 15% of its federal highway funding. Currently, all states and the District of Columbia have a 21-year-old drinking age.

What effect has this legislation had on motor vehicle fatalities? The answer is a very favorable one; it is estimated that there has been a 12% reduction in fatal-crash involvement of drivers under age 21. Annually, the minimum drinking-age laws (MDAs) save over 1000 lives.

Though the news about MDA laws has been very positive over the past 8 years, a recent disturbing trend has been noted. Alcohol related deaths for men in the 21-24 age group have remained relatively stable; however, there has been a significant increase in the number of females, age 21-24, who are involved in alcohol-related motor vehicle fatalities.

Responsible drinking and driving. Even with the raising of the legal drinking age, stricter traffic enforcement, and harsher penalties for the drunk driver, people are still going to drink and drive. Perhaps one answer to the drinking and driving problem is to teach people how to drink sensibly.

Of course, the best piece of advice is: "Don't drink if you're going to drive, and vice versa." Doing so does not mean that you can't party and be socially active. Here are some safe and practical suggestions:

1. *Designated driver:* If a group is going to an athletic event, bar, or concert, appoint a designated driver. This person will handle the driving chores for the evening but will abstain from drinking. The next week a different member of the group becomes the designated driver. Such an alternative is especially wise if you must travel very far.

2. *TAB, TAC, or W:* These are practical alternatives for the city dweller—"take a bus, take a cab, or walk." Let someone who is sober do the driving. The fare that you will pay is certainly cheaper than a license suspension and court costs for a DWI conviction.

3. *Stay overnight:* Responsibility for the safety of guests at a party is that of the host or hostess; in some states a party host can be held liable for the injuries caused by a drunken guest who is later involved in a motor vehicle accident. If some of your guests have had too much to drink, have them stay overnight. What's wrong with having 18 people sleep on the floor of your apartment? In the morning when they are sober, they can be on their way.

Although even small amounts of alcohol can have an effect on the central nervous system, most drinkers who have a relatively low BAC (0.01 to 0.03) will experience little or no impairment of mental functions and motor skills. If people are going to drink and drive, it is imperative that they do so with the utmost caution.

The body can handle one 12-ounce beer, or one glass of wine, or one mixed drink per hour without there being an increase in the blood alcohol level. Trouble occurs when a person rapidly consumes three or four drinks in a short period; this often happens when bars offer "happy hour" drink prices such as two for one. Because of the lag time between consumption of alcohol and its absorption into the bloodstream, a relatively sober individual may start to drive home; however, he will become increasingly intoxicated as more alcohol is absorbed into the bloodstream. If people abided by the "one drink per hour" rule, we would not have the problem of the drunk driver. By the way, 13 states now ban "happy hour" drink promotions in bars and restaurants (see Table 7-1, Alcohol Legislation, pp. 212-213).

Other factors that must be considered include the body weight of the individual, amount of food in the stomach, and nonalcoholic substances in alcoholic beverages. The more a person weighs, the more it will take to elevate his or her blood alcohol level. The livers of larger individuals do not oxidize alcohol any faster than those of smaller individuals; however, larger people have a greater volume of body fluids in which to dilute the alcohol. That's why the 118-pound wrestler can drink two or three beers in an hour and have noticeable problems, yet his 270-pound teammate drinks four and feels nothing.

To slow down that increase in BAC people should eat while drinking. The presence of food in the stomach delays the absorption of alcohol by diluting its concentration. Nonalcoholic substances in beverages, such as water, sugars, and minerals, also work to dilute the concentration of the alcohol.

A word of caution to sparkling-wine and champagne drinkers—the carbon dioxide in these beverages may speed up alcohol absorption, causing a rapid increase in blood alcohol level. Have you ever been drinking champagne at a wedding reception when that increased BAC suddenly hits you? The CO_2 in the champagne relaxes the pyloric sphincter at the base of the stomach, allowing the alcohol to pass quickly into the small intestine and then into the bloodstream. Before drinking sparkling wines, make sure you have food in your stomach to slow down this process.

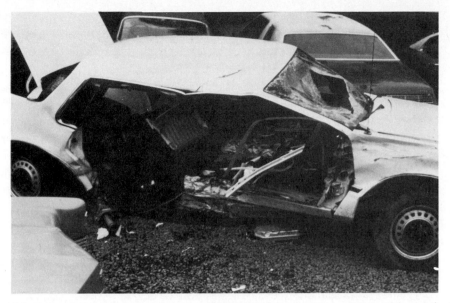

FIG. 7-8   On a spring break trip to Florida the drunk driver of this Oldsmobile Cutlass fell asleep and hit a guardrail on Interstate 95. He survived, but three fraternity brothers were killed.

Courtesy Mr. Paul Torpey.

A new approach in dealing with drinking and driving that has gained popularity in clubs and lounges has been the installation of coin-operated breath-testing devices. Similar to breathalyzers used by law enforcement personnel, these machines can give drinkers a relatively accurate estimate of their blood alcohol concentration. As a service to their customers, some bars even provide transportation home for those who fail the breath test.

Regardless of the innovations that are introduced to control drinking and driving, no one can make the decision but you! Ultimately such a decision is the individual responsibility of anyone who gets behind the wheel (Fig. 7-8).

ENVIRONMENTAL FACTORS IN VEHICLE ACCIDENTS

Environmental factors, both natural and man-made, account for less than 5% of vehicle accidents; however, when these factors are combined with a degree of human error, they become a significant factor in another 27% of accidents.[33] Unlike vehicle failure, which has a minimal effect on traffic accidents, environmental factors may play a role in nearly one third of these accidents.

Natural environmental factors such as rain, snow, wind, fog, and ice cannot be directly controlled or prevented, but they can be modified to some extent. Changes in roadway construction and drainage techniques have reduced the problem of water build-up on interstate highways during heavy rains. If water cannot be adequately drained from the roadway, drivers may experience a vehicle-handling problem known as "hydroplaning," in which the tires of the car break traction with the road surface. The development of multipurpose snow and rain tires has also reduced the negative effects of these weather factors on vehicle handling.

Another environmental modification for roadway surfaces has been the development of chemical agents that prevent ice build-up on bridges. Unlike most of the highway surface, which is insulated by the ground on which it sits, the bridge surface has no underlying insulation; consequently, when there is moisture on the roadway, the first surfaces to freeze are the bridgedecks.

Under situations of reduced visibility such as foggy weather and nighttime hours, auto headlamps provide a relatively restricted area of illumination. To aid in the perception of the contours of the roadway ahead, many highways are marked by yellow or white stripes along their edges. A variation to this has been the development of white and yellow center-lane reflective markers for two-lane roads.

Man-made environmental factors that may either contribute to or reduce motor vehicle accidents include roadway design, placement of road signs and traffic signals, roadside construction, and variation in traffic laws. Let's take a look at some of the positive and negative aspects of each of these factors.

Although it cannot always be avoided, a roadway design that forces vehicles to exit an expressway from the left side has a greater potential for accident causation, because the normal driver expectancy is to exit from the right. The same holds true for the sharply curving exit ramp; often a driver will enter the ramp from an interstate route and suddenly be confronted with a sharply curving roadway surface that requires quick deceleration to a speed of 15-20 mph. Time is needed to alert drivers to an unusual condition such as a left-side or sharply curving exit ramp; road signs warning drivers should be placed at selected intervals to alert them of these hazards. The addition of flashing lights near these exits may provide further protection.

Roadside construction, including signs, light poles, median barriers, and guardrails, does not always provide the protection for which it was designed. With the increasing push to make passenger cars more fuel efficient, it has become necessary to reduce the size and weight of these vehicles. Recent studies at the Texas Transportation Institute have indicated that roadside protective devices may not function adequately when small cars are involved.

Breakaway signs or light poles snap when hit by intermediate-sized or large cars, but they act like a wall when hit by a compact or subcompact model. The same holds true for **impact attenuators,** better known as crash cushions. These devices, consisting of sand- or water-filled barrels or overlapping sections of steel paneling, are installed in front of bridge abutments, guardrails, and overpass support columns. As a car hits them, the barrels collapse, thus gradually slowing the vehicle and dissipating the energy of its forward momentum. However, if the vehicle is too light, the crash cushion will act as a solid barrier instead of a collapsible one.

Although environmental factors can be controlled to a degree, they cannot be modified to the extent that everyone will be protected. Probably the most practical approach in dealing with the motor vehicle fatality problem lies in the areas of vehicle crashworthiness and passenger protection.

VEHICLE AND EQUIPMENT DESIGN HAZARDS

Another factor that must be considered in motor vehicle crashes is that of vehicle design or equipment malfunction. Improvements in vehicle characteristics and components such as braking, steering, mirrors, tires, and vehicle lighting enable the driver to handle the vehicle in a safer and more efficient manner.

With the enactment of the National Traffic and Motor Vehicle Safety Act, the NHTSA has been able to develop safety standards that require motor vehicles to attain a specific level of performance.[25] For example, Federal Motor Vehicle Safety Standard No. 105 (FMVSS No. 105), originally instituted in 1968, set limits for the stopping distance of passenger-car brake systems at various speeds; however, the standard did not include light trucks and vans. With the increasing popularity of pickups and vans in the late 1970s and early 1980s, there was a dramatic increase in fatal and serious injury accidents involving these vehicles. Research indicated that part of the reason for this increase was that trucks and vans were often involved in rear-end collisions with other vehicles. In 1983 NHTSA revised FMVSS No. 105. The new standard requires that light truck and van brake performance be similar to the existing standard for passenger cars.

In the 1990s a very positive vehicle-design change has been the addition of anti-lock braking systems to a variety of models of cars and light trucks. An anti-lock braking system (ABS) gives the driver better control over stopping, especially in emergency situations and under bad road conditions. The computerized ABS automatically pumps the brakes to reduce skids and loss of steering control.

Other NHTSA design standards that have dealt specifically with safe and efficient vehicle performance include reducing the amount of tinting in windshields to improve nighttime vision, minimizing blind spots by eliminating passenger-compartment obstructions, and improving vehicle visibility by instituting the use of high-mounted midline brake lights on all new cars and trucks since 1986. This latest NHTSA design standard has substantially reduced the incidence of rear-end crashes.

Recalls

Since the National Highway Traffic Safety Administration was created in 1966, 112 million vehicles have been involved in recall campaigns for the inspection and correction of safety-related defects. The purpose of the NHTSA recall program is to reduce motor vehicle injuries and deaths by correcting vehicle defects before they cause a serious problem and to encourage vehicle and vehicle equipment manufacturers to build products free of safety-related defects.

There are several ways in which safety-defect recalls are initiated. In the past the majority of recalls had been voluntarily initiated by manufacturers; however, in recent years the NHTSA has initiated nearly 50% of these actions. Defect investigations may be instituted through the Auto Safety Hotline or the yearly compliance inspections of new domestic and foreign vehicles. The **Auto Safety Hotline** (1-800-424-9393) provides consumers with a direct line of communication to the NHTSA. Information concerning potential safety-related defects is stored on computer tapes. If a preliminary analysis indicates a possible accident trend resulting from a defect, a formal investigation is started. The Hotline also provides information to callers concerning ongoing investigations or current recalls.

Another avenue used to identify vehicle defects is the NHTSA's annual compliance testing of selected new vehicle models. The tests are used to determine whether vehicle manufacturers have met the Federal Motor Vehicle Safety Standards established by the NHTSA. Imported motor vehicles must meet the same compliance standards as U.S. models. Test vehicle selections are made according to criteria that consider previous test results, accident data, owner complaints, and engineering evaluation of design features across all model lines. The existence of a compliance test program with public availability of the test results has been a strong inducement to manufacturers to improve their own safety monitoring programs.[25]

When a formal recall is instituted, manufacturers must notify owners directly, usually by registered mail. A recalled car or piece of equipment may be returned to any authorized dealer for correction and/or replacement. The manufacturer is responsible for fixing the defect, at no cost to the consumer, regardless of the time that has passed since the recall was announced. Effectiveness of these campaigns rests, in part, with the consumer; vehicles and equipment not returned to the dealer cannot be inspected and repaired.

Passenger Protection

The idea of protective packaging is not a new one; companies have frequently used various methods to ship fragile goods without significant damage, even when they receive rough treatment. **Crashworthiness** is the science of packaging people in automobiles so that when crashes inevitably occur the occupants are not unduly injured.

NHTSA researchers have taken two approaches in developing occupant crash protection. Special emphasis has been placed on the structural design of vehicles so that in a collision the passenger compartment will stay intact. The other area of emphasis involves the design of occupant restraints that are intended to prevent people from being thrown into the hard surfaces of the car's interior, including other people.[36]

Let's examine some of the structural design modifications that have helped vehicles better withstand the force of a crash. Since 1968 the Department of Transportation has tested cars to ensure that they meet minimum federal safety standards; over 50 of them have been enacted in that time. The safety standards require that all cars sold in the United States pass specified tests in 30-mph crashes (Fig. 7-9). In particular these tests attempt to measure how well vehicles can prevent occupants from

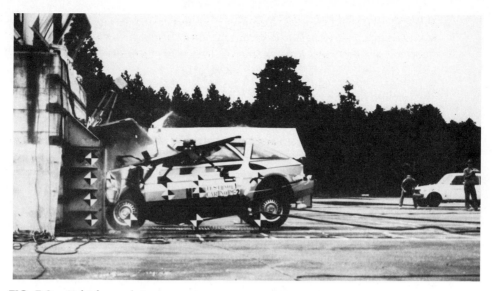

FIG. 7-9 Vehicle crash test.
Courtesy U.S. Department of Transportaion, National Highway Traffic Safety Administration.

being ejected, trapped, burned, or crushed in a collision. They also measure a vehicle's ability to absorb, control, or reduce crash forces on the occupants. Some of the specific safety standards that are evaluated in relation to a vehicle's structural integrity include:[14]

1. FMVSS–201: *Occupant protection in Interior Impact.* Since the development of this standard, safety measures have included the padded dash, padded armrests, and interior door and roof padding. Even vehicles manufactured in the mid-1960s had the solid metal dash boards that became blunt weapons when a person's head hit them. The advent of recessed gauges and instrument switches has also reduced the chances of puncture wounds if a person is propelled into the dash area.
2. FMVSS–203: *Impact Protection for the Driver from the Steering Control System.* After the initial impact of the vehicle, the driver's momentum will carry him into the steering wheel. To reduce the force of the driver/steering wheel collision, steering mechanisms on today's cars are designed to move forward under the impact, thus preventing a person from being impaled on the steering column.
3. FMVSS–204: *Steering Control Rearward Displacement.* At one time steering columns consisted of one solid piece of metal. If the column were hit during a frontal collision, it would be driven back into the passenger's seat. In essence, during a crash it acted like a solid metal spear going through whatever was in its way. For today's models, the maximum allowable rearward displacement is 5 inches; however, in a 30-mph crash, rearward displacement usually doesn't exceed 3 inches. This has been accomplished by using steering shafts made of multiple-joint segments that overlap on impact, thus shortening their overall length.
4. FMVSS–206: *Door Locks and Door Retention.* Since ejection from a vehicle during a crash puts a person at far more risk than any other condition, manufacturers have not only strengthened the latching and locking components of car doors, they have also redesigned and

relocated inside door handles. Before the enactment of this safety standard, door handles protruded into the passenger compartment and were operated by lifting upward. In collisions passengers often hit these handles, causing the doors to fly open and allowing passengers to be ejected. Another problem with the early doors was that they could be unlocked from the inside by lifting the door handle; consequently, a locked door in a collision didn't necessarily provide protection from being ejected.

Today's door handles are recessed so that they will not be activated as easily in a collision, nor will they be a source of injury if someone hits them. At the same time, rear door locks (where children are usually seated) can no longer be released when the handle is operated; the lock must be released before the door can be opened. Again, this has decreased the likelihood of accidental door opening during a crash.

5. FMVSS–214: *Side Door Strength.* Somewhat related to the factor of door retention is door strength. Statistics indicate that approximately 30% of the fatalities in motor vehicle accidents occur in side collisions. As smaller vehicles are being manufactured and emphasis is placed on weight reduction to increase fuel efficiency, the addition of steel support structures for doors and door frames is no longer practical. Potential solutions may include the use of polyurethane foam inside doors to provide a lightweight, energy-absorbing material and the improvement of seat design to cushion side-impact forces.

6. FMVSS–205: *Glazing Materials.* This standard involves the protective functions of wind-shields and side windows in motor vehicles. The most critical field of vision for a motor vehicle operator is the frontal view provided by the windshield. But a clear view is not the only thing that a windshield must provide. In a collision the windshield must also help to prevent passenger ejection from the vehicle.

The material that provides the least distortion is ordinary glass; however, on impact it breaks easily into daggerlike pieces that can cause severe lacerations. Safety glazing, on the other hand, is more resistant and does not break and shatter into large, jagged pieces. All of today's vehicle windshields are made from laminated glass (two layers of ordinary glass bonded to a middle layer of plastic). This provides a relatively strong impact-resistant barrier. If the glass does break, the pieces generally stick to the plastic and the plastic stretches to reduce chances of penetration. Although laminated safety glazing greatly reduces a passenger's chances of being ejected through the windshield, it can still cause severe lacerations. Currently NHTSA researchers are examining an alternative method of safety glazing used by European and some U.S. auto manufacturers in which a layer of polyurethane or a similar flexible plastic coating is applied to the inside of the windshield. If the passenger's face hits the windshield, this fourth layer prevents it from coming into contact with the broken glass. This four-layer system is known as antilacerative glazing.

A different type of safety glazing used in rear and side windows is tempered glass. It is heated and cooled in a special way to make it much stronger than ordinary glass. This relatively inexpensive glass crumbles into small pieces when broken, thus reducing the possibility of laceration. However, it is not as impact resistant as laminated glass and provides little protection in terms of ejection from the vehicle. A critical problem occurs in side-impact collisions or rollovers when these windows easily shatter and victims are partially ejected. Safety standards are now being considered to require side and rear windows to provide a greater amount of impact resistance.

7. FMVSS 301: *Fuel System Integrity.* One other area in which vehicles are evaluated in the 30-mph crash tests is that of fuel leakage after either frontal or rear collisions. As cars have been down-sized, the placement of vehicle fuel tanks has become a critical issue. In the past, larger vehicles—with their longer wheel base and structural dimensions—could provide a greater safe-area for tank placement. With today's lighter, shorter, and narrower cars there is a limited amount of space to provide for energy absorption and fuel tank protection in a crash.

Most safety engineers agree that placement of the fuel tank over the rear axle will allow for a significant amount of vehicle damage before the tank is involved. Other protective measures that have shown promise in maintaining fuel system integrity include the use of rubber bladders to line the gas tank, breakaway, self-sealing connectors, and telescoping fuel filler tubes. Rubber bladders were first used with Indianapolis-type racers to reduce the likelihood of postcrash fires. If fuel lines from the gas tank are severed, the connectors will seal over to prevent further fuel leakage. Many cars today are equipped with the telescoping filler tube. Depending on the forces of crash impact, the filler tube can either increase or decrease in length and still remain in contact with the gas tank.

It has been estimated that car manufacturers, by meeting the NHTSA 30-mph safety standards, could reduce a person's risk of death and serious injury in a severe crash by nearly 50%—*that is, providing vehicle occupants wear seat belts.*

In 1979 the Department of Transportation began an experimental crash test program to see which cars could exceed the 30-mph Federal Motor Vehicle Safety Standards.[24, 37] Cars were crashed into a concrete barrier at 35 mph; this is similar to two cars of the same size crashing head-on at 35 mph. Because a car's kinetic energy is equal to the mass times the velocity squared, it has been determined that the force of impact in a crash at 35 mph is 36% greater than in a crash at 30 mph.

Postcrash evaluations indicated that most cars could not provide protection at crash speeds 5 mph above the minimum standards, even though safety belts were used in all of the tests.

It was interesting to find that a number of subcompacts fared much better than some intermediate and large vehicles in fixed, rigid-barrier crashes. Not only were structural factors important to vehicle crashworthiness, but also the design and function of restraint systems seemed to be especially important for occupant safety. Many of the vehicles failed when their restraint systems allowed passengers' heads to hit the dash or steering wheel. However, the NHTSA felt that with minor changes in restraint design, test results would significantly improve.

The NHTSA crash tests have received mixed reviews from auto manufacturers; however, most highway safety specialists feel that the test results not only provide a useful means of comparing vehicles within the same weight class, but they also are useful in guiding the design of vehicle safety features.

Occupant Restraints

As NHTSA researchers and automotive engineers continue to improve the structural integrity and energy management capabilities of motor vehicles in crash situations, they must also continue their efforts to protect vehicle occupants. It makes no sense to design a car, truck, or van that can withstand massive crash forces in an initial vehicle collision if its occupants cannot survive a second collision with the vehicle's interior.

By studying automobile accidents, experts have found it is usually the second collision that injures or kills people. When one car hits another car or object, this is the first collision. The **second collision** occurs when unbelted occupants are thrown

What Happens in a Collision

1st, The Car Collision

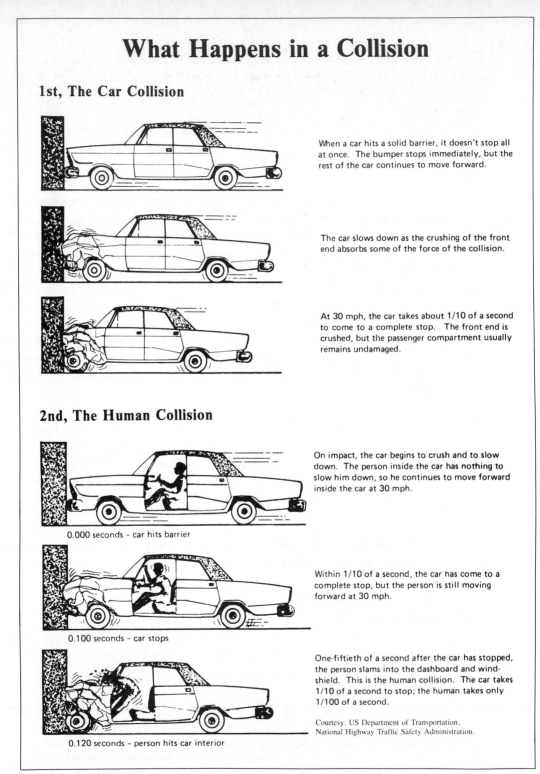

When a car hits a solid barrier, it doesn't stop all at once. The bumper stops immediately, but the rest of the car continues to move forward.

The car slows down as the crushing of the front end absorbs some of the force of the collision.

At 30 mph, the car takes about 1/10 of a second to come to a complete stop. The front end is crushed, but the passenger compartment usually remains undamaged.

2nd, The Human Collision

On impact, the car begins to crush and to slow down. The person inside the car has nothing to slow him down, so he continues to move forward inside the car at 30 mph.

0.000 seconds – car hits barrier

Within 1/10 of a second, the car has come to a complete stop, but the person is still moving forward at 30 mph.

0.100 seconds – car stops

One-fiftieth of a second after the car has stopped, the person slams into the dashboard and windshield. This is the human collision. The car takes 1/10 of a second to stop; the human takes only 1/100 of a second.

Courtesy: US Department of Transportation, National Highway Traffic Safety Administration.

0.120 seconds – person hits car interior

FIG. 7-10   What happens in a collision.
Courtesy U.S. Department of Transportaion, National Highway Traffic Safety Administration.

into the windshield, steering wheel, doors, dashboard, or other passengers (Fig. 7-10). These hard surfaces become instruments of death when people are thrown against them during any crash, including frontal, side-impact, and rear collisions as well as rollovers.

What is the answer to this problem? It's been around a long time—*the safety belt.* First appearing as a production option in Ford Motor Company automobiles in 1955, lap belts became standard equipment on all passenger cars in 1964. Since 1968 the combination lap-shoulder belt has been required in the front outboard seating positions of all cars sold in the United States. Although the lap belt prevents passenger ejection from a vehicle, unlike the lap-shoulder belt combination it doesn't adequately protect a person's head and chest from striking such hard surfaces as the windshield, dashboard, or steering wheel.

Investigations by the NHTSA and other organizations have indicated that the lifesaving effectiveness of lap and shoulder belts, *when they are worn,* is about 50%.[29]

Modifications to safety belts in the 1980s have added a further degree of comfort as well as protection for their users. To place the safety belt in the best position for crash protection, it should be pulled tightly across the occupant; however, for the sake of occupant comfort this is not practical. A pretensioning device has been developed that allows the safety belt to be worn loosely during normal driving conditions. If a crash occurs, the pretensioning sensors remove any slack in the belt and provide a snug fit. In high-speed crashes a second belt modification known as ''force limiting'' allows the safety belt to stretch gently under the force of a passenger's upper torso as he is thrown forward on impact. By allowing for some play or stretching in the safety belt the likelihood of broken ribs, broken collarbones, or injuries to internal organs is reduced. In the case of vehicle crashes involving side impact (30% of fatal accidents) and rear collisions or rollovers (10% of fatal accidents), the safety belt is the only occupant restraint that provides adequate protection (Fig. 7-11).

Despite the benefits of safety belts and their presence in nearly all passenger vehicles, the majority of American drivers and passengers have not used them. Safety-belt usage for all vehicles on the road in 1989 was 46%; roughly half of U.S. motorists do not wear safety belts.[5]

Let's take a look at some of the more frequently given reasons for such low usage rates and at the same time discuss why they are pretty flimsy excuses for not buckling up[7]:

Reason: ''I don't need a safety belt when I'm traveling at low speeds or going on a short trip.''
Fact: Of all fatal accidents, 50% involve impact speeds of less than 35 mph, 80% of all motor vehicle accidents occur at speeds less than 40 mph, and three out of four fatal crashes occur within 25 miles of the victim's house.

Reason: ''I might be saved if I'm thrown clear of the car in an accident.''
Fact: Statistically your chances of being killed are 25 times greater if you're ejected

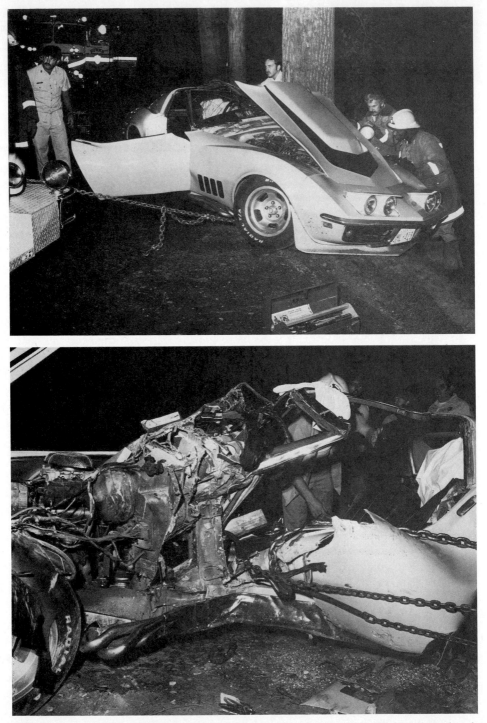

FIG. 7-11   The driver of this Corvette T-Top avoided serious injury when his lap-shoulder belt prevented him from being thrown out of the car.

Courtesy Fairfax County Fire and Rescue Department, Fairfax, Va.

from the car. Why? Because one of three things often happens: (1) The unbelted passenger is ejected through the windshield, (2) he is partially ejected and scraped along the ground as the car continues to move, or (3) he is thrown out the door and crushed by his own car.

Reason: "If I wear a safety belt, I might be trapped in a burning or submerged car."
Fact: Less than half of 1% of all motor vehicle collisions involve fire or submersion. Also, if you are protected by a safety belt, you are much less likely to hit the windshield or dashboard and be knocked unconscious. Your chances of escape are much better if you remain alert.

Reason: "It takes too much time and trouble to fasten my safely belt, and besides, I'm too uncomfortable and confined when I wear it."
Fact: It takes less than 10 seconds for most people to buckle up. Since 1980 vehicles have been equipped with flexible stiffeners that allow occupants to easily grasp safety belts and buckle them into place. At the same time new belt systems have eliminated the problems presented by automatic locking retractors. In older models a single, continuous movement of the safety belt was needed to buckle it into place. If a person stopped the belt, the retractor locked it into place and one would have to release it all the way and start over. Also, during normal driving the lap belt would tighten excessively; consequently, it became necessary to unbuckle and refasten the belt to relieve pressure on the abdomen. In today's models the belt does not have to be pulled across the body in a continuous motion; it can be extended in successive movements. Also, once connected into place, the safety belt will continue to move freely. It will lock into place only when there is a rapid forward pitch of the occupant as in the case of a sudden stop (Fig. 7-12).

Mandatory safety belt laws. Attempts to increase the voluntary usage of manual safety belts over the last two decades met with little success. Public information campaigns, incentive programs, and even safety-belt reminder devices in vehicles led to temporary increases in safety-belt usage at best.

On December 1, 1984, a landmark decision was made by the New York legislature. It became the first state to enact a mandatory safety-belt use law. As one legislator stated, "Freedom does not include the liberty to take unreasonable risks with one's own life or the lives of others. The preponderance of evidence shows that riding unrestrained in a motor vehicle is an unreasonable risk."[7]

In addition to the potential for reducing death, injury, and human suffering, an impressive argument for mandating safety-belt use is a substantial reduction in the economic costs of road trauma. The U.S. Department of Transportation estimates that the cost-benefit ratio of a safety-belt use law is of the order of 37.5 to 1.0. This means that for every dollar spent enforcing the legislation, society would save $37.50.

Since the passage of the New York legislation, 32 other states and the District of Columbia have enacted mandatory safety-belt use laws. Initial investigations of the effectiveness of these laws have shown impressive results; the various states have

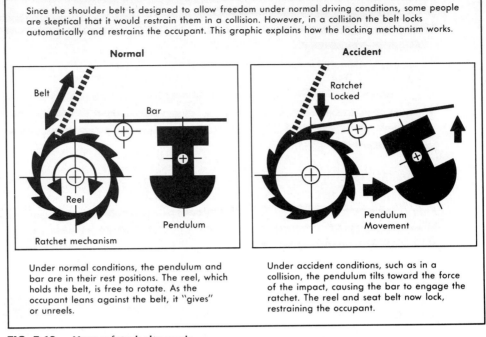

Since the shoulder belt is designed to allow freedom under normal driving conditions, some people are skeptical that it would restrain them in a collision. However, in a collision the belt locks automatically and restrains the occupant. This graphic explains how the locking mechanism works.

Normal

Belt

Bar

Reel

Ratchet mechanism

Pendulum

Accident

Ratchet Locked

Pendulum Movement

Under normal conditions, the pendulum and bar are in their rest positions. The reel, which holds the belt, is free to rotate. As the occupant leans against the belt, it "gives" or unreels.

Under accident conditions, such as in a collision, the pendulum tilts toward the force of the impact, causing the bar to engage the ratchet. The reel and seat belt now lock, restraining the occupant.

FIG. 7-12   How safety belts work.

Source. National Highway Traffic Safety Administration.

experienced decreases in motor vehicle occupant fatalities ranging from 7% to 10%. After initial safety-belt usage rates of as high as 70%, most states with mandatory belt laws are reporting that approximately 50% of motor vehicle occupants are consistently using safety belts. In those states without mandatory safety-belt laws only 33% of motor vehicle passengers use them.[26]

Automatic occupant protection (passive restraints). Are there alternatives to the manual safety belts now available? The answer is yes, and the truth of the matter is that they could have been available to the public as early as 1975. Two forms of automatic occupant protection that have been commercially developed and proven effective are air bags and automatic safety belts. Since they do not require the active participation of vehicle occupants, they are sometimes referred to as **passive restraints.**

Air bags are fabric cushions that inflate rapidly between the steering wheel and the driver, and the instrument panel and the front-seat passengers in the early part of a frontal crash. The air bags cushion the front-seat occupants from violent impact with the interior of the car as they move forward (Fig. 7-13).

Sensing devices in the dashboard and front bumper are designed to detect forces large enough to be harmful. Generally the bag will inflate at a barrier-equivalent impact speed of about 12 mph. When they are activated, the sensors send an electrical signal to the inflating modules, which fill the air bags within a fraction of a second to cushion the collisions of the occupants. To prevent the driver from sliding under the air bag coming from the steering wheel and to absorb lower body impact, knee restraints are located under the dashboard. On the passenger side of the vehicle one large cushion inflates at the time of a crash, protecting both the torso and lower body. Seconds after the impact the bags have completely deflated.

Invented in the 1950s, air bags were first developed in the late 1960s. Working with the Ford Motor Company, the Eaton Corporation produced the first practical air bags and successfully tested them in passenger cars in 1969. In the early 1970s General Motors further refined air bags under the name ''air cushion restraint system.'' As early as August 1970 General Motors pledged that air bags would be standard equipment on all its cars by 1975; however, this never came to pass.

Although it was never publicized, air bags were a special option in the 1972 Mercury Monterey and the 1973 Chevrolet Impala. They were also offered on GM's full-size luxury cars (Buick, Cadillac, and Oldsmobile) for model years 1974 to 1976.

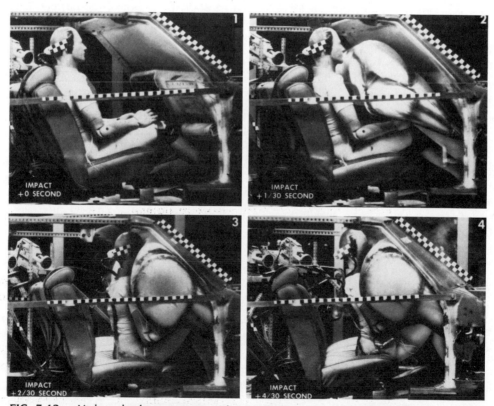

FIG. 7-13   Air bag deployment test with an unbelted passenger. Note the elapsed time in the four photographs.

Courtesy U.S. Department of Transportation. National Highway Traffic Safety Administration.

A total of approximately 12,000 cars equipped with air cushion restraint systems were sold from 1972 to 1976. More recently the federal government purchased 5000 1985 Ford Tempos equipped with driver air bags for use in government fleet vehicles.

How have they performed? To date, there have been over 300 crashes in which the air bags have been deployed. Compared with unrestrained occupants in similar cars, the passengers of the air bag-equipped vehicles have suffered 50% to 60% fewer deaths and injuries. Detailed investigations of each of these accidents have indicated that air bag systems have never failed to deploy and have seldom inflated in noncrash situations. With an estimated reliability of 99.995%, air cushion restraint systems are among the most reliable safety components in a car; in several of the crashes the air bag-equipped cars were more than 10 years old. Although they offer little protection during side impact or rear-end collisions or rollovers, air bags are highly effective in severe frontal crashes, which account for over 60% of all fatalities and serious injuries.

Probably the greatest advantage that air bags have over other occupant restraints is that they are inconspicuous and completely automatic, and they in no way inhibit or reduce occupant movement. If all vehicles were to have air bags as a standard safety feature, the usage rate would be *100%*—instead of the current 33% in states without mandatory safety belt laws and approximately 50% in states with mandatory laws.[26]

Marketing studies have indicated that nearly 70% of the driving population prefer air bags over any other occupant restraint system, even if this means an additional $400 to $500 being added to the sticker price of a new car. Although auto manufacturers claim that air cushion restraint systems would cost $500 to $800, air bag manufacturers and the Department of Transportation have estimated the cost for mass production to be from $100 to $300 per unit.[21]

During the early 1970s the stimulus of future government policies requiring automatic occupant crash protection resulted in substantial innovation in the technology of passive restraint systems. Along with the development of various air cushion restraint systems was the introduction of a passive restraint known as the automatic safety belt. In 1973 the Volkswagen Company demonstrated an experimental shoulder belt-knee bolster system that required no manipulation of belts or buckles. As a person enters the vehicle and closes the door, a shoulder belt moves automatically into place across the occupant's chest. The knee bolster is a padded panel that fits across the bottom of the dashboard and restrains the lower body in a crash.

In recent years a substantial amount of developmental work has produced a variety of automatic safety belt designs. Many of the newer models consist of both shoulder and lap belts. In most cases the belts are attached to the door frame at two different points; thus the occupant has to do nothing more than open and close the door. When the door is opened, the belts extend away from the wearer's body, and when the door is closed the belts deploy around the occupant for protection (Fig. 7-14).

Probably the most widely used and best accepted automatic safety belt is the motorized two-point system. When the door opens, a motor on the door frame moves the shoulder belt up and forward out of an entering passenger's way. When the door

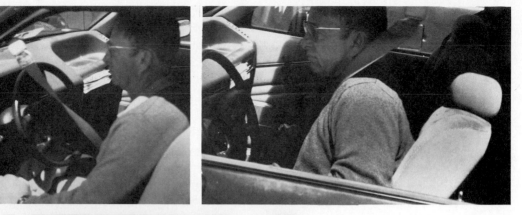

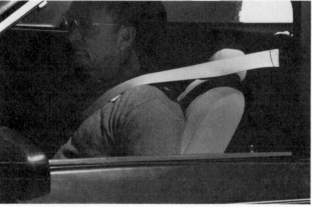

Fig. 7-14   Automatic safety belt.
Courtesy U.S. Department of Transportation,
National Highway Traffic Safety Administration.

is closed, the motor moves the belt around the door frame and into position. The passenger then manually operates the lap belt. Usage rates for automatic belts are approximately 85%.[29]

It is clear that modern occupant restraint systems, *(manual safety belts, automatic safety belts, and air bags),* are equally effective—when used. The difference in usage rates between manual safety belts and passive restraint systems is far more important than differences in crash protection offered by these three systems. On the basis of usage level, the air cushion restraint system—with its automatic deployment capabilities—would be in use virtually 100% of the time. With the supplemental use of a safety belt, the air bag system provides occupants with additional protection in rollover crashes and side-impact or rear-end collisions.

So why has it taken so long for passive restraints, either air bags or automatic belts, to be implemented if they have been available for such a long time? The answer: *politics and money.* On June 30, 1977, the U.S. Secretary of Transportation announced that beginning with model year 1982 (September 1981), all full-sized passenger cars manufactured for sale or use in the United States must be equipped with automatic restraint systems to protect front-seat occupants from serious injury in frontal crashes. In model year 1983 intermediate and compact cars were to be equipped with passive restraints and by model year 1984 (September 1983) all passenger cars would be required to have automatic crash protection.

However, in April 1981 the first step of the passive restraint ruling was delayed for a year from September 1981 to September 1982. Then in October 1981 the National Highway Traffic Safety Administration issued an order to cancel the automatic occupant protection regulation, citing as its reasons: (1) uncertainty about public acceptance and use of automatic safety belts that would be easy to disconnect permanently and (2) increased vehicle prices, which would affect both consumers and the slumping auto industry.

What about air bags? The auto manufacturers planned to install air cushion restraint systems in no more than 1% of their new cars; instead, vehicles would be provided with automatic safety belts of the easy-to-defeat variety. Facing stiff competition from foreign auto manufacturers in recent years, the U.S. car makers felt that the increased price of air bag-equipped vehicles would further reduce their sales and that safety belts with use-compelling features would also have a negative effect, especially if competitors offered vehicles with automatic belts that were easy to disconnect.

Immediately after the cancellation of the automatic-restraint requirements, consumer groups and insurance companies began litigation to overturn NHTSA's ruling. Thanks to the efforts of these organizations, the National Highway Traffic Safety Administration's decision was overturned by the U.S. Supreme Court on June 24, 1983. In its findings the Court held that the agency had been too quick in dismissing the benefits of detachable automatic safety belts; it further ordered NHTSA to reconsider its decision and to develop an alternative plan.

On July 11, 1984, the Department of Transportation issued an amended occupant crash-protection standard. It requires automatic occupant protection in all passenger automobiles manufactured on and after September 1, 1989.

Since 75% of occupant fatalities and injuries occur to drivers and most of the remainder involve passengers in the right outboard seat, these seating positions are covered by the standard. The center front passenger position and the rear seats are exempt from automatic protection. In addition, the passive restraint standard does not apply to trucks, tractors, or multipurpose vehicles such as jeeps.

The outlook for automatic occupant protection in the decade of the 1990s is good. To ensure that passive restraints will be a reality, many of the states enacting mandatory safety-belt usage laws say they will rescind the laws if an attempt is made by the federal government to no longer require automatic occupant protection. We have waited long enough; every year of delay has cost the nation at least 5000 lives, 70,000 critical injuries, and untold anguish for thousands of families. Automatic occupant protection is not a luxury—it's a necessity.

Child restraint systems. With the sudden deceleration that occurs in a motor vehicle collision, the unrestrained child becomes a human missile, even if he is being held on the lap of a restrained adult. The inertial forces produced by an infant in a frontal collision are three to four times greater than the grasping strength of any adult. So regardless of how tight you think you can hold your little one, it won't be enough in a collision. Even when a car is involved in a panic braking situation with no collision, small unrestrained children can be thrown forward, whereas a heavier adult stays in the seat.

By far the largest percentage of severe or fatal injuries occur when the child's head hits the dashboard and compartment hardware. Hardware includes the glove box, knobs, heater and air conditioning ducts, and add-on equipment, such as C.B. radios and gauges. A significant number of infants and toddlers receive fatal injuries when they are crushed by unrestrained adults who were holding them.

Another area in which child protection can be improved is passenger ejection. One fourth of the children killed in auto crashes are ejected from the vehicle. The introduction of hatchback vehicles has brought a special hazard to children in rear seats. On side or rear impact, hatchback doors tend to pop open, permitting ejection of unrestrained children.

For proper protection infants and small children need special seats that can be anchored by the vehicle's safety belts (Fig. 7-15). Infant carriers allow children under 1 year of age to be placed in a semireclining position facing the rear of the car. The carrier is lined with soft padding and has an internal harness to keep the baby in the

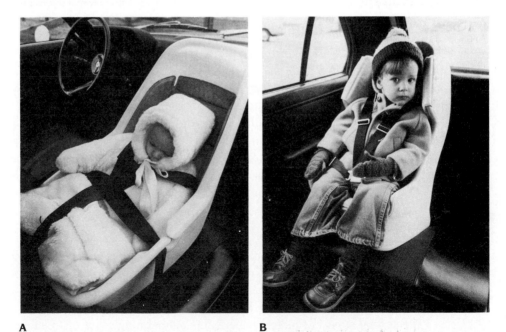

A   **B**

FIG. 7-15   Child restraints. **A,** Infant carrier. **B,** Child safety seat.

restraint; this device is anchored to the car seat with the vehicle's safety belt. In a crash the infant's back, rather than its chest and abdomen, absorbs the force.

For toddlers (ages 1 to 4), several restraints are available. The child safety seat is a mini-bucket seat in which the child is supported by a safety harness. This device is held in place by the car's seat belt and a top tether strap attached to the rear window shelf.

Another device, the child seat with shield, is a foam-padded plastic shell that closely covers a child's legs and abdomen and then bends away from the chest and face. It is held in place by the car's safety belt. The advantage of this model is that it allows the child freedom of movement. He can crawl into or out of the device by himself. Its disadvantage is that while you are driving the little one may not stay in the shield and then its effectiveness is defeated.

Various other booster seats and chairs are used in combination with lap and/or shoulder belts to provide protection for older children. Until a child is at least 4 feet 9 inches tall, it is recommended that the adult shoulder belt be used with some type of seat elevation. The key here is to have that small front-seat passenger protected. Often children and shorter adults will complain that the shoulder belt rubs the side of the neck. Though this may be slightly uncomfortable, it presents little hazard. In a crash situation the lap/shoulder belt combination provides the greatest protection. Adequate restraints have been developed to protect children; the trick is to get parents to utilize these devices.

All 50 states and the District of Columbia now have laws requiring the protection of young children (4 years and under) riding in passenger vehicles. Over the past 4 years it is estimated that nearly 1000 lives (250 children per year) have been saved as a result of this legislation. Although this is certainly good news, it must be tempered by the fact that only 80% of the children riding in automobiles during that time used a safety seat. What about the other 20% of these children from newborn to 4 years of age? You guessed it; they went unrestrained.[28]

To ensure the best protection for your child, use the safety seat according to the manufacturer's directions. Selecting a safety seat that is easy to use and to fasten into your car, as well as comfortable for your child, will help you to use it consistently and correctly. If we could get all passengers up to 4 years of age in correctly used safety seats, an additional 200 children could be saved annually.[28]

MOTORCYCLE SAFETY

A motorcycle can provide an economical and pleasurable means of transportation. With few exceptions it costs less to purchase, less to repair, and less to operate than an automobile. A 500 cc motorcycle can travel about 50 miles on a gallon of gasoline; smaller motorcycles will average close to 75 miles per gallon.

The special appeal of motorcycling is the exhilarating sense of freedom one gets from riding in the open. However, with the advantages of motorcycling there is a price to pay; this includes less weather and crash protection than that provided by an automobile. Consequently, motorcyclists must take certain measures if they are to maximize their enjoyment while minimizing their risks.

Motorcycle Accident Factors

What makes motorcycling dangerous? In an analysis of 900 motorcycle accidents, the University of Southern California's Traffic Safety Center found that 51% of all motorcycle accidents were precipitated by a vehicle operator other than the motorcyclist.[23] In other words, the cyclist's right of way had been violated by "the other guy." Of the 667 accidents in which the motorcycle struck or was struck by another vehicle, the driver of the other vehicle was at fault 65% of the time. Of the 233 single-vehicle motorcycle crashes, another motor vehicle was responsible for the accident in nearly 40% of the cases. Environmental factors such as weather, vehicle malfunction, and roadway surface played a role in less than 10% of all accidents analyzed.

Most motorcycle accidents occurred when the other vehicle driver did not see the motorcyclist. The motorcyclist's **conspicuity** (ability to be seen) was very low or absent in 46% of the accidents in which another driver violated the motorcycle right of way. This problem is often compounded when the motorcyclist assumes that the other vehicle driver sees him.

Most of the accident-involved riders had no formal motorcycle training; only 7% of them were trained through organized programs. This lack of proper training becomes more evident when we observe the evasive actions taken by riders in trying to avoid accidents. In those cases where avoidance actions were attempted, 76% of them were not properly executed. Skidding from overbraking was the most common execution problem that resulted in a loss of control of the motorcycle. Another braking problem that frequently occurred was the use of only the rear brake instead of both brakes while attempting to avoid a collision.

Nearly one third of the 900 riders took no evasive actions before their crashes. Several reasons have been suggested. Rider distraction was said to have accounted for part of this. Such things as surrounding traffic, nontraffic items, and motorcycle operation was cited as reasons why riders' attention was diverted from the roadway. As in the case with automobile accidents, alcohol plays a significant role in motorcycle mishaps. Approximately 55% of the riders severely injured or killed in motorcycle accidents have some alcohol or drug involvement.[20] Since the time a rider has to react properly to avoid a collision is usually 3 seconds or less, it would not be surprising to find that an alcohol-impaired person would have taken little evasive action to avoid an accident.

Demographics of motorcycle accidents. Now that we know some of the reasons how and why motorcycle accidents occur, let's take a closer look at persons involved in these accidents. Most of the riders are male (96%) and the majority of them are 17 to 26 years of age. Seventeen percent of them carry passengers. Almost half of the riders who carry passengers have little or no experience in doing so; likewise, 53% of the passengers are riding for the first time or have seldom ridden on a motorcycle.

75%

Collision contact areas on motorcycles very closely approximate those of passenger cars. Frontal collisions occur in 62% of the crashes, while side impacts account for 32% of the collisions. The threat of being struck from the rear is very low, occurring in only 6% of the accidents.

Crash severity in motorcycle accidents, as well as auto accidents, increases as speed increases. Most minor and moderate injuries occur between 11 and 20 mph; more serious injuries result from impacts at speeds of 21 to 30 mph; and the bulk of fatal accidents involve crash speeds in the 31 to 40 mph range. Remember the pictures of the 30-mph passenger-car crash tests? Can you imagine going through the same test on a motorcycle?

Needless to say, most motorcycle accidents (88%) result in rider injuries. Nearly 800 of the 900 riders involved in accidents during the University of Southern California study required some type of treatment. Injuries to the extremities were most common; however, trauma to the head and chest areas had the greatest potential for critical or fatal results. Riders wearing helmets received half as many head and neck injuries as unhelmeted riders. This becomes extremely important when one realizes that head injuries are the major cause of death in motorcycle accidents.

Rider protection. Unlike auto manufacturers, the motorcycle industry cannot do much in terms of vehicle design to increase rider crash protection. There are no side doors or steering columns to strengthen; no external structure surrounding the motorcycle to prevent passenger ejection; and no passenger restraint systems.

Nowhere is the term "defensive driving" more important than in the case of the motorcyclist. The first line of protection for the rider must be his ability to anticipate movements of other vehicles and to take the correct evasive actions when necessary. Motorcycle operator training can be one of the most effective measures for reducing these accidents. The Motorcycle Safety Foundation, a nonprofit organization sponsored by leading motorcycle manufacturers, developed a beginning rider course in 1974 that has been used widely throughout the United States. The course provides the rider with independent study activities, classroom instruction, and on-cycle exercises and drills under the supervision of a teacher. Instructional content includes such areas as: basic motorcycle maneuvers, riding on the street, and techniques for crash avoidance. The goal of this and other programs sponsored by the Motorcycle Safety Foundation is to reduce motorcycle accidents and injuries through rider education, licensing improvement, public information, and research programs.

Even the well-trained, highly motivated, and attentive rider can have an accident. To reduce the likelihood of injury from a spill, protective gear should be worn whenever a person is on a motorcycle. These items include a helmet, an eye protection device, jacket and pants, gloves, and footwear (Fig. 7-16).

1. Helmet: The most important piece of personal equipment for motorcycle riding is the helmet. As the USC study indicated, wearing a helmet significantly reduces the risk of serious head injury from violent impacts with such things as the pavement and other vehicles in an accident. Not surprisingly, it has been found that the newer "full-facial coverage" models provide considerably more protection

against injury to the face and eyes than the traditional helmets open at the chin.

Before a helmet can be sold in the United States, it must meet minimum standards for resistance to impact and penetration and for the strength of its chinstrap assembly. Helmets that conform to acceptable safety standards may be marked in a variety of ways:

a. DOT—means that the helmet meets the federal safety standards set by the U.S. Department of Transportation.

b. ANSI Z90. 1-1971 or ANSI Z90. 1a-1973—represent impact tests performed by the American National Standards Institute that meet DOT specifications. ANSI A90. 1b-1979 means that the helmet exceeds federal standards.

c. Approved by Snell Memorial Foundation—helmets with this label have successfully passed tests that are much more stringent than the federal standards.

An important thing to remember when you make a purchase is that helmets of the same basic design provide almost the same amount of protection against death or injury in typical road mishaps; an expensive helmet doesn't necessarily provide greater protection.

2. *Eye-protection devices:* To ride safely one must be able to see clearly. Goggles, a face shield, or a windshield can all provide adequate protection against wind, dust, bugs, rocks, and other foreign objects. Regular eyeglasses, however, will not provide the necessary protection, especially against wind and rocks. Many states now require motorcycle operators to wear eye-protection devices.

3. *Jacket and pants:* Proper clothing serves a number of purposes. It can protect one from the elements. It affords protection from bumps or abrasions during a slide along the pavement after a spill. It can increase one's chances of being seen by oncoming traffic.

Even in warm weather constant exposure to the wind can lower body temperature, producing both discomfort and slower reflexes. A long-sleeved, zippered jacket with snugfitting cuffs and waist will help to alleviate this problem. Both the jacket and pants of a rider should be of a durable material, leather or heavy denim, to provide maximum protection in the event of a spill.

Motorcyclists wearing high-visibility color clothing will greatly increase their conspicuity. Day-glow colors such as yellow, orange, and green, which are used to increase the visibility of emergency vehicles, will provide similar benefits for the motorcycle rider. Special riding vests in these colors can be worn over other garments.

4. *Gloves:* Good protection, as well as a better grip, can be obtained from leather gloves. However, they should not be too thick, or they will reduce one's ability to operate hand controls. In cold weather gauntlet-style gloves that fit over the bottom of coat sleeves will provide added warmth by preventing cold air from going up the sleeves.

5. *Footwear:* Heavy-soled leather boots that fit over the ankle will provide both protection and support for the motorcyclist. This footwear gives the rider a steady base to support himself and the motorcycle when stopped at an intersection. Boots

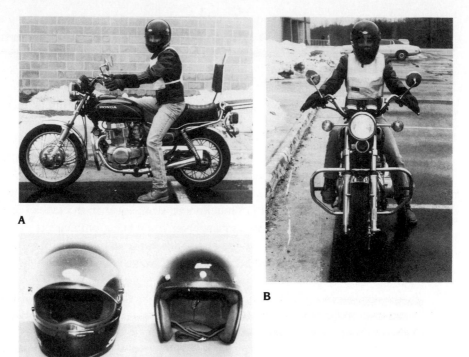

FIG. 7-16 Protection for the motorcycle rider. **A,** Essentials: helmet, face shield, leather jacket, heavy denim pants, leather gloves, and boots. **B,** To add to her conspicuity this rider is wearing a dayglow vest and using the motorcycle's headlamp during daylight hours. **C,** Notice the added protection provided by the full-face helmet.

with steel toes will further protect the rider in the event that a spill occurs or debris is kicked up from the road surface.

Since visibility of riders seems to be a major problem in motorcycle accidents, anything that can be done to increase their conspicuity should be attempted. While its major purpose is to illuminate the roadway at night, a motorcycle headlamp can produce more visibility for the rider who is coming toward traffic, even in daylight hours.

Correct positioning of your motorcycle in traffic and on the open road is another way to improve other road users' awareness of you. The left tire track of an automobile is probably the best location in which to ride. It allows you to see oncoming traffic more easily, and at the same time drivers can see you when a vehicle is in front of you. Also, the driver ahead will see you more easily in his rearview mirrors. One other advantage of this riding position is that it discourages other vehicles from crowding into the same lane with you.

Again, the bottom line for the safe operation of a motorcycle is to *drive defensively.* Assume that you are invisible and that motorists will not give you the right of way. Always try to look 10 to 12 seconds ahead so that you will have time to anticipate driver actions. Be especially alert when approaching an intersection; if you don't think the other driver has seen you, slow down and be ready to take evasive action.

Never focus on one vehicle or area for an extended period; keep your eyes moving. Be aware not only of what is in front of you but what is at the side or behind you. Head checks (glances over the shoulder) and frequent use of mirrors will keep you aware of the surrounding environment.

One other action that can give a motorcyclist that extra margin of safety is to allow for an adequate following distance. While a 3-second distance between the vehicle in front and the following rider is preferred, heavier traffic may make it necessary to reduce that to 2 seconds. Do not compromise yourself by reducing that following distance. In case there is trouble ahead, you will need that 2 seconds to react. The greatest danger for motorcyclists comes from traffic in front of them. Remember the three A's when riding your motorcycle: *Be alert, aware, and always under control.*

Helmet laws: yes or no? Since the early 1940s investigators have demonstrated repeatedly that helmets significantly reduce the odds of a motorcyclist's being severely or fatally injured in a crash. The results so impressed the Congress that in 1966 the Highway Safety Act included a mandate that all states establish legislation requiring motorcycle riders and passengers to wear helmets. States that did not comply with this regulation would not receive certain highway construction funds. In 1966 only three states had helmet laws in force; by 1975, 47 states had developed mandatory helmet laws. The fatality rate for motorcyclists declined from 12.8 to 6.5 deaths per 10,000 registered motorcycles during this 10-year period.[38]

However, the good news was not to continue. Three states, California, Illinois, and Utah, failed to meet the federal requirements. California and Illinois had no laws and Utah's applied only to riders traveling over 35 mph. Since they were going to lose millions of dollars in federal highway funding, these states began to lobby for a repeal of the federal helmet mandate. They were joined by groups such as the American Motorcycle Association and ABATE (A Brotherhood Against Totalitarian Enactments), which were opposed to mandatory helmet laws on the grounds of personal freedom. The basis of their appeal was that no one should be forced to take protective measures if the negative outcome would affect only the individual decision maker. The standard line went something like this: "It's my life and if I want to risk it, that's my business. After all, I'm the only one who will suffer in an accident. Let those who ride decide." The same misguided thinking is used today by people who refuse to wear safety belts in their passenger cars.

Tragically, the campaign was successful and Congress overtured its decision in 1976. No longer could the Department of Transportation withhold funding from states that did not have mandatory helmet laws. In rapid succession states began to repeal their helmet laws or modify them to apply only to riders under 18 years of age. By 1980, 28 states had made these changes. There was another dramatic change in rider death rates; this time it wasn't favorable. Fatality rates climbed from 6.5 to 8.9 per 10,000 registered motorcycles by 1981; throughout the 1980s the fatality rate has

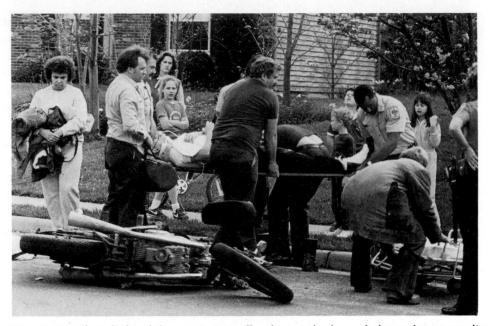

FIG. 7-17 Though his bike was minimally damaged, the unhelmeted motorcyclist received a serious injury, when his head hit the curb.
Courtesy Fairfax County Fire and Rescue Department, Fairfax, Va.

remained constant at approximately 8.5. With almost 6 million registered motorcycles in the United States, that higher death rate means that nearly 1500 more people die each year because of the repeal of the helmet laws.[20] This figure would be higher if it weren't for the fact that 22 states have retained their helmet laws (Fig. 7-17).

The documentation is clear that helmet use and helmet-use laws contribute substantially to lower head-injury and death rates. A 1984 study of the effect of helmet-law readoption in the state of Louisiana found that the first year the new law went into effect there was a 30% reduction in motorcycle fatalities. This significant reduction in deaths occurred during a time when motorcycle registrations increased by 6%.

Recently Texas published an extensive study documenting the differences in mortality between helmeted and unhelmeted riders. Between 1977 and 1985 over 500 additional motorcyclist deaths occurred on Texas roadways as a result of the repeal of its motorcycle helmet law.[6] By the way, Texas reenacted its helmet law in 1989.

Dummy—you're a *dummy* if you think those who don't wear helmets are the only ones to suffer when they have accidents! What about the mothers, fathers, brothers, sisters, wives, husbands, and children of motorcyclists who are killed or severely injured because they didn't wear a helmet? In a cost-benefit analysis of motorcycle helmet-law repeals, researchers at Pennsylvania State University estimated that an additional $18 million for medical care and rehabilitation will be expended annually in each of those 28 states no longer requiring helmet usage. Over 60% of these medical care costs will be paid by public funds.[6] Unless motorcycle helmet laws are reinstated, increased motorcycle usage will mean additional deaths and suffering for riders and their families as well as an additional monetary burden for the rest of society.

What About Mopeds? During the post-World War II years of the late 1940s, automobiles, motorcycles, and fuel were in short supply on the European continent; however, bicycles were in abundance. The enterprising Europeans, using available resources, developed the motorized bicycle, better known as the moped. It quickly began to play a major role in the transport systems of many countries; even today one in three French motor vehicles is a moped.

Before 1974 mopeds were classified as motorcycles in the United States. Since they lacked foot brakes, bright lights, and turn signals (standard features of U.S. motorcycles), they were not allowed to be sold here. In 1974 NHTSA relaxed these standards so that mopeds could be imported for sale. By 1977 the Vehicle Equipment Safety Commission, an organization of state transportation officials, established minimum construction requirements for mopeds, thus separating them from motorcycles. The Moped Association of America, sponsored by the various manufacturers, promoted the development of ''moped laws'' in each state, which would allow these vehicles to be sold and used on streets and roadways (Fig. 7-18).

Although they have become popular, with over 1 million registered vehicles in the U.S., mopeds are something of a mixed blessing. Too many Americans consider mopeds to be no more than glorified bicycles.

Engine displacement limitations restrict the maximum speed of these vehicles to 30 mph or less. This lack of power and inability to keep up with traffic is one of the moped's many hazards. At the same time a speed of 30 mph is more than adequate to produce severe or fatal injuries in a moped collision. One other factor related to the

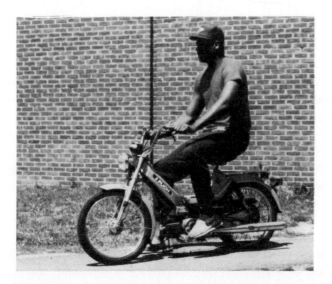

FIG. 7-18 The apparel of this moped operator offers him little protection in case of an accident.

lack of power in a moped is that carrying a passenger frequently overloads the vehicle so that it will not accelerate or handle properly.

Since many moped riders are young and relatively inexperienced, one of their biggest problems is bringing the vehicle to a stop, especially when the road surface offers minimal traction. Experienced moped riders depend on the rear brake for ordinary stopping, while a combination of front and rear brakes is used if the rider must come to a quick stop. To coordinate the brakes takes a certain amount of dexterity, achieved only when a rider has been willing to spend the practice time developing this skill.

Probably the two most important tips for a moped rider are:

1. Develop the skills necessary to handle the vehicle. Before attempting to operate the moped in traffic, be sure that you have trained sufficiently in an off-road setting. Since many moped riders are 16 years of age and under, courses in moped driver education in junior high schools are a realistic training alternative. This idea becomes even more relevant after reading recent NHTSA research findings concerning moped accidents. Unlike motorcyclists whose right of way is impeded by another vehicle, moped riders are at fault the majority of the time. Failure to yield the right of way and improper signaling by the moped rider cause the greatest number of accidents. The moped is a motorized vehicle, not a bicycle; consequently, riders must realize their responsibility for proper operation.

2. When operating a moped, use all available protective measures. Wear proper safety gear; helmets, eye-protection devices, and durable clothing can provide significant protection in a crash. The use of headlamps and high-visibility clothing will increase one's chances of being noticed in traffic. As in the case of the motorcyclist, the moped rider may not be seen easily; so always drive defensively.

PEDESTRIAN SAFETY

Annually, pedestrian fatalities account for approximately 17% of motor vehicle-related deaths. Each year more than 7000 pedestrians are killed and an additional 100,000 are injured. Not surprisingly, two age groups are particularly vulnerable: the very young and the elderly. Studies in the United States and England have indicated that while the highest motor vehicle death rates were recorded for those between 15 and 44 years of age, pedestrian death rates were highest for those under 10 and over 65 years of age.[22]

Young children often lack the ability to adequately judge vehicle distances, and they do not have an adequate understanding of traffic signs and signals. This is very likely the reason why children in primary grades (6 to 9 years of age) are involved in three times as many pedestrian accidents as children ages 11 to 14. Small children told to look to the left and right before they cross the street may not realize that they must be looking for moving vehicles when they do this. Because they do not fully understand the meaning of this action, the children will look both ways and then proceed into traffic.

Another problem that lessens with age involves the ability to anticipate vehicle movement. How do you cross a busy roadway that has no intersections or traffic signals? Do you not look for gaps in the traffic flow and then use them to cross the street? Most of us will cross close behind the last car before a vehicle gap; however, this requires a certain amount of timing and anticipation. Young children can perceive distances between cars, but they have trouble using these distances and judging when to cross the roadway.

Elementary school traffic-education programs can be valuable in helping children to better understand rules of the road. However, the ability to judge vehicle motion and spatial relationships seems to develop over time and cannot be presented easily in the school setting. Therefore, emphasis must be placed on the child's crossing streets only at intersections or with an adult.

The problems with elderly pedestrians differ from those of the very young; older pedestrians understand the dangers of crossing streets and the responsibilities involved, but aging takes its toll on a person's sensory abilities and motor capabilities. Failing eyesight may hamper one's ability to detect approaching traffic, while problems with movement will increase the time it takes to get across the street.

A misconception held by many elderly persons is that vehicle drivers recognize their vulnerabilities and thus will accommodate older persons attempting to cross a street. It is sad to say, but older Americans do not receive that respect. In a study of pedestrian right of way at marked crossings, it was found that drivers were more likely to stop for young, attractive women than any other group—not a surprising finding in a youth-oriented nation.

Causes of Pedestrian Accidents

Nearly 60% of pedestrian accidents involve attempts to cross a street or roadway either at an intersection or between intersections. The overwhelming majority of the time it is the fault of the pedestrian, not the vehicle operator. The victim makes a poor choice of where and when to cross the street or fails to make an adequate visual search of the roadway before crossing.

Probably the most common occurrence is the midstreet dart-out. An example of this is the young child who runs into the street from between two parked cars. A vehicle operator is immediately put at a disadvantage for two reasons: There is a very short time available for responding, and the driver is not expecting to encounter a pedestrian in the middle of the street. A similar problem that often involves adults is the intersection dash, in which a person suddenly attempts to cross the street as oncoming traffic is approaching or as the traffic signal is changing. In this last-second dash, drivers are not expecting pedestrians whom they had noticed earlier to suddenly attempt a crossing.

An environmental factor that plays a significant role in many pedestrian accidents is vehicle obstruction. Delayed detection of a pedestrian by a car or truck driver is often the result of another vehicle parked along the traffic route. This includes parked cars, buses stopped to discharge passengers, and ice cream or food vendors. On four-

and six-lane roadways, other moving vehicles may block a driver's view of a pedestrian attempting to cross.

Other pedestrian accidents involve persons jogging, standing, walking, or working in or near the roadway. As with motorcycle and moped riders, the pedestrian presents a visibility problem. The contrast of the pedestrian with the background is a key to visibility in daylight hours. That is why construction workers, police, and other personnel working in or near the roadway should wear high-contrast colors such as orange or yellow.

In the evening or nighttime hours, the ability of clothing to reflect headlight illumination will increase a pedestrian's chances of being seen. Colors that absorb light such as gray, black, and brown greatly reduce pedestrian visibility. An Indiana study of nighttime pedestrian accidents revealed that in 87% of the cases drivers claimed they failed to see victims until it was too late to stop. Later laboratory studies indicated that drivers traveling 40 mph or faster will fail to detect pedestrians at least 55% of the time.[30]

The importance of wearing reflective clothing at night cannot be overemphasized. White clothing works well because of its ability to reflect light; however, reflectorized strips that can be attached to clothing will provide even more pedestrian illumination for an oncoming driver.

A discussion of any type of traffic accident involvement would not be complete without the mention of alcohol and its role. And yes, pedestrian fatalities show a considerable victim involvement with alcohol. Department of Transportation figures indicate that approximately 60% of fatally injured adult pedestrians had measurable blood alcohol levels and nearly half of this group had BACs of .20 or more.[30,31] Pedestrian accidents related to alcohol consumption were found to be more frequent among males 19 to 49 years of age and tended to occur more often on weekends and at night. This group appears to be significantly overrepresented in dart-and-dash accidents, in which the person suddenly leaves the curb and quickly moves into the path of an oncoming vehicle. A reduction in the ability to judge distances and a lack of motor coordination can be as fatal for the intoxicated pedestrian as for the vehicle driver.

An innovation that has created further hazard for pedestrians in recent years is the miniaturized stereo radio-tape player with a headset attachment. A person can walk down the street and drown out all sounds but the music being played. Sirens, honking horns, and screeching brakes, which could alert the pedestrian to imminent danger, will not be heard by a person wearing headphones. How many people do you know who wear these devices while walking to classes or work or while they are jogging or rollerskating?

Countermeasures for Pedestrian Safety

One of the best ways to reduce the hazard of pedestrian-vehicle confrontation would be to separate the two groups. Several approaches may be taken to accomplish this goal. The design and construction of pedestrian overpasses and underpasses is a practical alternative in areas of dense traffic. This allows people in the neighborhood to move around freely without stopping vehicle movement.

A somewhat different alternative that still separates pedestrians and vehicles is the construction of pedestrian malls in which no vehicle traffic is allowed. This has become very popular in areas undergoing urban redevelopment. The pedestrian mall not only provides a safe environment for those on foot but also allows for the development of an aesthetically pleasing environment that may stimulate renewed interest in cities. Other communities have compromised and limit vehicle traffic during certain hours or days of the week. In areas where there are many children, the community should provide safe play areas away from traffic.

When pedestrians and vehicles cannot be completely separated, the use of well-marked crosswalks seems to provide a certain amount of protection for the person on foot. The widely spaced white markings of the crosswalk are designed to attract the attention of vehicle operators and pedestrians alike. However, a person crossing the street in a marked crosswalk needs to maintain an awareness of approaching vehicles, since it may be impossible for motorists to stop in some situations.

Variations of the crosswalk design have shown some success in European countries. At specific crosswalk locations in British cities, flashing yellow lights have been added. Whenever a pedestrian is in one of these crosswalks, all oncoming traffic must stop. They have proved especially effective in locations with a high amount of pedestrian traffic, such as schools and universities.

Another design used in a number of countries is the pedestrian guardrail, which extends from the end of the crosswalk several hundred feet down the block. This fencelike structure forces people to go to the intersection to cross the street and reduces the likelihood of persons darting into the roadway in front of unsuspecting motorists.

Pedestrians traveling along or near the roadway should take further protective measures. The key is to see and be seen. By walking or jogging on the side of the road against traffic, a person will be able to anticipate problems from oncoming vehicles and have the time to react appropriately. A good rule to follow is never to assume that drivers see you. Whether during daylight or darkness, the pedestrian needs to be highly visible to oncoming traffic.

MOTOR VEHICLE INSURANCE

Next to a home, a motor vehicle is the most substantial investment that many people will make. It may be no more than a means of transportation or it may be your pride and joy. Whatever the case, *it must be insured!*

Coverages may vary from company to company, but basic policies are similar. They should provide specific protection against financial losses caused by injury to you, damage to your car, injury to others, and damage by your car.

Bodily Injury and Property Liability

Bodily injury and property damage liability coverage will pay for personal injury you might do to other people or for damage to their property in the event of a motor vehicle accident in which you are at fault. If the injured parties decide to sue, the policy provides legal defense and/or payment of damages up to the policy's limit.

Medical Payments

Up to the limits you choose, the **medical payments** coverage of your policy will pay medical expenses for you and passengers in your vehicle, regardless of who was at fault. This coverage extends to vehicles other than your own, provided you have received permission to operate them.

Uninsured Motorists

Most states require that vehicle operators have insurance protection; however, that doesn't guarantee that everyone will purchase it. **Uninsured motorist** coverage will pay the amount that insured policyholders should have collected for bodily injury or vehicle damage caused by a person who has no insurance or who is underinsured. This coverage will also protect you if you are the victim of a hit-and-run driver who cannot be identified. While injury payments involve no deductible fee, vehicle damage is subject to a deductible.

Optional Coverages

Unlike the above coverages, which are required in most states, collision and comprehensive vehicle coverages are optional. **Comprehensive coverage** refers to loss of or damage to a vehicle caused by something other than a collision. Fire, theft, vandalism, hail, or water are just a few of the perils that may damage your vehicle. Personal property you may have left in a car or truck will be covered only to $100; personal belongings such as clothing, cameras, and sports equipment should be covered on a homeowner's or renter's policy.

Collision coverage pays for damage to your car when you have been at fault in an accident. This is an especially important coverage to have if your vehicle is relatively new.

With both comprehensive and collision coverages there is usually a deductible fee that the policyholder will have to pay in the event of a claim. The insurance company will pay those expenses above the deductible.

SUMMARY

By far the greatest number of accidental deaths occurs yearly on our nation's streets and highways, accounting for nearly 50% percent of the total. It is even more tragic that 28% of the fatalities involve drivers 15 to 24 years of age.

Factors contributing to motor vehicle fatalities include human error, vehicle design or mechanical malfunction, and the environment, both manmade and natural. Human error accounts for the majority of fatal motor vehicle accidents. Speeding, failure to yield, driving left of center, and tailgating are just a few of the incorrect driving skills that lead to accidents. Often these problems are compounded by the drinking and/or drug-taking driver.

Because of the potential lethality of the drinking driver, law enforcement agencies have found it necessary to become more aggressive in identifying and prosecuting drunk drivers. Groups such as Mothers Against Drunk Driving support the enactment of stronger drunk-driving legislation as well as the return of the legal drinking age to 21 in all states.

Regardless of the legislation that is enacted, it must be realized that people will continue to drink and drive. Therefore, some practical suggestions such as appointing a designated driver, taking a cab, or staying overnight when you are going to drink heavily may be a more realistic approach.

To reduce the effects of environmental forces on vehicle control, highway engineers have developed roadway drainage systems to prevent water build-up on road surfaces and chemical agents to prevent freezing of bridge surfaces. Other design innovations include breakaway signs and multiple crash barriers that help to protect a vehicle's occupants from man-made environmental hazards along the roadway.

While improvements in components such as braking, steering, and lighting have led to fewer malfunctions, better handling, and improved crash avoidance, a critical aspect that must be considered with motor vehicles is that of design and crash protection.

Crashworthiness is determined by how well a vehicle can absorb, control, or reduce crash forces on its occupants. Federal safety standards require that all cars sold in the United States pass specified tests in 30-mph collisions.

By studying films of these test collisions, experts have found that occupant fatalities most often result when passengers strike hard surfaces inside the vehicle. The best way to prevent this from occurring is use of the combination lap and shoulder belt, which has been standard equipment on passenger cars since 1968.

Both the air bag and the automatic safety belt have proved highly effective in the real-world crash situation. Their rates of effectiveness are very similar to those of standard lap-shoulder belt systems. The advantage of automatic systems is that they have the capability of significantly increasing usage levels. Because they are unobtrusive and do not restrict passengers in any way, air bags have received the highest ratings in consumer polls.

Associated with the issue of occupant protection is that of child restraint. As with adults, few infants and small children are properly restrained in motor vehicles. For proper protection, infants and small children need special seats that can be anchored by the vehicle's safety belts.

Since 1970 motorcycle registration in the United States has doubled; however, rider fatalities have also nearly doubled during the same period. Although it has many advantages, the motorcycle has one major disadvantage—it offers little protection in a crash. To increase their safety, motorcyclists must be concerned with becoming highly visible, wearing proper protective gear, and developing evasive action skills.

First imported to the United States in 1974, the moped has become a popular means of transportation among the young; however, its lack of power and inability to keep up with traffic is one of the moped's more serious hazards. The moped operator must be conspicuous in traffic, wear protective gear including a helmet, and develop the skills necessary to handle the vehicle.

A group that often has trouble interacting with motor vehicles is the pedestrian population. Those at greatest risk are persons under 10 and over 65 years of age. The young often have an inadequate understanding of traffic signs, signals and movement, while the elderly have reduced sensory and motor capabilities.

One of the best ways to reduce the hazards of pedestrian-vehicle confrontation is to separate the two groups through the use of traffic overpasses, pedestrian malls, and safe play areas.

Next to a home, a motor vehicle is the most substantial investment many persons will make. To protect yourself and your investment, insurance is a necessity. The major coverages should include bodily injury and property damage liability, medical payments, and uninsured motorist protection. Most states require vehicle owners to have these coverages in a policy.

Key Terms

Auto Safety Hotline   Provides consumers with a direct line of communication to the National Highway Traffic Safety Administration (1-800-424-9393).

Blood alcohol concentration (BAC)   The quantity of alcohol (a percentage expressed as a decimal) that is in the bloodstream.

Blood alcohol level (BAL)   A term synonymous with BAC.

Bodily injury and property damage liability   Insurance that pays for personal injury to others or for property damage in the event of a motor vehicle accident in which you are at fault.

Collision coverage   Insurance that pays for damage to your car when you have been at fault in an accident.

Comprehensive coverage   Insurance that covers loss or damage to a vehicle caused by something other than a collision.

Conspicuity   Ability to be seen.

Crashworthiness   A vehicle's ability to protect passengers in the event of a crash.

DUI   Driving under the influence (of alcohol).

DWI   Driving while intoxicated.

Impact attenuators   Usually sand- or water-filled barrels or overlapping sections of steel paneling; on impact they collapse, gradually slowing the vehicle and dissipating the energy of its forward momentum. Also known as ''crash cushions.''

Medical payments   Insurance that covers medical expenses for you and passengers in your vehicle.

Passive restraints   Protective devices that do not require active participation of vehicle occupants (automatic safety belts, air bags).

Second collision   Occurs when unbelted occupants are thrown into the car's windshield, steering wheel, doors, dashboard, or other passengers after the car has hit another car or object (the first collision).

Uninsured motorist   Insurance coverage that pays the amount that insured policyholders should have collected for bodily injury or vehicle damage caused by a person who has no insurance.

References

1. Blatt, J.: Program activities associated with safety belt use, Washington, D. C., Feb. 1989, National Highway Traffic Safety Administration.
2. Camp, L. W.: Here's how the supplemental air bag works, Dealer World 7(8):6, Oct. 1986.
3. Cerrelli, E. C.: Older drivers, the age factor in traffic safety, Washington, D. C., Feb. 1989, National Highway Traffic Safety Administration.
4. Fell, J. C.: Alcohol involvement rates in fatal crashes: a focus on young drivers and female drivers, DOT HS 807 184, Washington, D. C., Sept. 1987, National Highway Traffic Safety Administration.
5. Gurin, D. B.: Overrepresentation of safety belt non-users in North Carolina traffic crashes, Washington, D. C., Feb. 1989, National Highway Traffic Safety Administration.
6. Hertz, E. S.: The effect of helmet law repeal on motorcycle fatalities a four year update, Washington, D. C., Sept. 1989, National Highway Traffic Safety Administration.
7. Highway Users Federation/Automotive Safety Foundation: The safety belt proponent's guide, DOT HS 806 683, Washington, D. C., Jan. 1985, U.S. Department of Transportation.
8. Kahane, C. J.: An evaluation of child passenger safety: the effectiveness and benefits of safety seats, DOT HS 806 890, Washington D. C., Feb. 1986, U.S. Department of Transportation.
9. Muller, A.: Evaluation of the costs and benefits of motorcycle helmet laws, American Journal of Public Health 70(6):586, 1980.
10. National Highway Traffic Safety Administration: Drinking age 21: facts, myths and fictions, DOT HS 806 704, Washington, D. C., Jan. 1985, U.S. Department of Transportation.
11. National Highway Traffic Safety Administration: Effect of raising the legal drinking age on driver involvement in fatal crashes. the experience of thirteen states, DOT HS 806 902, Washington, D. C., Nov. 1985, U.S. Department of Transportation.
12. National Highway Traffic Safety Administration: An evaluation of child passenger safety: the effectiveness and benefits of safety seats summary, DOT HS 806 889, Washington, D. C., Feb. 1986, U.S. Department of Transportation.
13. National Highway Traffic Safety Administration: Fatality trends: motorcycles, Washington, D. C., Sept. 1986, U.S. Department of Transportation.
14. National Highway Traffic Safety Administration: Federal motor vehicle safety standards and procedures, DOT HS 805 674, Washington, D. C., April 1985, U.S. Department of Transportation.
15. National Highway Traffic Safety Administration: Guide for detecting drunk drivers at night, ed. 2, DOT HS 805 711, Washington D. C., Jan. 1982, U.S. Department of Transporation.
16. National Highway Traffic Safety Administration: Highway safety '84: a report on activities under the Highway Safety Act of 1966, Washington, D. C., 1985, U.S. Department of Transportation.
17. National Highway Traffic Safety Administration: The national accident sampling system, DOT HS 806 583, Washington, D. C., Sept. 1990, U.S. Department of Transportation.
18. National Highway Traffic Safety Administration: Reducing highway crashes through administrative license revocation, DOT HS 806 921, Washington, D. C., April 1986, U.S. Department of Transportation.

19. National Highway Traffic Safety Administration: State and community program area report: alcohol countermeasures, Washington, D. C., Sept. 1986, U.S. Department of Transportation.
20. National Highway Traffic Safety Administration: State and community program area report: motorcycle safety, Washington, D. C., Sept. 1986, U.S. Department of Transportation.
21. National Highway Traffic Safety Administration: State and community program area report: occupant protection, Washington, D. C., Sept. 1986, U.S. Department of Transportation.
22. National Highway Traffic Safety Administration: State and community program area report: pedestrian safety, Washington, D. C., Sept. 1986, U.S. Department of Transportation.
23. National Highway Traffic Safety Administration: Summary of results: motorcycle accident factors study, No. 341-428/331, Washington, D. C., Sept. 1980, U.S. Government Printing Office.
24. National Highway Traffic Safety Administration: Testing how well new cars perform in crashes, Washington, D. C., 1986, U.S. Department of Transportation.
25. National Highway Traffic Safety Administration: Traffic safety '84: a report on activities under the national Traffic and Motor Vehicle Safety Act of 1966 and the Motor Vehicle Information and Cost Savings Act, Washington, D. C., 1986, U.S. Department of Transportation.
26. National Safety Council: Accident facts, 1990 ed. Chicago, 1990, The Council.
27. Night Riding Tradeoffs, Driver, September 1981, p. 18.
28. Partyka, S. C.: Lives saved by child restraints from 1982 through 1987, DOT HS 807 371, Washington, D. C., Dec. 1988, National Highway Traffic Safety Administration.
29. Partyka, S. C.: Lives saved by selt belts from 1983 through 1987, Washington D. C., August 1988, National Highway Traffic Safety Administration.
30. Partyka, S. C.: Papers on victim age-pedestrians and occupants, DOT HS 807 292, Washington, D.C., June 1988, National Highway Traffic Safety Administration.
31. Podolsky, D.. Alcohol, other drugs, and traffic safety, Alcohol Health and Research World 9(4):16, Summer 1985, p. 16.
32. Prudential Property and Casualty Insurance Company: Family auto insurance, Holmdel, N. J., 1980.
33. Richardson, H. A.: Risk of death from motor vehicle crashes, Washington, D. C., June 1987, National Highway Traffic Safety Administration.
34. The ABC's of winter driving—accelerating, braking, cornering, Family Safety, Winter 1982, p. 4.
35. Trumble, J., and Walsh, J. M.: A new initiative for solving age-old problems, Alcohol Health and Research World 9(4):2, 1985.
36. U.S. Department of Transportation: Automobile occupant crash protection: progress report no. 3, DOT HS-805 474, Washington, D. C., July 1980.
37. U.S. Department of Transportation: The car book, Stock No. 0-335-248, Washington, D.C., Jan. 1981, U.S. Government Printing Office.
38. Watson, G. S., Zador, P. L., and Wilks, A.: The repeal of helmet use laws and increased motorcyclist mortality in the United States, 1975-1978, American Journal of Public Health 70(6):579, June 1980.
39. Williams, A. F., and others: Drugs in fatally injured young male drivers, Public Health Reports 100:19, 1985
40. Wilson, D.C.: The effectiveness of motorcycle helmets in preventing fatalities, Washington, D. C., March 1989, National Highway Traffic Safety Administration.
41. Womble, K. B.: The impact of minimum drinking age laws on fatal crash involvements—an update of the NHTSA analysis, Washington, D. C., Jan. 1989, National Highway Traffic Safety Administration.

Resource Organizations

Alliance for Traffic Safety
c/o Hazel McKee
370 Wakeforest Drive, #89
Houston, TX 77098

American Association for Automotive
Medicine
40 Second Avenue
Arlington Heights, IL 60005

American Automobile Association
1000 AAA Drive
Heathrow, FL 32745

American Pedestrian Association
P O. Box 624, Forest Hills Station
Forest Hills, NY 11375

American Seat Belt Council
P. O. Drawer F
300 Buckelew Avenue
Jamesburg, NJ 08831

American Trucking Associations
2200 Mill Road
Alexandria, VA 22314

Automobile Occupant Protection Association
PO. Box 289
Glenview, IL 60025

Center for Auto Safety
2001 S Street N. W., Suite 140
Washington, DC 20009

Federal Highway Administration
400 7th Street S. W.
Washington, DC 20590

Highway Users Federation for Safety and
Mobility
1776 Massachusetts Avenue N. W.
Washington, DC 20036

Insurance Institute for Highway Safety
1005 Glebe Road
Arlington, VA 22201

Japan Automobile Manufacturers Association
1050 17th Street N. W.
Washington DC 20036

Moped Association of America
130 East Main Street
Malone, NY 12953

Mothers Against Drunk Driving
669 Airport Freeway, Suite 310
Hurst TX 76053

Motorcycle Industry Council, Inc.
3151 Airway Avenue, Building P-1
Costa Mesa, CA 92626

Motor Vehicle Manufacturers Association of
the United States
7430 2nd Ave, Suite 300
Detroit, MI 48202

Motorcycle Safety Foundation
5525 Twin Knolls Road, Suite 330
Columbia, MD 21045

National Association of Women Highway
Safety Leaders
3008 North 16th Drive
Phoenix, AZ 85015

National Highway Traffic Safety Administration
400 7th Street S.W.
Washington, DC 20590

National Motorcycle Commuter Association
P. O. Box 3371
Reston, VA 22090

Remove Intoxicated Drivers
P. O. Box 520
Schenectady, NY 12301

Tire Industry Safety Council
National Press Building
529 14th Street N. W., Suite 844
Washington, DC 20045

Vehicle Equipment Safety Commission
4660 Kenmore Avenue
Alexandria VA 22304

CHAPTER 7

Applying What You Have Learned

1. Take a close look at your car or truck and determine which of the following safety features it has:

Year _____ Make _____ Model _____

a) Airbags
   Driver Side ☐
   Passenger Side ☐
b) Anti-lock brakes ☐
c) Automatic safety belts ☐
d) Center high-mounted
   brake light ☐
e) Energy absorbing bumpers ☐
f) Four-wheel drive ☐

g) Head restraints
   Front ☐
   Rear ☐
h) Padded dashboard ☐
i) Radial tires ☐
j) Rear-seat shoulder
   harnesses ☐
k) Right side mirror ☐
l) Anti-lacerative windshield
   glazing ☐

2. Examine your motor vehicle insurance policy. Which of the following policy endorsements do you have, and what is the cost for each endorsement?

a) Bodily injury/property liability ☐ $ _____
b) Medical payments ☐ $ _____
c) Uninsured motorist ☐ $ _____
d) Comprehensive coverage ☐ $ _____
e) Collision coverage ☐ $ _____
f) Towing ☐ $ _____
g) Temporary vehicle replacement ☐ $ _____
      (post-accident car rental)
            Total Premium Payment $ _____

8 Occupational Safety

Since nearly one third of a person's adult life is spent on the job, it is not surprising to find that the working environment has a vital impact on one's health.

A. A. Coetzee: Toxic pollution: its effects on health, National Safety and Health News

AN ACT

To assure safe and healthful working conditions for working men and women, by authorizing enforcement of the standards developed under the Act, by assisting and encouraging the States in their efforts to ensure safe and healthful working conditions; by providing for research, information, education, and training in the field of occupational safety and health; and for other purposes.*

With these words Congress prefaced the enactment of the Occupational Safety and Health Act of 1970, the most comprehensive legislation ever developed for worker safety. In this chapter we will investigate the development of occupational safety in the American workplace. Some of the questions that will be addressed are: What measures have been taken by government and industry to protect workers against occupational illnesses and injuries? What protections are available to the worker who has been injured or who has developed an occupational illness? What does the future hold for the occupational safety and health movement?

HISTORICAL PERSPECTIVE

Much of the safety movement in America has been based on the influence of industrial safety programs. The first trade societies, developed in the 1790s (Chapter 1), provided compensation for members who were injured on the job. Worker safety was considered a personal responsibility. If a person was hurt on the job and could not continue working, his or her family and friends would become the only means of financial support.

By the mid-nineteenth century mechanization in industry not only increased productivity, it also presented hazards of a type and magnitude previously unknown to

---

*Occupational Safety and Health Act of 1970 Public Law 91–596, 91st Congress 5.2193 December 29,1970.

the American worker. Crushing injuries and amputations were common in mining, railroading, and steel production.

Women received no more protection than men in the industrial setting. In the textile mills of the Northeastern United States, women frequently lost hands and fingers in spinning machines. Concerned with the public outcry that something be done, Massachusetts legislators in 1877 passed the first law requiring that protective guards be placed on hazardous machinery.[2] By the early 1900s most industrial states had enacted similar legislation.

Although machine guarding reduced some of the hazards in the workplace, men and women continued to be killed or permanently injured all too often in work-related incidents. Most people came to accept injury and death as conditions of progress.

In an attempt to gain some type of relief for workers, Alabama and Massachusetts passed employer-liability acts in the late 1880s, which allowed employees to sue their employers for damages resulting from injuries. However, few claimants were successful, since most courts allowed employers to use three basic defenses:

1. Contributory negligence: If employers could prove that the worker had contributed in some way to his or her injury, they were not held liable.

2. Assumption of risk: All work involves certain risks, and employees were expected to know beforehand about the particular risks of their jobs.

3. Negligence of a fellow worker: If the employer could show that a fellow worker's actions had contributed to the accident, then the employer could not be held responsible for the injuries that had been incurred.

At the turn of the century no one had a clear idea of how many workers were injured or killed in industrial accidents. One of the first comprehensive surveys of industrial injuries was the Pittsburgh Survey of 1906 to 1907. Investigators in Allegheny County, Pennsylvania (the greater Pittsburgh area), recorded 526 on-the-job fatalities and 500 permanently disabling injuries between July 1, 1906, and July 1, 1907. This survey was the impetus for the development of industrial safety in America.[33]

Following the publication of the Pittsburgh Survey in 1907, the Association of Iron and Steel Electrical Engineers (AISEE) was organized. Considered the first national industrial safety group to be established in America, the AISEE was formed to evaluate the problems and hazards of the relatively new profession of electrical engineering.

After a series of disastrous mine accidents between 1900 and 1910, the U.S. Bureau of Mines was created in 1910. The objectives of the Bureau were to investigate mine accidents, study health hazards, and seek some means of correcting the situation.

In 1911, the passage of the first workers' compensation law in Wisconsin had a profound effect on the direction of the industrial safety movement in America. The law provided (1) medical care to injured workers, (2) compensation for workers during the period of disability, and (3) benefits to their survivors in case of death.[5]

The most important provision of this legislation was that it eliminated the question of fault for the injury; regardless of the cause, the injured worker would be covered. Between 1911 and 1915, 30 other states enacted similar legislation. These laws provided a financial incentive for employers to prevent accidents, since more injuries would mean higher premiums for compensation insurance.

In October of 1913 the National Safety Council (NSC) opened its first office in Chicago. Since its inception, many industries have become associated with the NSC in an effort to improve the safety of the American worker. An estimate of work-related fatalities during the National Safety Council's first year was 23,055 for a working population of 38 million. The fatal accident rate was 61 per 100,000 workers. In 1989 NSC statistics indicated that 10,400 work-related deaths occurred in a workforce of 117 million people; the death rate was 9 per 100,000 workers.[21] For nearly 80 years the National Safety Council has provided leadership in promoting the safety of Americans in the workplace.

Influenced by public concern for worker safety, the federal government established the Department of Labor in 1913 "to foster, promote, and develop the welfare of wage earners of the United States."[13] To assist the Department of Labor, a Bureau of Labor Statistics was created to collect and tabulate data concerning occupational injuries. In 1926 the Bureau began compiling records regularly for a significant number of industries.

Many of the advances in industrial safety during the 1920s and 1930s involved the development of safety standards and codes. Published by groups such as the American Standards Association, the American Society of Safety Engineers, and the National Safety Council, these standards and codes spelled out the procedures for safely performing work skills and using protective equipment. The Walsh-Healey Public Contracts Act of 1936 required companies working under federal contracts of $10,000 or more to follow specific safety codes and standards. During this time H. W. Heinrich proposed that many job-related accidents were the result of workplace stress. Because of his insight there was a new focus on worker attitudes, training, and unsafe behavior.

During World War II and the Korean conflict, expansion of the work force and increased working hours led to increased work-related deaths and injuries. However, with a return to peacetime, accident rates began another steady decline through the 1950s.

Safety engineers and managers could not determine whether it was because of an increasingly inexperienced work force (resulting from the post–World War II baby boom) or rapid changes in production and technology, but the trend of the 1960s was an increase in occupational injuries and illnesses. The increasing costs of medical care and compensation for disabled workers and the financial losses to industry through lost production were staggering. In 1964, President Lyndon B. Johnson convened the President's Conference on Occupational Safety to appraise the status of industrial safety in the American workplace. This conference marked a renewal of federal commitment to worker protection. In 1970, the culmination of President Johnson's efforts was the enactment of the Occupational Safety and Health Act, probably the most widely sweeping piece of legislation to affect both industry and workers alike.

OSHA: THE ACT AND ITS ADMINISTRATION

Coverage of the Occupational Safety and Health Act extends to all employers and employees in all 50 states, including the District of Columbia, Puerto Rico, and all other territories under federal government jurisdiction. The act does not cover self-employed persons, farms on which only immediate members of the owner's family are employed, and workplaces already protected by other federal statutes (for example, miners are protected under the federal Mine Safety and Health Act of 1977).

Under the Occupational Safety and Health Act, the **Occupational Safety and Health Administration (OSHA)** was created within the Department of Labor. To accomplish the goal of assuring working men and women of a safe and healthful environment, the agency was given a number of responsibilities:[26]

1. Maintenance of a reporting and recordkeeping system to monitor job-related injuries and illnesses.
2. Development of mandatory job safety and health standards and their effective enforcement.
3. Research in occupational safety and health.
4. Establishment of training programs to increase the number and competence of occupational safety and health personnel.
5. Provision for the development, analysis, evaluation, and approval of state occupational safety and health programs.

In the following sections we will attempt to clarify each of these OSHA responsibilities.

Recordkeeping and Reporting

Statistical data are vital to the monitoring and solving of problems in the workplace. Recognizing this need, the Occupational Safety and Health Administration, in collaboration with the Department of Labor's **Bureau of Labor Statistics (BLS)**, established a record-keeping and reporting system with which employers covered by the act must comply. Although virtually all employers in the Private sector are covered by the act, to ease the record-keeping burden on small businesses, federal regulations exempt employers having 10 or fewer employees from the OSHA reporting requirements.[26]

Employers of 11 or more employees must maintain records of occupational injury and illness. Recordable cases consist of all occupational deaths and illnesses and those nonfatal injuries that result in one or more of the following: loss of consciousness, one or more lost workdays, restriction of work or motion, transfer to another job, or medical treatment other than first aid.[24] As defined by OSHA, an **occupational illness** is any abnormal condition or disorder, other than one resulting from an occupational injury, caused by exposure to environmental factors associated with employment; included are acute and chronic illnesses that may be caused by inhalation, absorption, ingestion, or direct contact with toxic substances or harmful agents.[8] Damage to muscles, nerves, tendons and joints as a result of repetitive motion over an extended period of time would be considered an occupational illness rather than an injury. An **occupational injury** is any injury, such as a cut, fracture, sprain, or amputation, that results from a work-related accident or from exposure involving a single incident in the workplace.

Forms that are used to maintain these data are the OSHA No. 200—Log and Summary of Occupational Injuries and Illnesses, and the OSHA No. 101—Supplementary Record of Occupational Injuries and Illnesses. All records must remain in a place of business for 5 years after their initial posting.

OSHA No. 200 and the annual survey of occupational injuries and illnesses. Within 6 days of an accident, all recordable injury and illness cases must be noted on OSHA form number 200 (Fig. 8-1).[4, 25] Minor injuries such as small cuts and bruises do not have to be logged on this form. Other information that is tabulated includes the number of injuries and illnesses without lost workdays, the number of injuries and illnesses involving lost or restricted workdays, and the number of days away from work or requiring restriction of activity.[25]

At the end of each calendar year, the data are summarized on the log sheets. This information serves three purposes: (1) It helps OSHA compliance officers get a better picture of plant safety during an inspection (employers are required to have logs available at all times in their establishments), (2) it provides employees with information about safe or unsafe conditions in their workplace (log summaries must be posted for employee inspection during February each year), and (3) it is used by the Bureau of Labor Statistics in its Annual survey of occupational injuries and illnesses.

The survey data are then used by OSHA to determine injury and illness trends in the various private-sector industries (Table 8-1). Intraindustry comparisons can further delineate particular types of establishments that may need special emphasis in terms of OSHA safety inspections or safety-related research. Notice in Table 8-1 that incidence rates are based on 100 full-time equivalent workers (100 workers x 40 hours per week x 50 weeks per year = 200,000 hours). Utilizing this formula, a small company of 50 workers could compare its record with a much larger corporation having 5000 or 6000 workers. Companies using different manufacturing techniques and producing totally different products can still be compared using incidence rates.

The Supplementary Data System. Because employers report injuries and illnesses to the Bureau of Labor Statistics using only summary data from OSHA form number 200, the Annual Survey of Occupational Injuries and Illnesses contains no information about worker characteristics, type of illness or injury, or source of the illness or injury. Nevertheless, for every recordable case the Occupational Safety and Health Act requires that an employer identify this specific information.

Recognizing that uniformity of data among states was essential for the development of a reliable data base, the BLS developed the **Supplementary Data System (SDS)** in 1978. Under this voluntary program, participating states process information

Bureau of Labor Statistics
Log and Summary of Occupational
Injuries and Illnesses

For Calendar Year 19 _____

U.S. Department of Labor

Company Name

Establishment Name

Establishment Address

Form Approved
O.M.B. No. 1220-0029

NOTE: This form is required by Public Law 91-596 and must be kept in the establishment for 5 years. Failure to maintain and post can result in the issuance of citations and assessment of penalties. *(See posting requirements on the other side of form.)*

RECORDABLE CASES: You are required to record information about every occupational death; every nonfatal occupational illness; and those nonfatal occupational injuries which involve one or more of the following: loss of consciousness, restriction of work or motion, transfer to another job, or medical treatment (other than first aid). *(See definitions on the other side of form.)*

Case or File Number	Date of Injury or Onset of Illness	Employee's Name	Occupation	Department	Description of Injury or Illness
Enter a nonduplicating number which will facilitate comparisons with supplementary records.	Enter Mo./day.	Enter first name or initial, middle initial, last name.	Enter regular job title, not activity employee was performing when injured or at onset of illness. In the absence of a formal title, enter a brief description of the employee's duties.	Enter department in which the employee is regularly employed or a description of normal workplace to which employee is assigned, even though temporarily working in another department at the time of injury or illness.	Enter a brief description of the injury or illness and indicate the part or parts of body affected. Typical entries for this column might be: Amputation of 1st joint right forefinger; Strain of lower back; Contact dermatitis on both hands; Electrocution—body.
(A)	(B)	(C)	(D)	(E)	(F)

Type, Extent of, and Outcome of INJURY

Extent of and Outcome of INJURY

Fatalities	Nonfatal Injuries				
Injury Related	Injuries With Lost Workdays				Injuries Without Lost Workdays
Enter DATE of death.	Enter a CHECK if injury involves days away from work, or days of restricted work activity, or both.	Enter a CHECK if injury involves days away from work.	Enter number of DAYS away from work.	Enter number of DAYS of restricted work activity.	Enter a CHECK if no entry was made in columns 1 or 2 but the injury is recordable as defined above.
Mo./day/yr.					
(1)	(2)	(3)	(4)	(5)	(6)

Type, Extent, and Outcome of ILLNESS

Type of Illness							Fatalities	Nonfatal Illnesses			
CHECK Only One Column for Each Illness *(See other side of form for terminations or permanent transfers.)*							Illness Related	Illnesses With Lost Workdays			Illnesses Without Lost Workdays
Occupational skin diseases or disorders	Dust diseases of the lungs	Respiratory conditions due to toxic agents	Poisoning (systemic effects of toxic materials)	Disorders due to physical agents	Disorders associated with repeated trauma	All other occupational illnesses	Enter DATE of death.	Enter a CHECK if illness involves days away from work, or days of restricted work activity, or both.	Enter a CHECK if illness involves days away from work.	Enter number of DAYS away from work.	Enter number of DAYS of restricted work activity.	Enter a CHECK if no entry was made in columns 8 or 9.
(a)	(b)	(c)	(d)	(e)	(f)	(g)	Mo./day/yr.				
							(8)	(9)	(10)	(11)	(12)	(13)

PREVIOUS PAGE TOTALS

TOTALS (Instructions on other side of form.)

Certification of Annual Summary Totals By _____ Title _____ Date _____

OSHA No. 200

POST ONLY THIS PORTION OF THE LAST PAGE NO LATER THAN FEBRUARY 1.

INJURIES

ILLNESSES

FOLD

FIG. 8-1 OSHA Form No. 200

Source: U.S Department of Labor, Occupational Safety, and Health Administration

Table 8-1   BLS estimates of occupational injury and illness incidence rates by industry, 1987–1988

| Industry Division | Incidence Rates[c] | | | | | |
| | Total Recordable Cases[d] | | Lost Workday Cases | | Nonfatal Cases Without Lost Workdays | |
	1984	1983	1984	1983	1984	1983
Private Sector[e]	8.0	7.6	3.7	3.4	4.3	4.2
Agriculture, forestry, and fishing[e]	12.0	11.9	6.1	6.1	5.9	5.8
Mining	9.7	8.4	5.3	4.5	4.3	3.9
Construction	15.5	14.8	6.9	6.3	8.6	8.5
Manufacturing	10.6	10.0	4.7	4.3	5.9	5.7
Transportation and public utilities	8.8	8.2	5.2	4.7	3.6	3.5
Wholesale and retail trade	7.4	7.2	3.3	3.1	4.2	4.1
Finance, insurance, and real estate	1.9	2.0	0.9	0.9	1.0	1.1
Services	5.2	5.1	2.5	2.4	2.7	2.7

Source: Bureau of Labor Statistics, U.S. Department of Labor.   See footnotes below.

OSHA Definitions (See OSHA form No. 200 and Recordkeeping Requirements, Revised 1978):

Occupational injury is any injury such as a cut, fracture, sprain, amputation, etc., which results from a work accident or from an exposure involving a single incident in the work environment.

Occupational illness of an employee is any abnormal condition or disorder, other than one resulting from an occupational injury caused by exposure to environmental factors associated with employment. It includes acute and chronic illnesses or diseases which may be caused by inhalation, absorption, ingestion, or direct contact.

Lost workdays are those days which the employee would have worked but could not because of occupational injury or illness. The number of lost workdays should not include the day of injury or onset of illness. The number of days includes all days (consecutive or not) on which, because of injury or illness: (1) the employee would have worked but could not or (2) the employee was assigned to a temporary job, or (3) the employee worked at a permanent job less than full time, or (4) the employee worked at a permanently assigned job but could not perform all duties normally connected with it.

Recordable cases are those involving an occupational injury or occupational illness, including deaths. *Not* recordable are first aid cases which involve one-time treatment and subsequent observation of minor scratches, cuts, burns, splinters, etc., which do not ordinarily require medical care, even though such treatment is provided by a physician or registered professional personnel.

Nonfatal cases without lost workdays are cases of occupational injury or illness which did not involve fatalities or lost workdays but did result in: (1) transfer to another job or termination of employment, or (2) medical treatment, other than first aid, or (3) diagnosis of occupational illness, or (4) loss of consciousness, or (5) restriction of work or motion.

Source and footnotes for table above and on page 31.
Source: Bureau of Labor Statistics, U.S. Department of Labor, survey involving a nationwide sample of approximately 280,000 units.
[a]Industry division 2 and 3 digit SIC code totals include data for industries not shown separately.
[b]Standard Industrial Classification Manual, 1972 Edition, 1977 Supplement.

[c]Incidence Rate = $\dfrac{\text{(No. of injuries \& illnesses} \times 200{,}000) \text{ OR (No. of lost workdays} \times 200{,}000)}{\text{Total hours worked by all employees during period covered}}$

200,000 = base for 100 full-time equivalent workers (working 40 hours per week, 50 weeks per year).
[d]Includes fatalities. Because of rounding, the difference between the total and sum of the rates for lost workday cases and nonfatal cases without lost workdays may not reflect the fatality rate.
[e]Excludes farms with less than 11 employees.

Source: Accident Facts 1991 Edition, National Safety Council (1990), Chicago.

from employers' first reports of injury submitted to their industrial commissions or workers' compensation agencies. Depending on a state's requirements, employer injury reports may consist of insurance forms, worker compensation forms, or OSHA No. 101. To alleviate confusion, the Bureau of Labor Statistics requires states to code cases in the same manner using a standard format. Variables included in the information system are worker occupation, industry, sex of worker, nature of the injury or illness, body part or parts affected, and source of injury. This material is provided to the Bureau of Labor Statistics by each of the 37 participating states.

Although it does not directly identify the causes of accidents, the SDS can be used to identify areas where problems exist. Fig. 8-2, Fig. 8-3, and Fig. 8-4 are examples of data that can be generated from the Supplementary Data System. Fig. 8-2 illustrates the nature or kinds of injuries and illnesses that occurred, while Fig. 8-3 specifies the body parts that were affected. Fig. 8-4 takes these data one step further and combines the information so that we can tell how body parts are most often damaged.

A more recent development by the Bureau of Labor Statistics has been the Work Injury Report Survey Program (WIR), which encompasses special surveys of occu-

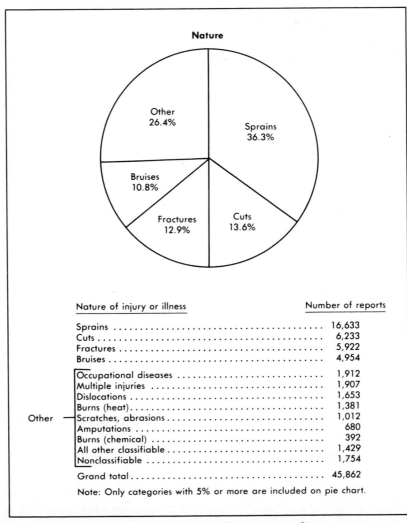

FIG. 8-2 Nature of occupational injuries and illnesses in Indiana.

Source: The Department of Statistics, Division of Labor, State of Indiana (1990).

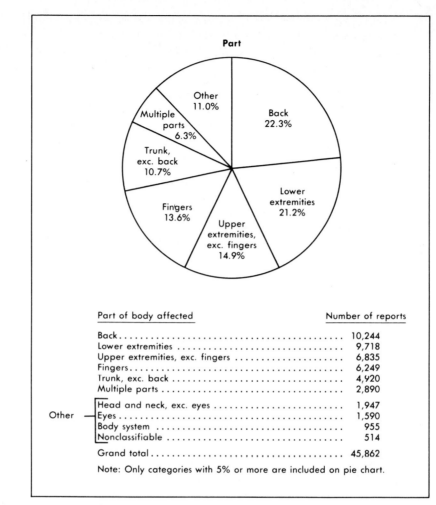

FIG. 8-3 Parts of the body affected by occupational injuries and illnesses in Indiana.
Source: The Department of Statistics, Division of Labor, State of Indiana (1990).

pational injuries to obtain causal information tailored to specific problem areas that are identified by the Supplementary Data System. These surveys include questions relating to how a particular injury occurred, what work and environmental factors were involved, and the extent of training and work experience of the injured worker.

Workers who have been involved in the type of accident that is under investigation are sent detailed questionnaires by state industrial commissions participating in the program. The resulting data are processed and analyzed by the Bureau of Labor Statistics. Final reports are used by OSHA and the National Institute for Occupational Safety and Health in the development of industry compliance standards and employee training programs.

With the Annual Survey of Occupational Injuries and Illnesses, the Supplemen-

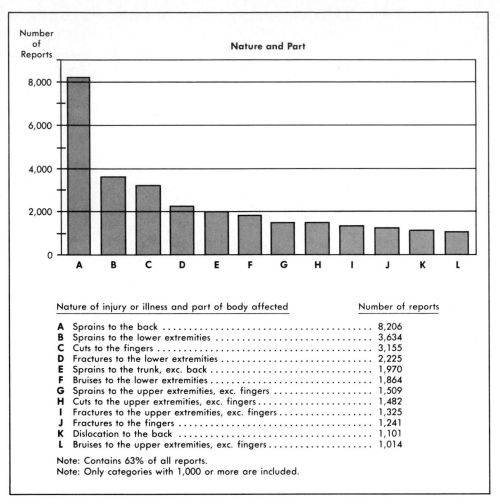

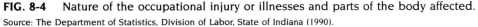

Nature of injury or illness and part of body affected	Number of reports
A Sprains to the back	8,206
B Sprains to the lower extremities	3,634
C Cuts to the fingers	3,155
D Fractures to the lower extremities	2,225
E Sprains to the trunk, exc. back	1,970
F Bruises to the lower extremities	1,864
G Sprains to the upper extremities, exc. fingers	1,509
H Cuts to the upper extremities, exc. fingers	1,482
I Fractures to the upper extremities, exc. fingers	1,325
J Fractures to the fingers	1,241
K Dislocation to the back	1,101
L Bruises to the upper extremities, exc. fingers	1,014

Note: Contains 63% of all reports.
Note: Only categories with 1,000 or more are included.

FIG. 8-4   Nature of the occupational injury or illnesses and parts of the body affected.
Source: The Department of Statistics, Division of Labor, State of Indiana (1990).

tary Data System, and the Work Injury Report Program, the Occupational Safety and Health Administration has a variety of methods for collecting data that can be used to improve the process of standards development and enforcement.

OSHA Job Safety and Health Standards

In carrying out its duties OSHA is responsible for promulgating legally enforceable standards. The intent of these job-safety standards is to ensure that employers adopt a variety of means and methods to protect their workers.

Today, OSHA uses a four-step process for setting worker health standards:[3]
1. The first step in the process of regulation is to determine that a particular practice or substance poses a ''significant risk'' to workers.

2. Once a ''significant risk'' is verified, a way to substantially reduce that risk must be developed.

3. Next, OSHA will look at the best available data to set the most protective exposure limit that is both technologically and economically feasible.

4. The final consideration deals with how employers can meet the proposed safety standard in the most cost-effective way. In this manner, workers will be provided with effective protection from job hazards without severely penalizing the employer's earning or profit potential.

A primary source of recommendations for standards is the **National Institute for Occupational Safety and Health (NIOSH)**; however, only OSHA, which is part of the Department of Labor, can *set* and *enforce* health and safety standards. State and local governments, standards-producing organizations such as the National Fire Protection Association, labor unions, industry representatives, or interested persons may also make proposals for the development of standards.

To assist businesses and the public in keeping current with OSHA standards, the OSHA subscription service was developed. Available through the Superintendent of Documents, this service provides listings of recently adopted industry standards or changes that have appeared in the *Federal Register*. Other ways of keeping current with rules and regulations include trade association newsletters and private publications such as *Safety management* and *The OSHA compliance letter*.

Enforcement of standards. To enforce its standards, the Occupational Safety and Health Administration is authorized to conduct workplace inspections; however, with 1200 inspectors, only 1% to 2% of the 3 million workplaces covered by OSHA can be visited annually. For this reason a system of inspection priorities has been established.

Imminent danger situations are given top priority. An imminent danger in a workplace occurs when there is a reasonable certainty that serious injury or death may occur to workers if the condition is not corrected immediately. When an OSHA office receives a request from employees or an authorized representative (for example, a union) for an inspection, the area director reviews the information and determines whether the allegation warrants an inspection. On inspection, if an imminent danger is found, the employer must remove affected employees from the danger area and make immediate corrections. If the employer fails to take the appropriate actions, OSHA has the authority to shut down that section of the workplace where the danger exists.

A second priority is given to those situations where a fatality has occurred or an accident has resulted in the *hospitalization* of five or more employees. In either of these cases, employers are required by law to report details of the incident within 48 hours to OSHA. The post-accident investigation is used to determine whether OSHA standards were violated.

Employee complaints to OSHA that do not represent imminent danger or documented serious injury are third on the list of priorities; inspectors will be sent to the worksite at some later date. In all cases where an employee has filed a complaint with

OSHA, his or her name will be withheld from the employer if the agency is requested to do so. This protects the worker from possible employer retaliation.

Because some industries are more dangerous than others, OSHA has established as its fourth priority the inspection of high-hazard workplaces. Industries are selected for inspection on the basis of death, injury, and illness incidence rates determined from the BLS Annual Survey. Businesses involved in the exposure of employees to toxic substances also fit into this category. High-hazard industries include roofing and sheet metal construction, longshoring, logging contractors, and meat processing. Hazardous substance industries involve the use of cotton dust, lead, and silica, to name a few.

The final inspection priority for OSHA is that of low-hazard industries, such as the wholesale and retail trade, hospitals, and educational services. Whereas the inspection ratio for high-hazard industries is approximately 1 out of 21, the inspection ratio for low-hazard groups is 1 out of 1300.

Citations, penalties, and hazard abatement. If violations are found during an inspection, the OSHA compliance officer has authority to issue citations at the worksite after receiving approval from the area director. Citations inform employers and employees of regulations and standards that have been violated. The citation also specifies the amount of time that has been allotted to correct or abate the problem. In conjunction with citations that are issued, various fines may be proposed.

A major complaint of businesses in the past was that OSHA personnel would cite violations but failed to offer assistance about how the problems could be corrected. Today OSHA compliance personnel not only identify hazards in the workplace, but they are now responsible for assisting employers in identifying ways to abate these hazards at the time the violations are discovered; thus correction of problems can occur much sooner.

Assistance for Implementing Safety Programs

A program authorized by Congress in the late 1970s and which OSHA now provides is a free on-site consultation service in every state. Unlike an OSHA inspection, there are no citations or penalties issued for violations discovered during the on-site consultation; however, it is required that serious hazards be corrected.

In most states this consultative service is provided by a state agency; for example, the Virginia Department of Labor and Industry has a Division of Voluntary Compliance and Training, which provides on-site consultations at the request of an employer. The Division also holds conferences and offers safety training courses throughout the year. When a state agency does not provide this service, private contractors have been authorized to conduct the on-site consultations.

Other sources of assistance in developing safety programs may come from insurance carriers, which offer periodic inspections to evaluate hazards; and trade associations, which offer specific information to member companies. Many unions are willing to offer safety and health expertise to industries, since both groups are interested in worker safety. The National Safety Council also has a broad range of information services available to a variety of businesses.

State OSHA Programs

In an effort to reduce duplication of resources and services provided by the federal government and state agencies, the Occupational Safety and Health Act permits any state to develop and enforce its own occupational safety and health program. Currently, 25 states have their own OSHA programs, with sole inspection authority in the industries they cover.

State OSHA programs offer a number of advantages over the federal system. State agency personnel are more likely to be familiar with the specific needs and problems of local businesses and industries. Whereas the federal Occupational Safety and Health Act provides for worker health and safety in private industry only, state OSHA programs can cover everyone in the state, including state and county employees as well as persons in agriculture.

Research in Occupational Safety and Health

Although it does not fall under the direct responsibility of the Occupational Safety and Health Administration, occupational safety and health research is a major component of Public Law 91–596, the Occupational Safety and Health Act. The act gives the Department of Health and Human Services the responsibility for developing a research agency; thus, the National Institute for Occupational Safety and Health (NIOSH) was created.[24] NIOSH is responsible for identifying occupational safety and health hazards, determining methods to control them, and recommending federal standards to limit these hazards.

''Why,'' you may ask, ''isn't NIOSH a part of the Department of Labor as is the Occupational Safety and Health Administration?'' Simply put, the answer is to prevent a conflict-of-interest situation. NIOSH is mainly concerned with scientific knowledge about hazards and the use of technology in eliminating them, while OSHA and the Department of Labor must consider the financial condition of industry in terms of setting and enforcing standards. Consequently, it was believed that if NIOSH was under the control of the Department of Labor, occupational safety research would be slanted in favor of the financial considerations of industry, rather than toward the well-being of workers.

As part of the Department of Health and Human Services' Public Health Service, NIOSH has focused on the effects of exposure to hazardous substances in the workplace, methods for analyzing and measuring the levels of exposure, and recommendations for worker exposure limits.[14]

EXPOSURE TO OCCUPATIONAL HAZARDS

Injury, death, and disease resulting from occupational hazards create one of the nation's most serious, yet preventable, public health problems. Data from the National Safety Council and the Bureau of Labor Statistics indicate that approximately 10,400 persons died in work-related accidents in 1989, while an additional 1.7 million workers lost workdays as a result of occupational injuries or illnesses.[21]

While occupational injuries are often dramatic and easy to identify, occupationally related disease information is elusive. The recording and reporting of illnesses present many measurement problems. Employers and physicians are often unable to recognize illnesses as work-related because signs and symptoms may not occur until some time after a person has retired or changed employment. The time between exposure and onset of disease symptoms presents a serious problem regarding accountability; employers are often reluctant to accept liability for a work-related disease that may have originated under a different employer. At the same time, a number of chronic diseases (lung disorders, cancer) may involve multiple factors, including age of the worker, diet and nutrition, smoking, and environmental exposures as well as the job-related hazards. Lack of employee awareness regarding hazardous work exposures increases the difficulty of identifying a disease as occupational, since physicians often rely on patient information to make a diagnosis.

As technology has increased, so have the potential problems. We are only now realizing the impact of some of these hazards. Although certain occupations present greater risk in terms of illness or injury, almost every job has a certain number of hazards associated with it.

Two programs that have been available in identifying occupational hazards are the Bureau of Labor Statistics' Supplementary Data System and NIOSH's Hazard Evaluation and Technical Assistance (HETA) program.[7] The information from the 37 states participating in the SDS has been used to develop a reliable data base concerning characteristics of work-related illness and injury. These descriptions have been used to identify the conditions that most frequently expose workers to a higher risk of illness or injury and to set priorities for future research activities.

The HETA program has been particularly valuable to small businesses that have been unable to afford the professional services needed to uncover and correct problems in their workplaces. The evaluations are conducted by NIOSH personnel at the request of employers. Not only do the evaluations help to identify new hazards, they provide workers and employers with methods for correcting the hazardous situations. It is not surprising to find that blue-collar workers (laborers, operatives, and craftworkers) account for the majority of injuries in the American workplace. Blue-collar workers make up 40% of the workforce but have 77% of the work-related illnesses and injuries. White-collar workers (professionals, technicians, and salesworkers) make up 48% of employment but account for only 12% of the illnesses and injuries. The other group, service workers (educational, hospital, and food-service personnel) account for 12% of the labor force and 11% of work-related illnesses and injuries.[32]

Let's take a look at some of the workplace hazards that have been uncovered by NIOSH investigators, especially those that have implications for the future. Most of the problems that we will discuss are considered occupational illnesses. The determinant for distinguishing work-related illnesses from injuries is the "single incident concept." Contact with a hot surface or caustic chemical, which produces a burn in that single exposure, is an injury. Likewise, a single blow that damages tendons in the hand is also considered an injury. However, if tissue damage results from prolonged exposure to a hazardous substance or environmental factor, or occurs after repeated movement over a period of time, it is considered an occupational illness.

Back Injuries

Although back injuries were known to be common in certain occupations that required the lifting of heavy objects, it wasn't until the late 1970s that information about these injuries identified how widespread the problem was. At least one third of all jobs require the lifting or moving of heavy objects. Workers' compensation data indicate that material-handling tasks are the leading cause of injuries and lost-time accidents in industry.[14,16]

Excessive application of force from lifting can put a severe strain on the musculature of the lower spine, especially when awkward postures are required. It is not uncommon to find nurses, fire fighters, and ambulance personnel who have become disabled while attempting to rescue or move accident victims. Fatigue from attempting to handle heavy objects also contributes to accidents involving crushing injuries of the hands and feet. The muscles used to maintain grip show evidence of fatigue first; thus grip strength may be a key factor in developing lifting standards.[14]

Since there are currently no OSHA standards regulating lifting in the workplace, NIOSH researchers are attempting to establish limits on maximum load and reach distance for workers. At the same time they are developing a battery of dynamic strength tests that can be used to predict worker capabilities for lifting tasks. The strength tests can be used to identify workers who may be susceptible to injuries associated with lifting. The lifting standards will reduce the likelihood of workers lifting materials that would put an excessive strain on the musculoskeletal system.

Wear and Tear Syndrome

Have you ever worked in a factory or on an assembly line where you performed the same task repeatedly? Maybe it was tightening several bolts or screws on a dishwasher, soldering wires on a radio, or cutting fabric of varying lengths. How many bolts were tightened, wires soldered, and pieces of fabric cut during the 8- or 10-hour shifts that you worked? Now multiply that times 5 days per week and 50 weeks per year. A lot of wear and tear on muscles, ligaments, tendons, and joints, wouldn't you say?

That small amount of trauma every day adds up. Jobs requiring highly repetitive motions of the hands and arms cause irritation, swelling, and inflammation of tissues and joints. Biomechanical hazards that have been identified by NIOSH investigators include excessive wrist flexion and extension, reaching overhead, pinch gripping, and wrist and arm torque.[7,34] Because the individual traumatic events do not result in immediately observable injuries, several years may elapse before the worker begins to have problems. Diseases resulting from this chronic physical abuse include bursitis, tendonitis, and **carpal tunnel syndrome (CTS)**. CTS is a disorder that occurs when inflamed tendons and membranes in the wrist swell, damaging nerves that control finger and hand movement. High incidences of these disorders may occur in the following occupations: small component assembly, meat cutting, letter sorting, and garment and upholstery work.

Current research indicates a low level of employer and employee awareness about many of the chronic effects of repeated trauma. Annually, about 23,000 cases of "wear and tear" disorders, which account for 250,000 lost workdays, are reported to the Occupational Safety and Health Administration. However, NIOSH researchers estimate that because of this lack of awareness, a more accurate figure would be more than 230,000 cases annually.[14]

Another type of chronic trauma that may affect a great number of workers is "occupational vibration." It is estimated that approximately 6.8 million American workers are exposed daily to "whole-body vibration," including truck drivers, heavy equipment operators (bulldozers, tractors), and even flight attendants.[14,16] These people have one thing in common: They work in environments where there is a constant state of vibration. To date, no studies have shown a relationship between whole-body vibration and a particular disease or injury.

The same cannot be said for the 1.2 million workers who are exposed to "hand-arm vibration." Hand-arm vibration (sources of which include pneumatic, electrical, and gasoline-powered tools) has been causally linked to a disease of the hands known as **Raynaud's phenomenon** or vibration white fingers (VWF).[15] This progressive disease involves, in most cases, irreversible occlusion of the blood vessels in the fingers. In its terminal stages, it can result in gangrene and loss of fingers. Recent studies completed on miners and construction workers who used pneumatic drilling and chipping tools found that nearly 50% of the miners and 39% of the construction workers exhibited symptoms of this disease.[16]

Have you ever used a chain saw, power drill, or other vibrating equipment? Do you remember the tingling sensation and numbness you felt in your hands after using it? Think about the men and women who use those tools 8 hours a day; you can imagine the wear and tear to which their hands and arms are subjected.

You say you've never worked in construction, never worked on an assembly line, and never operated any type of vibrating tool. Well, have you ever typed, used a key punch, or worked on a video display terminal? Office work can also be a very repetitive operation, and can lead to problems similar to those just mentioned.

Studies of key-punch operators and typists have shown that the constant repetition of the typing activity may lead to painful wrist problems. The resulting condition is known as **tenosynovitis**, the inflammation and swelling of tendons in the wrist.[9,14]

In the 1990s, the computer has become an essential piece of equipment in the workplace. In 1978 there were approximately 1 million computers in use in the United States; in 1992 the number is expected to reach more than 30 million.[36] An essential component of any computer is its video display terminal (VDT), an electronic device that displays information on a screen. The computer provides its user with a quick and easy way to input and access large amounts of data. Records management, billing, proposal writing, manuscript editing, and graphics production are just a few of the tasks that have been simplified by this device.

As with any new technology, misperceptions by the public and inappropriate use of such equipment can present problems in the workplace. In the late 1960s, national attention was drawn to the emission of ionizing radiation (x-rays) from color television sets. Quick action by the electronics industry and the development of solid-state circuitry eliminated this problem in the early 1970s.

In the 1980s, questions arose about low frequency electromagnetic field emissions from VDTs. As electricity flows through a computer monitor, it generates electromagnetic fields (charged particles of radiating energy) (EMFs) at differing frequencies. Though high frequency radiation (which can damage cellular tissues) is produced by the monitor, it does not escape; however, very low frequency (VLF) and extremely low frequency (ELF) electromagnetic fields escape from the screen and cabinet of a video display terminal.[30] Concern about these low-level EMFs came to the forefront when laboratory studies of human cells revealed abnormal structural changes after exposure to them.

Several investigations in the mid-1980s suggested that low-level EMFs might be linked to an increased incidence of miscarriage in women who worked at video display terminals more than 20 hours per week. With nearly 20 million women utilizing VDTs in the workplace, these findings, if true, had far reaching implications about the use of computers. In 1984 the National Institute for Occupational Safety and Health launched a large-scale, long-term study to investigate these claims.

Findings of the NIOSH study, published in 1991, indicated that there were no significant differences in the miscarriage rates of women who used VDTs and those who did not.[27] In fact, the miscarriage rate of women using VDTs was slightly lower than that of the control group. However, it was noted that VDT operators (word processing and information specialists) had significantly higher levels of visual and musculoskeletal problems than control groups. They also tended to exhibit higher levels of anxiety and irritability than people who do not operate VDTs. Further investigation indicated that the repetitive nature of the occupation (that is, working at a keyboard and display screen 8 hours a day and 5 days a week) plus work-station problems, such as screen glare, improper keyboard and screen placement, inadequate table and chair heights, and excessive noise levels, appeared responsible for most of the problems.[15]

If you use a VDT regularly, keep the following points in mind[6,36]:

1. Many VDT operators experience eyestrain because they need corrective lenses.

2. Fluorescent lighting and sunlight can make a VDT difficult to read; locate equipment away from large windows and protect screens from bright overhead lights.

3. For easier viewing, the screen should be 18 to 20 inches from your eyes and the screen face should be tilted back 10 to 20 degrees.

4. Ideal working posture should permit a 90-degree angle between the upper and lower arm, leaving the forearm horizontal. This will take the strain off the upper back

and shoulders. In addition, the angle between the upper and lower leg should be 90 degrees or slightly more to provide maximum seated comfort.

5. Regular interruptions from VDT work, requiring operators to walk and stretch, are needed to maintain comfort and productivity.

6. Impact or dot-matrix printers, which are used with computer operations, can create noise levels in the 90 dBA range. (At this level OSHA standards require hearing protection for employees.) Attenuating covers and acoustic pads should be used with these printers to reduce sound levels to a more acceptable (60 dBA) range.

As we have seen, ''wear and tear'' syndrome can occur in a variety of occupations, from heavy construction to clerical work. A scientific approach often used by occupational safety and health specialists to correct such job-related disorders is known as **ergonomics**. This problem-solving technique looks at how the workplace, job practices, and equipment design features interact to affect the well-being of employees.

When specific tools are used, the problem often involves positioning or design. If a worker must stand or sit in an awkward position to use equipment, repositioning of tools or perhaps raising or lowering a workbench may be all that is necessary to correct the situation. Meetings may need to be held with tool manufacturers to redesign equipment. In the case of high-vibration, hand-held equipment, investigations have centered on better insulation to reduce vibration.

In occupations where redesigning or repositioning of equipment is not feasible, a modification of work practices is the most likely alternative. Strategies for rotating workers in and out of particularly stressful operations can maintain production levels while protecting the quality of the employees' lives. Modification of the work-rest regimen could also have beneficial, long-term effects. By providing more relief time, an employer can reduce the likelihood of a worker's developing a ''wear and tear'' disorder; this, in turn, is likely to prevent a decline in worker productivity.

Another means of affecting work practices is through education and training of personnel. Too often an employee learns the correct method of equipment operation through a trial and error process in which errors translate into injuries. Workers who are aware of the possible difficulties that may arise are more likely to avoid stressful and hazardous work practices; they are also better prepared to recognize the signs and symptoms of a disorder in its earliest and most easily treatable stages.

Farm Safety

Because it is a highly mechanized and rapidly evolving industry, farming constantly presents new hazards for workers. The term *agriculture* includes not only production of livestock and crops, but forestry, fishing, and services related to farming, such as grain storage and fertilizing. In 1989, there were 1300 agricultural work-related deaths, of which 700 involved farm residents doing farm work and 600 involved nonfarm residents working in industries classified as agricultural.[21]

Although the largest number of farm work injuries are associated with falls, the most severe consequences are the result of tractor and agricultural machinery-related accidents. Tractor accidents account for only 8% of agricultural injuries, yet they are responsible for more than one third of all farm-related deaths. Likewise, agricultural machinery plays a role in only 16% of farm accidents, but the resulting injuries account for 52% of farm-related permanently disabling injuries and 20% of worker deaths.

Tractors present three primary risks for operators: (1) overturns, which account for nearly half of the tractor fatalities; (2) cases in which operators are run over by their vehicles when they fall from the tractor; and (3) cases in which the power takeoff of the tractor is used to operate other machinery.

In the majority of tractor accidents, victims either fail to recognize the danger involved in the operation of these vehicles or they do not have the necessary skills to handle a tractor under adverse conditions. Three design changes that were implemented in the 1970s have the potential to significantly reduce these fatalities, provided farm personnel use them. The design of a wider front base for newer tractors lowers their center of gravity, thus decreasing the chance of vehicles overturning. The addition of roll cages, similar to those used in car racing will protect the driver from being crushed should the tractor tip over. However, to receive the maximum protection from a roll cage, the tractor operator must remain in the cab of the vehicle; this requires the use of a safety belt, a modification that can be added to most tractors.

The power takeoff of a tractor presents a special hazard for the operator. The power takeoff is an attachment on most tractors that can be used to operate a variety of machinery including bushhogs, snowblowers, and augers. Through a series of gears, power from the tractor's engine is used to operate this equipment, often at relatively high revolutions per minute (RPM). If loose clothing, such as a jacket, shirt sleeve, or glove, is caught by one of the revolving drive shafts, a person's hand, arm, or body can be drawn into the machinery quickly—and there will be no way for this person to shut down the device. To prevent such a tragedy, any moving drive shaft should be covered to lessen the chances of being caught. At the same time, no fewer than two people should use the power takeoff on a tractor. When operating machinery with a power takeoff, someone should be standing by to shut off power immediately should a problem arise. Any time there are machinery malfunctions, attempts to repair them should take place only when the power is off and all moving parts have stopped.

In the 1990s there has been an increasing sophistication, not only of farm machinery, but in those methods used to attain high crop yields. Major advances have occurred in the development of fertilizing agents and pesticides; however, the use of chemical methods to increase both the quality and quantity of crops has been a mixed blessing for agricultural workers. Although the benefits of spraying fields and crops with a vast array of fertilizers, weed killers, and pesticides is obvious in terms of increased yield, little is known about the long-term effects of the absorption and inhalation of these substances by farm workers; however, the association between pesticides and adverse health effects has been demonstrated clearly during their formulation and manufacture.

In the late 1970s, the production of the pesticides dibromochloropropane (DBCF) and kepone was curtailed when they were found to produce such side effects as sterility and severe neurological disorders in workers handling them.[23] It is likely that similar problems might occur in agricultural workers who handle a wide variety of chemicals. It is essential that these individuals utilize the appropriate protective gear when applying such agents.

Chemicals in the Workplace

Today you would be hard pressed to find an occupation that did not expose you to some type of chemical hazard. Even persons who do not work directly with hazardous materials can be exposed to them in the work environment. Contact with chemical hazards most often occurs through inhalation of gases or fine, particulate matter. Some materials can be absorbed through the skin and affect internal organs, while others may damage the skin surface directly.

The effects of chemical contact may be either localized or systemic. A **localized effect** means that the action of the chemical takes place at the point of contact. Many of the chronic lung diseases are the result of localized damage. Exposure to cotton dust over a period of time is likely to result in a condition known as **byssinosis** or brown lung disease. A condition that is well documented in the coal-mining industry is **pneumoconiosis** or black lung disease. Both of these illnesses result from workers inhaling large amounts of cotton or coal dust, leading to the obstruction of air passages.

A **systemic effect** means that the action of the hazardous substance occurs somewhere other than the point of entry. Vinyl chloride, a gas used in the production of plastics, has been linked with a rare form of liver cancer known as **angiosarcoma**. Although it is inhaled into the lungs, the actual site of damage is the liver. Organic solvents used in the manufacture of paints, resins, and varnishes have a similar systemic effect; they are inhaled or absorbed through the skin and can cause liver or kidney damage. Many of these substances may cause cancer in animals and humans and are called **carcinogens**.

A substance that has been shown to cause both localized and systematically adverse health effects is asbestos. Since this fibrous material is fire- and wear-resistant and demonstrates a high degree of strength, it is not surprising to find that asbestos has been widely used as an insulating material for the last 60 years in ships and buildings.

Asbestos insulating material that is in good condition presents little environmental risk to a building's occupants; however, if the insulation is disturbed on a regular basis through vibration or human contact, it will release microscopic fibers into the air. As these fibers are inhaled into the lungs over a period of years, obstructive deposits known as ''asbestos bodies'' form and block breathing passages. This chronic lung condition, known as ''asbestosis,'' is an example of a localized adverse effect. A systematic disease associated with the ingestion of asbestos fibers is mesothelioma, a form of cancer affecting the lining of the chest cavity, and the abdominal wall. Asbestos fibers may penetrate the lungs and imbed in the pleural wall or continue into the abdomen to do their damage.[11,22]

Is exposure to toxic or hazardous substances in the workplace a new phenomenon? Definitely not! Although standards development for occupational exposure to hazardous substances gained widespread attention in the 1970s with the passage of the Occupational Safety and Health Act, descriptions of the dangers of exposure to materials in the workplace were recorded as early as the eighteenth century, when English physicians reported the classic signs of byssinosis (brown lung disease) in mill workers who were exposed to cotton and flax dust. Similar historical literature reported the plight of English coal miners and their signs of pneumoconiosis, better known as black lung disease.[19]

Workers in the mills and mines would initially develop a tightness in the chest accompanied by some breathing difficulty. The longer they worked under these conditions, the more severe the symptoms became. Incessant coughing, shortness of breath on exertion, and the development of a "barrel chest" were trademarks of these occupations. The prolonged irritation of the coal and cotton dusts that were inhaled for 15 to 20 years led to the progressive obstruction of lung tissues, and ultimately work in the dusty atmosphere of the cotton mill or coal mine would become impossible. Seldom did these people live beyond 50 years of age.

In the 1800s, there was an increasing recognition of the hazards associated with exposure to lead.[20] Its low melting point, malleability, and weather resistance allowed this metal to be used without the need for complex equipment; however, it was found that lead vapors produced during the heating process were inhaled and easily absorbed into the blood stream. Plumbism or lead poisoning was shown to be responsible for loss of finger movement in printers who were exposed to hot lead type. Bouts of intense abdominal pain (known as "lead colic") were also linked to exposure to lead. Because the kidneys were involved in filtering lead from the bloodstream, prolonged absorption of lead was responsible for progressive and irreversible loss of kidney function in some workers.

Benzene is a solvent that was first used in the rubber industry at the turn of the century; it still has numerous applications in chemical and petroleum manufacture. As early as 1909 there were numerous reports of fatal cases of benzene poisoning resulting from workplace exposure. Deaths have occurred from both acute and chronic exposures. Acute benzene poisoning has led to worker deaths when vapors were inhaled in enclosed spaces, such as tanks containing residues.

By far the more common problem with benzene is chronic poisoning. The early uses of benzene resulted in the widespread exposure of workers to vapor levels in excess of 1000 ppm (1000 parts per million parts of air). This particular figure doesn't mean much until you realize that current workroom air standards developed by the Occupational Safety and Health Administration limit worker exposure to no more than 10 ppm (10 parts per million parts of air).[18] The major effects of exposure to benzene vapor over prolonged periods of time involve the body's blood-forming system, including reductions in white and red blood cell counts as well as bone marrow changes. These changes have been shown to occur in workers exposed to concentrations of no more than 60 ppm. Generally the removal of employees from the benzene environment for extended periods (4 to 8 months) have resulted in a correction of the blood cell difficulties. However, the literature indicates significant evidence that chronic benzene exposure may produce leukemia in susceptible individuals. The National Institute for Occupational Safety and Health estimates that 2 million persons in the workforce have potential exposure to benzene.[18]

Coal dust, cotton dust, asbestos, lead, and benzene are but five of the thousands of substances that can cause harm to those in the workplace. Each of these hazards has been around for some time, allowing researchers to document the problems with which they are associated and to establish safe worker exposure limits. What about the nearly 1000 new chemicals that are introduced into the workplace annually? For example, do you know some of the hazards associated with trichloroethylene, polychlorinated biphenyls (PCBs), polyvinyl chloride (PVC), or ethylene oxide? For that matter, do you know whether you are working with any of these in your job?

As we have seen, exposure to chemicals in the workplace can pose a variety of serious problems. It is estimated that as many as 25 million American workers are exposed to one or more chemical hazards regularly. In addition, NIOSH's yearly investigations of occupational illnesses indicate that a substantial number of them result from workplace exposures to hazardous chemicals.

Because of the seriousness of these safety and health problems and the lack of chemical hazard information available to many employees and employers, OSHA issued a new standard in November 1983. The standard, entitled *Hazard communication* (29 CFR 1910), was implemented to reduce the incidence of chemical-related illnesses and injuries in the workplace by providing employees with information they need to protect themselves and ensuring that their employers are providing them with adequate protection.[37]

Hazard communication starts with chemical manufacturers and importers. They must provide available scientific data concerning the hazards of the chemicals they import or produce. Each chemical is evaluated for its potential to cause adverse health effects and its potential as a physical hazard such as flammability. Companies may do their own research, or they may use findings from governmental agencies or private research groups.

Information obtained from hazard evaluations is used by chemical manufacturers, importers, and distributors to develop container labels and material safety data sheets (MSDS) for each chemical produced. Every container of hazardous chemicals that is shipped must have a label that identifies the following:[37]

1. Chemical name.
2. Name, address, and emergency phone number of the chemical manufacturer or importer.
3. Physical hazards: Is it flammable? Corrosive? Explosive?
4. Health hazards: Is it carcinogenic? Will it irritate the skin?
5. Storage and handling instructions.
6. Protective clothing or equipment to be used when handling the chemical.

If the chemicals are transferred to other containers at the worksite of the purchaser, that company becomes responsible for labeling any new containers.

A more detailed hazard communication tool, which must be supplied to purchasers by chemical manufacturers and importers, is the material safety data sheet (MSDS). The MSDS (see Fig. 8-5) provides detailed information about the following:[29, 37]

1. Identity of the manufacturer.
2. Hazardous and worker exposure limits* to the chemical.
3. Physical characteristics of the chemical—boiling point, specific gravity, appearance, and odor, etc.
4. Fire and explosion data—ignition temperature, flash point, and special firefighting procedures.
5. Health hazard data—effects of exposure, emergency care procedures.
6. Reactivity data—conditions to avoid, incompatible chemicals, hazardous decomposition products.
7. Spill or leak procedures.
8. Special protection information—personal protective equipment that may be needed for handling.

Copies of material safety data sheets for hazardous chemicals to which workers are likely to be exposed must be readily available to them.

This new OSHA standard also requires employers to develop a written hazard-communication plan and an employee training program. The written plan basically spells out the specifics of container labeling, the use of material safety data sheets, employee training, and the listing of hazardous chemicals in each work area.

In their employee training programs, employers are required to discuss the new hazard-communication standard, explain the use of container labels and MSDSs, identify the location of specific hazardous chemicals in the workplace, and demonstrate the methods used to protect workers from these chemical hazards.

Rather than directly control exposure levels in the workplace, the hazard-communication standard is designed to enhance employer and employee awareness of the safety and health hazards associated with chemical substances. Ultimately, this should result in increased worker use of personal protective devices, improved work practices, and a reduction in the incidence of chemical-source injury and illness.

Women in the Workplace

With the passage of the Civil Rights Act of 1964, discrimination based on race, religion, sex, or national origin was made illegal. In particular, Title VII of the Civil Rights Act struck down laws that discriminated in terms of employment opportunities.[35] Restrictive regulations, such as limitations on the amount of weight a woman could lift on the job, were overturned; thus, job opportunities for women took on a

---

*Two exposure limits that you may see are the American Conference of Governmental Industrial Hygienists (ACGIH) Threshold Limit Values (TLVs) or the Occupational Safety and Health Administrations's Permissible Exposure Limits (PELs). Usually measured in parts per million (ppm), these exposure limits represent chemical concentrations under which it is believed nearly all workers may be exposed day after day with no adverse effects.

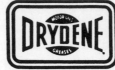

MATERIAL SAFETY DATA SHEET

Date Issued: 02/14/90

Section A — IDENTIFICATION & EMERGENCY INFORMATION

Manufacturer's Name: **DRYDEN OIL COMPANY**
Emergency Telephone Number: **301-574-5000**
800-777-1466

Address: **9300 Pulaski Highway**
Baltimore, Maryland 21220

Product Name: DRYDENE STEEL CUT MEDIUM (SCM), STEEL CUT HD (SCH)

Chemical Name:
PETROLEUM LUBRICATING OIL

CAS Number (For Finished Product):
COMPLEX MIXTURE
CAS Number Not Applicable

Product Appearance & Odor:
CLEAR, DARK BROWN LIQUID
MILD PETROLEUM ODOR

HAZARDOUS MATERIALS IDENTIFICATION SYSTEM (HMIS)

Health	1	Flammability	1	Reactivity	0

HAZARD RATING: Least-0 Slight-1 Moderate-2 High-3 Extreme-4

SECTION B — COMPONENTS & HAZARD INFORMATION

COMPONENTS	CAS NO. OF COMPONENTS	APPROXIMATE CONCENTRATION
Lubricating Oil Base Stock	64741-88-4	GREATER THAN 80%
Proprietary Additives	Mixture	LESS THAN 20%

Exposure Limit for Total Product: 5mg/m^3 oil mist   Basis: OSHA Reg 29 CFR 1910.1000

THIS PRODUCT IS *NOT* CONSIDERED HAZARDOUS BY OSHA IN ACCORDANCE WITH 29 CFR 1910.1200 OSHA COMMUNICATION STANDARD

This product does not contain any chemical listed as a carcinogen or potential carcinogen by OSHA, IARC, Monographs or the National Toxicology Program.
U.S. TSCA Inventory: All components are included on the U.S. TSCA Inventory.
CERCLA: Under the Comprehensive Response, Compensation, and Liability Act, (CERCLA), certain release to air, land, or water may be reportable to the National Response Center at 800-424-8802. Circumstances surrounding the release and cleanup determine reportability. This product is not subject to CERCLA reporting requirements.
SARA Sections 301-304: Threshold Planning Quantity (TPQ), EPA Regulation 40 CFR 355 SARA 301-304 not applicable.
SARA Sections 311-313: Toxic Chemical Release reporting, EPA Regulation 40 CFR 372 SARA Sections 311-313 not applicable.

SECTION C — PHYSICAL DATA
THE FOLLOWING DATA ARE APPROXIMATE OR TYPICAL VALUES.

Boiling Range: Not Determined

Specific Gravity (H$_2$O=1): .880..895 APPROX.

Pour Point: -18.C

Viscosity: 100.F CST 25/35

Solubility in Water: Negligible, Below 0.1%

Percent Volatile by Volume: NEGLIGIBLE
Vapor Pressure: NEGLIGIBLE
Vapor Density: GREATER THAN AIR
Evaporation Rate: NEGLIGIBLE

SECTION D — FIRE PROTECTION INFORMATION

FLASH POINT & METHOD: Min. ASTM D-92 C.O.C. ºC,(ºF.)
176(350)

AUTOIGNITION TEMPERATURE:
NOT DETERMINED

NATIONAL FIRE PROTECTION ASSOCIATION (NFPA) — Hazard Identification
Health —1
Flammability —1
Reactivity —0
Basis: Recommended by Dryden Oil Co.
HAZARD RATING (NFPA):
4-Extreme 3-High 2-Moderate
1-Slight 0-Insignificant

UNUSUAL FIRE & EXPLOSION HAZARDS:
NONE

FLAMMABLE LIMITS or EXPLOSIVE LIMITS: (Approximate Percent By Volume In Air)
THESE ARE *ESTIMATED* VALUES.
LOWER FLAMMABLE LIMIT— 0.9%   *UPPER* FLAMMABLE UNIT— 7%

Form No. MSDS 1.0   67   (01)   BALTIMORE, MARYLAND   341   (OVER)
6560

FIG. 8-5 A material safety data sheet for petroleum lubricating oil.

Source: City of Fairfax Fire and Rescue Service, Fairfax, Va.

SECTION D — FIRE PROTECTION INFORMATION (Continued)

HANDLING PRECAUTIONS: Use product with caution around heat, sparks, pilot lights, static electricity and open flame.

DECOMPOSITION PRODUCTS UNDER FIRE CONDITIONS: Fumes, smoke, carbon monoxide, sulfur oxides, aldehydes and other decomposition products, in the case of incomplete combustion.

EXTINGUISHING MEDIA & FIRE FIGHTING PROCEDURES: Foam, water spray (fog), dry chemical, carbon dioxide and vaporizing liquid type extinguishing agents may all be suitable for extinguishing fires involving this type of product, depending on the size or potential size of fire and circumstances related to the situation. Plan fire protection and response strategy through consultation with local fire protection authorities or appropriate specialists.
The following procedures for this type of product are based on the recommendations in the National Fire Protection Associations' *Fire Protection Guide on Hazardous Materials.*

Use water spray, dry chemical, foam or carbon dioxide. Use water to keep fire-exposed containers cool. If a leak or spill has not ignited, use water spray to disperse the vapors and to provide protection for men attempting to stop a leak. Water spray may be used to flush spills away from exposures. Use supplied air breathing equipment for enclosed or confined spaces or as otherwise needed.

EMPTY CONTAINER WARNING: "Empty" containers retain residue (liquid and/or vapor) and can be dangerous. DO NOT PRESSURIZE, CUT, WELD, BRAZE, SOLDER, DRILL, GRIND OR EXPOSE SUCH CONTAINERS TO HEAT, FLAME, SPARKS OR OTHER SOURCES OF IGNITION: THEY MAY EXPLODE AND CAUSE INJURY OR DEATH. Do not attempt to clean since residue is difficult to remove. "Empty" drums should be completely drained, properly bunged and promptly returned to a drum reconditioner. All other containers should be disposed of in an environmentally safe manner and in accordance with governmental regulations.

SECTION E — PROTECTION & PRECAUTIONS

RESPIRATORY PROTECTION: No Special Requirements under ordinary conditions of use and with adequate ventilation.
VENTILATION: No Special Requirements under ordinary conditions of use.
PROTECTIVE GLOVES: Use chemical resistant gloves, if needed, to avoid prolonged or repeated skin contact.
WORK PRACTICES / ENGINEERING CONTROLS:
Keep containers and storage containers closed when not in use. Do not store near heat, sparks, flame or strong oxidants.

EYE PROTECTION: Use splash goggles or face shield when eye contact may occur.
PERSONAL HYGIENE: Remove contaminated clothing: launder or dry clean before reuse. Remove contaminated shoes and thoroughly clean before reuse; discard if oil-soaked. Clean skin thoroughly after contact, before breaks and meals, and at end of work period. Product is readily removed from skin by waterless hand cleaners followed by washing thoroughly with soap and water.

SECTION F — SPILL OR LEAK PROCEDURE

ENVIRONMENTAL IMPACT: Report spills as required to the appropriate authorities. U.S. Coast Guard Regulations require immediate reporting of spills that could reach any waterway including intermittent dry creeks. Report spill to the Coast Guard toll free number 800-424-8802.
PROCEDURES IF MATERIAL IS RELEASED OR SPILLED: Recover free product. Add sand, earth, or other suitable absorbent

material to the spill area. Minimize breathing vapors. Minimize skin contact. Open all windows and doors. Keep product out of sewers and watercourses by diking or impounding. Advise authorities if the product has entered or may enter sewers, watercourses, or extensive land areas.
ASSURE CONFORMITY WITH ALL APPLICABLE REGULATIONS.

SECTION G — REACTIVITY

STABILITY:	HAZARDOUS POLYMERIZATION:	CONDITIONS & MATERIALS TO AVOID:
Stable	Will Not Occur	Avoid heat, open flames and oxidizing materials.

HAZARDOUS DECOMPOSITION PRODUCTS:

Thermal decomposition products are highly dependent on the combustion conditions. A complex mixture of airborne solid, liquid, particulates and gases will evolve when this material undergoes combustion. Carbon monoxide and other unidentified organic compounds may be formed upon combustion.

SECTION H — Emergency & First Aid Procedures and Primary Routes of Entry

EYE CONTACT:
If splashed into the eyes, flush with clear water for 15 minutes or until irritation subsides. If irritations persists, call a physician.
SKIN CONTACT:
In case of skin contact, remove any contaminated clothing and wash skin thoroughly with soap and water.
INGESTION:
If ingested, DO NOT induce vomiting; call a physician immediately.

INHALATION:
Vapor pressure is very low. Vapor inhalation under ambient temperature conditions is not normally a problem. If overcome by vapor from hot product, immediately remove from exposure and call a physician. Administer oxygen, if available. If over-exposed to oil mist, remove from further exposure until excessive mist oil condition subsides.

SECTION I — Effects of Overexposure

Skin: Prolonged or repeated skin contact may cause skin irritation.   **Eye:** Slight irritation.   **Ingestion:** Relatively non-toxic.

THE PRECISE COMPOSITION OF THIS MIXTURE IS PROPRIETARY INFORMATION. A MORE COMPLETE DISCLOSURE WILL BE PROVIDED TO A PHYSICIAN OR NURSE IN THE EVENT OF A MEDICAL EMERGENCY.

UNDER THE PENNSYLVANIA RIGHT TO KNOW ACT 35 P.S. 7311 (a), the specific chemical identity is being withheld as a trade secret, except in the event of a medical emergency.

FIG. 8-5 cont'd   A material safety data sheet for petroleum lubricating oil.

new dimension. No longer would the working woman be limited to the stereotyped jobs of the "weaker sex"; for example, clerical work, retail sales, nursing, and teaching.

In the 28 years since the passage of the Civil Rights Act, a new generation of women has moved into a wider range of industrial occupations that expose them to silica, lead, coal dust, and a variety of unknown toxic chemicals.

In the twentieth century a question has arisen: "Do women and men react differently to job stresses and toxic substances?" As early as 1902, the medical literature indicated that women were more readily affected by toxic substances than were men.[19] This was further supported by a 1908 congressional investigation of women working in the phosphorus match industry. Many of these women had suffered from "phossy jaw," a degenerative bone disease that caused a marked deformity of the lower jaw. However, because the majority of workers in this industry were women, it was not surprising to find that more women than men suffered from this condition. If the incidence of phossy jaw in men working in the match industry had been investigated, researchers would have discovered that men exposed to phosphorus were just as likely to develop the disease. However, this was not done, and the theory that women were the "weaker sex" gained credence.

This myth was reinforced after the Triangle Shirtwaist Factory fire in 1912. Because of blocked or nonexistent fire escapes, 154 women and young girls died. The disaster had a twofold effect: It made the public aware of the need to enforce fire safety codes in the workplace and it reconfirmed the fragile and delicate nature of women, since many of the victims were trapped in the fire when they could not move equipment away from exit doors.

These tragedies led many states to enact protective legislation concerning where, how, and when women should work, thus effectively blocking them from better paying jobs and an opportunity to compete with men in the workplace. Although Congress created a Women's Bureau within the Department of Labor in 1920 to promote employment opportunities for women, nothing was done to dispel the myth of female inferiority.[35]

The first detailed study of women in the workplace was completed during World War II. Because a large portion of the male population was involved in the war effort, women were needed to replace men in the workforce to maintain productivity at home. Women worked in steel mills, foundries, and factories—everywhere that men worked.

During the early 1940s, Dr. Anna Baetjer of Johns Hopkins University, with U.S. Army funding, investigated the capabilities of women in the performance of certain jobs and their susceptibility to job-related injuries and diseases. Her report, *Women in industry: their health and efficiency*, concluded[9,31]:

> There is no reliable evidence to support the generally accepted view that women are more susceptible than men to occupational hazards. At present there is no reason why normal women should be restricted anymore than men from working at jobs which involve the use of toxic substances.

Her conclusions have been quite accurate. The belief that women are unable to do many of the jobs performed by men seems to lack scientific foundation. Women are no more susceptible to hazards, such as temperature extremes and toxic agents, than are men. Comparisons of the relative frequencies of injuries and diseases occurring in both men and women in the same occupations and industries indicate that work activity, not the gender of the worker, is a more significant determinant. In fact, men in traditionally female occupations suffer injuries common to their female counterparts and with the same frequency.[31]

Although the average strength of women is approximately two thirds that of men, it should not be assumed that women cannot perform heavy, manual labor. Strength differences between working men and women are less significant than the differences between working and nonworking women. It has only been in recent years that strength training has become a socially acceptable endeavor for women. Hiring policies for positions requiring strenuous work should be based on meeting specific job criteria, regardless of whether the applicant is a man or a woman.

Nonetheless, Dr. Baetjer did have a word of caution for pregnant women. She stated that since major physiological changes take place during pregnancy, there was the possibility that exposure to toxic substances might affect both the mother and her developing child.

In the 45 years since Dr. Baetjer's study, only minimal research has been completed on the effects of job exposures on the developing fetus. It wasn't until the 1960s and the tragedy of the "Thalidomide babies" that the public became aware of the potential of a chemical's crossing the placental barrier and affecting the fetus. Thalidomide is an example of a **teratogen**, an agent that interferes with the development of the unborn child. Many of the children born to mothers who took this sedative early in pregnancy had either missing or deformed arms and legs.

In the early 1970s, studies of pregnant women and their work-related exposures to toxic substances indicated that a wide variety of chemicals could have a devastating effect on the fetus. Epidemiologic studies of women regularly exposed to anesthetic gases (doctors, dentists, nurses, and technicians) found that these women have two to three times as many miscarriages as nonexposed personnel. Also, there was an increase in the incidence of birth defects in children born to women working with anesthetic gases.[9]

Other potentially teratogenic substances, which may cause miscarriages, stillbirths, and birth defects when pregnant women are exposed to them, include polyvinyl chloride (PVC), one of the most commonly used plastics; and trichlorethylene and methylene chloride, used as degreasing and dry cleaning agents.

Many of these chemicals may also be present in the breast milk of mothers who are exposed, thus posing a very real threat to newborns and their chances for development. Just as the first 3 months of pregnancy are a critical time in which exposure to toxic materials can severely harm the fetus, the first 2 years of a child's life are important in terms of organ development. It has been theorized that affected brain centers may be responsible for later behavioral problems and learning disabilities as the exposed child gets older.

With the findings from these studies, it would be difficult to dispute Dr. Baetjer's concern for the pregnant woman and her unborn child. The answer seems to be simple: Women of child-bearing age should be excluded from occupations that involve exposure to potentially toxic substances. Right? Wrong! First, this policy would be highly discriminatory. It has been estimated by NIOSH that as many as 30% of the jobs women now hold may have some potential for exposure to toxic substances.[9] However, loss of these job opportunities for women could have a tremendously negative impact on the economic situations of many American families.

Second, what about the fertile male and the effects of his exposure to the same toxic substances? In many cases, research has indicated that men exposed to such toxic agents as lead, vinyl chloride, benzene, ethylene oxide, and chlorinated hydrocarbons have suffered from a number of reproductive problems, including infertility, abnormal sperm development, and genetic disorders.[17,18,20] Since these chemicals can cause a change or mutation in the genetic material of a living cell, they are called **mutagens**. The study involving women who worked with anesthetic gases also investigated the effects on men. The study found that the risk of miscarriage for wives whose husbands were exposed to anesthetic gases was twice that of women whose husbands were not exposed. A similar finding indicated that the incidence of birth defects in the children of exposed male operating-room personnel was almost twice that of children whose fathers were not exposed. Another investigation demonstrated that women whose husbands worked in the vinyl chloride and plastic industries had a significantly higher incidence of miscarriages and stillbirths than the rest of population.[9]

What is the answer? Ideally, it would be to establish OSHA exposure limits that would protect both men and women during their reproductive years, as well as their developing offspring. However, since many of the exposure limits for toxic substances have not been determined, a more realistic policy might include some of the following alternatives for women:
1. Transferring pregnant workers to jobs that have reduced exposures.
2. Allowing the use of sick-leave and maternity benefits during pregnancy.
3. Establishing a temporary leave policy without a loss of seniority and other benefits on returning to work.

Some people may argue that the above policies are exclusionary for women workers; however, if we look more closely, they only exclude the pregnant worker. Since a number of substances, including benzene, polychlorinated biphenyls (PCBs), and lead, have been shown to be more toxic to a fetus than to an adult, it seems reasonable that a pregnant worker should be protected from such an environment.

What would you do, if you were the director of health and safety in a battery plant that exposed a number of pregnant workers to high levels of lead? Would you use one of the alternatives that were mentioned, or would you leave this decision to your pregnant employees?

As of March 20, 1991, you would have no say in this matter. On that day the Supreme Court ruled that employers cannot exclude women of child-bearing age from jobs that pose reproductive hazards, even if they are actually pregnant. To do so would constitute illegal sex discrimination.[12]

In their majority decision, the Justices stated that ''decisions about the welfare of future children must be left to the parents who conceive, bear, support, and raise them, rather than to the employers who hire those parents. Women as capable of doing a job as their male counterparts may not be forced to choose between having a child and having a job."[12]

As we move through the decade of the 90s, a controversy that is likely to arise is the issue of liability for children injured in the womb by workplace hazards. If a company warns women of the risks involved and does its best to minimize them, will it later be held liable for such injuries?

Workers' Compensation

Each year nearly 2 million members of the nation's workforce are injured on the job or develop occupational illnesses that result in lost workdays.[21] Almost 100,000 people in this group will be permanently disabled. Who will take care of these employees and their families? Today, that's an easy question to answer: It will be their states' workers' compensation programs. However, at the turn of the century, the answer would not have been so simple. Before 1911 and the passage of the first workers' compensation laws, employees had to sue for damages and prove that an employer had been negligent.

Now, all 50 states and the U.S. territories have workers' compensation programs. They provide benefits to workers and their dependents for injuries or illnesses directly related to their employment, regardless of who is at fault. Benefits may vary from state to state, but they generally cover all medical and rehabilitation costs incurred by workers. Income or cash benefits to replace an employee's lost income usually equals two thirds of his or her weekly or monthly wage.[5] In the case of a permanent disability, Social Security payments from the federal government will supplement the worker's compensation payments.

These programs are paid for by employers; employees do not contribute to the payment of this insurance. In essence, this system encourages employer interest in safety and rehabilitation. By preventing and controlling occupational injuries and illnesses, an employer can reduce claims payments and insurance premiums, thus reducing costs to the firm.

A COMPANY SAFETY PROGRAM: USING WHAT WE'VE LEARNED

Whether your company has 5000 employees or 50, the basis for any safety program is worker protection. In this section let's examine the basic elements needed to develop a profitable strategy for handling occupational safety and health: organization and planning, identifying and correcting hazards, equipment design, safety training, disaster planning, and program evaluation.

Organization and Planning

The success of the safety program depends on staff and management involvement; however, initially, a single person must have overall responsibility. At a larger plant this may be the director of safety, the industrial hygienist, or the head of personnel;

whereas in a smaller establishment the plant manager or a foreman may assume this position. As a first order of business, the safety coordinator must become familiar with those OSHA standards that apply to the particular plant's operations. In some cases, this may include an understanding of those rules and regulations of the Environmental Protection Agency (EPA) that apply to chemical and toxic waste disposal.

Supervisory personnel can provide valuable information to a safety manager about the various technical operations in the plant. For instance, maintenance foremen are likely to be aware of OSHA standards that apply to electricity, lighting, heating equipment, and housekeeping procedures, while the supervisor in electroplating would have an understanding of the caustic and corrosive chemicals being used in that department. In a small business, employees who have been with the company for a number of years would be the people who could supply needed technical information to a safety supervisor.

Most businesses come under OSHA's general industry standards, but if you are involved with construction or maritime operations, you will need the OSHA standards that apply to these classifications. Persons involved in mining operations also have a separate set of standards, but they are not regulated by OSHA; instead, they are under the auspices of the Mine Safety and Health Administration (MSHA), another agency in the Department of Labor.

Some states have developed their own OSHA-approved programs. They may have adopted the existing federal standards, or they may have established their own standards. If your business is subject to state enforcement, the OSHA area office can refer you to the appropriate state agency for further assistance. These offices and agencies should be able to answer any questions you may have concerning the applicability of standards in the workplace.

Using the OSHA standards that apply to your business, it may be advantageous to develop a safety manual to provide both general and specific information for employees. General information might include proper procedures for lifting materials, reporting accidents, or evaluating the plant. The more specific information in this manual would include such things as the type of personal protective equipment required in the various departments around the plant and detailed instructions for the safe operation of the plant's equipment and machinery. Provision of such a manual will simplify the processes of personnel training and hazard identification and abatement.

During the early stages of organizing and planning, it is critical that top management personnel clearly demonstrate their interest in safety and health. If the supervisors and crew chiefs know that the plant managers adhere to all hazard-control rules and regulations issued by the company, they will be more inclined to carry out their own safety responsibilities. Unfortunately, in some businesses, upper management has given only lip service to safety programs. When supervisors reported hazards in their operations, plant managers made excuses and did not correct the problems. In those cases, it is fairly certain that the negative feelings of supervisors who were not supported by upper-level management were quickly communicated to other employees, and the safety programs failed. Only when there is active leadership, direct participation, and enthusiastic support by both management and nonmanagement personnel will a company's safety program succeed.

Identifying and Correcting Hazards

To maintain a safe and healthful workplace, a company needs to do two things: (1) identify workplace hazards that exist currently or that may develop, and (2) install procedures to control these hazards, eliminating them if possible.

Several approaches can be taken to identify workplace hazards. A review of past injury and illness records will enable a safety manager to locate those high-risk areas to which immediate attention must be directed. Records that are most likely to be available include OSHA form number 200 (the Annual Survey of Injuries and Illnesses) and state Workers' Compensation reports. These statistics can also be used by a company to compare its injury or illness rates with those of other companies in the same industry.

Injury and illness reports may not be the only records a company must maintain. Certain OSHA standards that deal with toxic substances and hazardous exposures require records on the exposure levels of employees, physical examinations, and autopsy findings. These records are used to identify particularly hazardous operations and jobs in an industry.

A second approach to identifying job hazards is the use of a self-inspection checklist. The checklist should be based on the OSHA standards that apply to your business. If your company has a safety manual, it may be worthwhile to include the checklist in that manual. For plants that have several operations, each department should have its own self-inspection checklist. The box on p. 294 lists some sample questions that pertain to general plant safety procedures.

Once hazards have been identified, it is time to institute control procedures. This may include equipment design, machine guarding, and the use of personal protective equipment to control unsafe conditions, or it may entail extensive employee training to eliminate unsafe worker practices.

Equipment Design

Design of the workplace and the equipment used in it not only reduces the incidence of illnesses and injuries, but it also gives employees a sense of confidence and security. Equipment should be designed so that it will make it difficult for a worker to be exposed to danger. In the auto industry large presses used to produce fenders, hoods, and door panels require operators to have both hands on control buttons before the machine can be activated. If the operator's hand is removed from one of these buttons, the press will immediately stop, thus eliminating the risk of the operator reaching into the machine and possibly losing a hand or arm.

All machines or operations that expose employees to rotating parts, pinch points, flying chips, particles, and sparks should be guarded. This may be no more elaborate than placing a shatterproof plastic shield or metal screen in front of the moving parts.

Employee Protection

	OK	Action Needed		OK	Action Needed
1. Is there a hospital, clinic, or infirmary for medical care near your business?	☐	☐	8. Are approved respirators provided for regular or emergency use where needed?	☐	☐
2. If medical and first aid facilities are not nearby, do you have one or more employees trained in first aid?	☐	☐	9. Is all protective equipment maintained in a sanitary condition and readily available for use?	☐	☐
3. Are your first aid supplies adequate for the type of potential injuries in your workplace?	☐	☐	10. Where special equipment is needed for electrical workers is it available?	☐	☐
4. Are there quick water flush facilities available where employees are exposed to corrosive materials?	☐	☐	11. When lunches are eaten on the premises, are they eaten in areas where there is no exposure to toxic materials, and not in toilet facility areas?	☐	☐
5. Are hard hats provided and worn where any danger of falling objects exists?	☐	☐	12. Is protection against the effects of occupational noise exposure provided when the sound levels exceed those shown in Table G-16 of the OSHA noise standard?	☐	☐
6. Are protective goggles or glasses provided and worn where there is any danger of flying particles or splashing of corrosive materials?	☐	☐			
7. Are protective gloves, aprons, shields, or other means provided for protection from sharp, hot, or corrosive materials?					

Develop your own checklist. These are only sample questions.

Source: U.S. Department of Labor, Occupational Safety and Health Administration: OSHA *Handbook for Small Businesses*, Washington, D.C., U.S. Government Printing Office.

Operations that expose employees to hazardous air contaminants such as coal dust, cotton dust, or lead particles may require a more complex and expensive ventilation system to provide adequate protection.

Depending on the type of workplace hazard, personal protective equipment may be rather elementary or quite complicated. Safety glasses and face shields provide facial and eye protection from flying particles, sparks, and splashing chemicals; hard

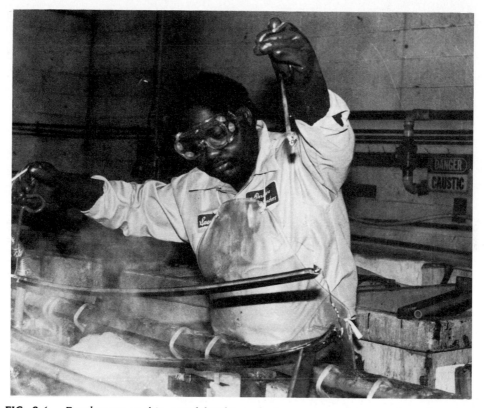

FIG. 8-6   Employees at this metal-finishing plant are exposed to caustic and corrosive chemicals on a regular basis. In addition to rubber gloves and goggles, this man is wearing a chemically treated worksuit, which will protect him from spills and splashes. Courtesy: Alexandria Metal Finishers, Inc. Alexandria, Va.

hats offer protection from bumping into equipment or from falling objects; and gloves, boots, and aprons offer partial covering for the limbs and torso (Fig. 8-6). The use of respirators can be a complicated matter; certain filters and masks will only be effective when specific contaminants are in the air. In some cases, full-body suits and self-contained breathing apparatus must be worn to provide the necessary protection.

Safety Training

As mentioned earlier in this chapter, occupational injuries are likely to occur during the first months of employment. Workers fail to perceive warnings of danger or underestimate hazards because they are unfamiliar with the environment. When an employee tackles a job without a clear understanding of what to do or what might go wrong, accidents are likely to result.

Initial safety training of new employees involves three phases. The first phase is a general orientation to the work environment. It should cover the standard safety practices that apply to all workers in the plant. For instance, some companies require that all workers wear safety glasses and steel-toed safety shoes. Plants manufacturing explosives or highly flammable products may ban the carrying of incendiary materials (lighters, matches, cigarettes) by employees. Since back injuries are a common problem, proper techniques for lifting may also be included.

The next step in this training process is a discussion of the company's emergency procedures. Workers will need to know how and where to report injuries; they should be informed of the locations of safety features such as emergency exits, fire extinguishers, gas masks, showers, and eye baths; and they should be made aware of disaster or evacuation plans that have been established. The use of a company safety manual would be a handy way to provide information for these first two phases of safety training.

The final phase of safety training for new employees involves instruction from their immediate supervisors. Here, they are given the step-by-step safety procedures for their particular jobs. Supervisors demonstrate appropriate work methods and routine safety checks. This is followed by hands-on practice of the same job procedures and precautions by the new workers. At the completion of this third phase of training, the new employee should have the impression that *work* and *safety* are inseparable terms.

In addition to conducting initial training sessions for new employees, a growing number of safety managers conduct regular observations of all personnel. Reporting sheets, which spell out specific job hazards, act as training materials for employees as well as monitoring instruments for the company's safety program. Workers who fail to pass any of the safety observations are scheduled for retraining with their supervisors, while those observed practicing good safety techniques are rewarded with bonuses such as free passes to amusement parks or sporting events.

With the advent of lightweight videotaping equipment, television has become a handy tool for safety training. Videotaping of unsafe actions as they occur allows supervisors to use a form of ''instant replay'' to correct hazardous behaviors. Videotapes of an accident scene can be used not only to analyze the incident, but also to train personnel so that a recurrence can be prevented.

Although safety training programs for new employees may vary from company to company, safety training generally involves three essential elements: (1) demonstrations of appropriate work methods, (2) observations and evaluations of worker performance, and (3) follow-up, which may include either corrective measures to improve performance or positive reinforcement for a job safely done. Safety training is an ongoing process and must be conducted on a regular basis from the first day on the job to the last.

Disaster Planning

While equipment design and safety training can do much to reduce workplace hazards, there is always a potential for disaster. No matter how slim the chance of a catastrophe's occurring, a company must be prepared for such an event. OSHA

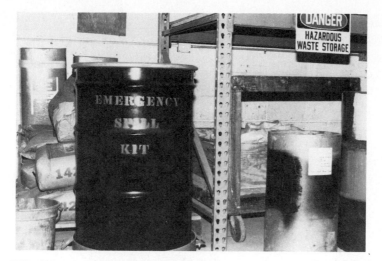

FIG. 8-7   Portable emergency spill kits like this one are located throughout the plant, and employees receive emergency spill training on a regular basis.
Courtesy: Alexandria Metal Finishers, Inc. Alexandria, Va.

defines a catastrophe as "any incident that either kills a worker or causes the hospitalization of at least five employees."[26]

The first step in the organization of an effective disaster plan is to identify the potential sources of disaster in the workplace. Each department in the plant should be examined. Are there areas where flammable liquids are stored? Are there operations in the plant that involve highly toxic chemicals, molten metals, or flammable liquids and gases? Are overhead cranes used to move heavy loads through the plant? Is your facility located in an area of the country where such natural disasters as tornadoes or flash floods might occur?

Once these potential trouble spots are identified, the next step is to evaluate the resources available to handle a major emergency. Does your community have a hospital, fire department, or rescue squad? Do you have in-plant equipment and personnel to control a fire or chemical spill? (See Fig. 8-7.) How many employees have first aid training?

The third and most important step is to organize and coordinate your resources. Interested plant personnel may be assigned to disaster teams. Employees who are volunteer fire fighters are likely candidates for a fire control team.

Other plant personnel who have first aid training could form the rescue team. Persons with special skills and interests could be responsible for chemical spills, salvage operations, or traffic control. Since employees are likely to be at the scene when a disaster occurs, they have the potential to significantly reduce the death and injury toll with a rapid, well-organized response (see Fig. 8-8).

Don't make the mistake that many companies do—they have disaster plans, but only on paper. Make sure the plan is realistic and workable. Conduct in-service programs throughout the year on various topics to give employees hands-on experi-

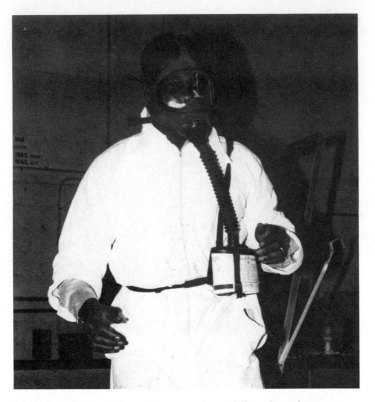

FIG. 8-8 This employee is a member of the plant disaster team, which uses a number of specialized pieces of equipment in its training sessions.

Courtesy: Alexandria Metal Finishers, Inc. Alexandria, Va.

ence in emergency procedures. It does no good to have a chemical-spill team if all members are not familiar with the chemicals that they are expected to handle in an emergency. Also, don't expect workers to know how to use fire extinguishers, gas masks, or other equipment if they have never operated them before.

With the internal resources in place, it is now time to coordinate them with the outside agencies (police, fire, and rescue services). The plant safety manager will need to work closely with these organizations in establishing a cohesive chain of command. In a time of disaster, there will be plenty for everyone to do, but all responsibilities should be planned in advance. Each of these agencies should be informed about the toxic materials and hazards that they may face. The more they know about your operations, the better prepared they'll be to help you when needed.

Now that your plan is in place, it is time to test it with a mock disaster drill. Although people will quickly realize that it's not the real thing, a disaster drill is useful in identifying the strong points and weak points of your program. In this way problems that may surface can be solved long before there is a need to use the disaster plan.

Program Evaluation

The final and perhaps most important component of a company's safety program is evaluation. Injury and illness reports that are used to identify high-risk occupations and dangerous work areas in a plant can also provide valuable information about the success or failure of innovations such as equipment design changes, personal protective gear, and employee safety training. For example, analysis of injury reports for a 6- or 12-month period *after* the implementation of corrective measures may indicate that the number of injuries has not decreased; however, the reports may show that the severity of injuries has been significantly reduced, thus decreasing the number of lost workdays. With such an evaluation, a company could determine the cost effectiveness of its program.

Another evaluation strategy is that of employee observation. Observation of randomly selected employees by plant managers and supervisors can be used to determine the effectiveness of safety training. Failure of employees to operate equipment safely may indicate that training procedures need to be modified. On the other hand, such observations may show that the training program is effective but certain employees may need special assistance or counseling. Regular evaluation of the safety program will ensure that working men and women receive the maximum in workplace protection.

A LOOK TO THE FUTURE

In the 1990s three factors will play a major role in influencing occupational health and safety in the workplace:

1. With a decline in the overall physical condition of workers and more women in the labor force, many tools, machines, and work practices will become increasingly hazardous, thus requiring major modifications. At the same time, the accelerated use of "robot technology" will require new strategies to avoid problems for personnel who operate, maintain, and service these systems. Because robots generally require more space than humans who perform the same task, workers will need to become aware of the dangers associated with the movement of the robot assembly.

2. An estimated 63,000 chemicals are believed to be currently in use in the United States, with an additional 1000 being added each year.[23] Many of these products have received little or no testing in terms of the hazards they may present during their manufacture and use. A major thrust in the chemical industry will be the production of genetically engineered organisms. Their role in new-product development will be heavily debated in the coming decade.

3. As the state of the art for identifying work-related diseases improves and the level of worker awareness to hazards in the workplace increases, a more reliable measure of occupational illnesses will result. This, in turn, will have two effects:

   a. It will increase compensation claims from workers for past exposures.

   b. It will stimulate employers and the government to provide better protection for the American worker.

RESPONSIBILITY FOR SAFETY AND HEALTH: A TEAM APPROACH

Too often the mention of "safety in the workplace" is like a call to battle. Immediately sides are chosen; it quickly becomes management versus labor, federal OSHA versus state OSHA, government intervention versus free enterprise, big business versus small business, or similar conflicts. However, this doesn't have to be so. In fact, a successful program will result only when all of these groups work together. At the federal level, it is the responsibility of OSHA and NIOSH to develop standards and guidelines for our nation's industries and to conduct occupational safety and health research to keep pace with the changing needs of the workforce. On the state level, industrial commissions, worker's compensation agencies, and state OSHA authorities are in a position to interpret the special needs of local industries while carrying out the federal provisions.

The key leadership role for safety lies at the company or management level. The attitude of supervisors toward job safety and health will be reflected in the attitudes of employees. Since top management (that is, owners, company presidents, vice-presidents) influences supervisor attitudes, the policy of safety starts at the top. Corporate responsibility must include the commitment of funds to provide the safest possible environment for employees.

When you consider responsibility for worker safety, don't forget to include the employees. Each worker has a responsibility to follow safety procedures and instructions in his or her job performance. This includes wearing personal protective devices, using the correct equipment-operations procedures, and not coming to work under the influence of alcohol or other drugs. Employees should identify hazards in their immediate production areas, including fellow workers, and take appropriate action to control them.

Trade unions can do much to assist management in providing for employee safety—and they do not have to play the role of adversary to accomplish this. Union personnel are in a position to monitor the adequacy of environmental protection provided by the company while observing worker behavior in terms of safe job performance. Many unions have safety and health expertise in specific worker hazards, which they are more than willing to share with companies. If there is an open line of communication between labor and management, coordinated company-union action can result in better worker protection and, in the long run, increased profit margins. It is a simple equation:

$$\text{Healthy workers} = \begin{array}{c} \text{Reduced insurance and} \\ \text{compensation payments} \\ \text{and increased productivity} \end{array} = \text{Increased profits}$$

SUMMARY

Much of the safety movement in America has been influenced by programs that were first established in the industrial setting. Today's insurance policies, which provide protection against illness, injury, and property damage, are the result of efforts that began in the early 1800s to protect both workers and the companies for which they worked.

In the 1990s occupational illnesses have become a prominent and costly industrial safety problem. Traditionally, sprains and strains of the back and injuries to the lower and upper extremities accounted for the most frequent and costly compensation cases. However, in recent years, NIOSH investigations have indicated a trend in occupational illnesses caused by prolonged exposure to hazardous substances or repetitious movements over a period of time. Conditions such as tendonitis, bursitis, and carpal tunnel syndrome result from repeated twisting or turning movements, which injure tendons, ligaments, muscles, and nerves. Work that involves partial or whole-body vibration may result in serious damage to blood vessels, muscles, or nerves over an extended period of time.

Chemicals in the workplace present problems after a worker has been exposed to their toxic effects for months or years. By no means is exposure to toxic substances a new phenomenon in the workplace. As early as the eighteenth century, physicians had identified illnesses that were caused by chronic exposure to cotton dust, coal dust, and lead particles.

Today, work-related exposure to toxic substances has become more widespread as the number of chemicals being used and produced rapidly increases. NIOSH researchers have also found that many chemicals, once thought to be safe, are likely to be carcinogenic if a worker has been exposed to them for 15 or 20 years. With an estimated 63,000 chemicals currently in use in the United States, extensive research is needed to keep the danger of exposure for workers at a minimum.

Ultimately, safety and health in the workplace is a team effort; government, private industry, and the labor force must work together. At the government level, federal and state agencies are responsible for collecting data, conducting research, and developing guidelines to keep pace with the changing needs of the workforce. At the management or company level lies the key leadership role. The development of a well-organized and planned safety program can maximize worker safety while increasing productivity and profits. At the worker level, each employee has a responsibility to follow safety procedures and instructions in his or her job. Only with these coordinated efforts can safe and healthful conditions be assured for the American worker.

Key Terms

Angiosarcoma   A rare form of liver cancer.

Bureau of Labor Statistics (BLS)   A recordkeeping and reporting agency that provides statistical data to monitor and solve problems in the workplace.

Byssinosis   Brown lung disease, caused by prolonged exposure to cotton dust.

Carcinogens   Substances that may cause cancer in animals or humans.

Carpal tunnel syndrome (CTS)   Inflamed tendons and membranes in the wrist swell, damaging nerves that control finger and hand movement.

Ergonomics   How the workplace, job practices, and equipment design features interact to affect the well-being of employees.

Localized effect The action of the chemical takes place at the point of contact.

Mutagen A substance that can cause a change or mutation in the genetic material of living cell.

National Institute for Occupational Safety and Health (NIOSH) Responsible for identifying occupational safety and health hazards, determining methods to control them, and recommending exposure limits.

Occupational illness Any abnormal condition or disorder, other than one resulting from an occupational injury, caused by exposure to environmental factors associated with employment.

Occupational injury Any injury that results from a work-related accident or from exposure involving a single incident in the workplace.

Occupational Safety and Health Administration (OSHA) Assures working men and women of a safe and healthful environment by setting and enforcing health and safety standards.

Pneumoconiosis Black lung disease, caused by prolonged exposure to coal dust.

Raynaud's phenomenon The narrowing of blood vessels in the fingers caused by constant, heavy vibration.

Supplementary Data System (SDS) A voluntary program in which participating states code accident and injury cases from their workers' compensation agencies. This information is given to the Bureau of Labor Statistics for the development of a reliable data base to identify where problems exist.

Systemic effect The action of the hazardous substance occurs somewhere other than the point of entry.

Tenosynovitis Inflammation and swelling of tendons in the wrist.

Teratogen An agent that interferes with the development of an unborn child.

References

1. American Society of Safety Engineers: The first 75 years, Des Plaines, Ill., 1986.
2. America's first industry: 200 years of safety and the glass industry, Safety Newsletter, Chicago, July 1976, National Safety Council.
3. Auchter, T. G.: An address to the Mountain States Employers Council, Denver, Jan. 28, 1982.
4. Bureau of Labor Statistics: Occupational safety and health statistics: concepts and methods, Report 518, Washington, D.C., 1978, U.S. Government Printing Office.
5. Cinney, J.: Workers' compensation: how it works, National Safety and Health News, July 1985, p. 30.
6. Computer and Business Equipment Manufacturers Association: Health and safety aspects of visual displays, Fact Sheet 1, Washington, D.C., 1985.
7. Habes, D. J., and Putz-Anderson, V.: The NIOSH program for evaluating biomechanical hazards in the workplace, Journal of Safety Research 16 (2): 49, 1985.
8. Hilaski, H. J.: Understanding statistics on occupational illness, Monthly Labor Review, March 1981, p. 25.
9. Hricko, A., and Brunt, M.: Working for your life: a woman's guide to job health hazards, The Labor Occupational Health Program, Berkeley, Calif., 1976, University of California.
10. Indiana Division of Labor, Department of Statistics: Characteristics of occupational injuries and illnesses in Indiana: 1988, Indianapolis, 1990.
11. Lungs are a vulnerable shortcut for contaminants to enter the body, Occupational Health & Safety, June 1986, p. 27.
12. Marcus, R.: Justices find bias in fetal protection, The Washington Post, March 21, 1991, pp. Al, A14-15.
13. Milestones, National Safety News, May 1963, p. 72.

14. National Institute for Occupational Safety and Health: NIOSH report on occupational safety and health under public law 91 -596: 1980, Washington, D.C., July 1981, U.S. Government Printing Office.
15. National Institute for Occupational Safety and Health: Health hazard evaluation summaries, Washington, D.C., May 1981.
16. National Institute for Occupational Safety and Health: The federal mine health program in 1980, Washington, D.C., Feb. 1981, U.S. Government Printing Office.
17. National Institute for Occupational Safety and Health: Occupational exposure to vinyl chloride, Washington, D.C., April 1977, U.S. Government Printing Office.
18. National Institute for Occupational Safety and Health: Occupational exposure to benzene DHEW (NIOSH) Publication No. 74-137, Washington, D.C., 1974, U.S. Government Printing Office.
19. National Institute for Occupational Safety and Health: Occupational exposure to cotton dust, DHEW (NIOSH) Publication No. 75-118, Washington, D.C., 1974, U.S. Government Printing Office.
20. National Institute for Occupational Safety and Health: Occupational exposure to inorganic lead, DHEW (NIOSH) Publication No. 73-11010, Washington, D.C., 1972, U.S. Government Printing Office.
21. National Safety Council: Accident facts: 1990 ed., Chicago, 1990, The Council.
22. National Safety Council: Asbestos: data sheet 1-709-86, National Safety and Health News, May 1986, p. 41.
23. NIOSH registry of toxic effects of chemical substances: 1985, Washington, D.C., 1986, U.S. Government Printing Office.
24. Occupational Safety and Health Act of 1970, Public Law 91-596, 91st Congress, S. 2193, Washington, D.C., 1970.
25. Occupational Safety and Health Administration: Record keeping requirements under the occupational safety and health act of 1970 (rev. 1978), G. P. O. 361-270/4935, Washington, D.C., 1981, U.S. Government Printing Office.
26. Occupational Safety and Health Administration: All about OSHA, OSHA 2056, Washington, D.C., 1980, U.S. Government Printing Office.
27. Okie, S.: No link found between VDTs, miscarriages, The Washington Post, March 14, 1991, pp. A1, A21.
28. Pendergrass, J. A.: VDTs—how real the hazard? National Safety and Health News, Dec. 1985, p. 43.
29. Pennsylvania Department of Labor and Industry: Pennsylvania worker and community right to know program, Harrisburg, Penn. Sept. 1986, Right to Know Office.
30. Roberts, M.: Computer waves, U.S. News and World Report, Sept. 10, 1990, pp. 83–87.
31. Root, N., and Daley, J. R.: Are women safer workers? A new look at the data, Monthly Labor Review, Sept. 1980, p. 3.
32. Root, N., and McCaffrey, D.: Targeting worker safety programs: weighing incidence against expense, Monthly Labor Review, January 1980, p. 3.
33. The safety revolution, National Safety News, May 1963, p. 37.
34. Srachta, B. J.: Job tenosynovitis is preventable, National Safety and Health News, July 1985, p. 50.
35. Stellman, J. M.: Women's work, women's health: myths and realities, New York, 1977, Pantheon Books.
36. Travers, P. H., and Stanton, B. A.: Office workers and video display terminals: physical, psychological and ergonomic factors, Occupational Health Nursing, Nov. 1984, p. 586.
37. United States Department of Labor, Occupational Safety and Health Administration: Hazard communication: final rule, Federal Register 48 (228)-53280, 1983.

Resource Organizations

AFL-CIO
Occupational Safety and Health
815 16th Street N.W.
Washington, DC 20006

American Industrial Health Council
1330 Connecticut Avenue N.W.
Washington, DC 20036

American Industrial Hygiene Association
475 Wolf Ledges Parkway
Akron, OH 44311

Bureau of Labor Statistics
Occupational Safety and Health Statistics
Department of Labor
200 Constitution Avenue N.W.
Washington, DC 20210

Industrial Health Foundation
34 Penn Circle W.
Pittsburgh, PA 15206

International Labor Organization
Occupational Safety and Health Section
c/o Washington Branch Office
1750 New York Avenue N.W.
Washington, DC 20006

Mine Safety and Health Administration
4015 Wilson Boulevard
Arlington, VA 22203

National Association of Manufacturers
Occupational Safety and Health Committee
1776 F Street N.W.
Washington, DC 20006

National Institute for Farm Safety
460 Henry Mall
Madison, WI 53706

National Institute for Occupational Safety
and Health
5600 Fishers Lane
Rockville, MD 20857

Occupational Health Institute
40 South Arlington Heights Road
Arlington Heights, IL 60005

Occupational Safety and Health
Administration
200 Constitution Avenue N.W.
Washington, DC 20210

Public Citizen, Inc.
P.O. Box 19404
Washington, DC 20036

Society for Occupational and Environmental
Health
2021 K Street N.W., Suite 305
Washington, DC 20006

Women's Occupational Health Resource
Center
School of Public Health
600 West 168th Street
Columbia University
New York, NY 10032

CHAPTER 8

Applying What You Have Learned

1. Utilizing the incidence rate formula that appears at the bottom of Table 8-1 on page 269, compare the lost-workday rates of the following three businesses:

	A	B	C
Number of lost workdays	480	204	1125
Total hours worked by all employees	1,2000,000	600,000	3,000,000
Lost-workday rate per 100 full-time workers	_____	_____	_____

a) Which of the businesses had the highest lost-workday rate per 100 full-time workers?

b) Which of the businesses had the lowest lost-workday rate?

c) Which of the businesses suffered the greatest number of lost workdays?

2. Discuss your reaction to the Supreme Court's ruling that women of child-bearing age cannot be excluded from jobs that pose reproductive hazards.

3. Who should be responsible for a child with severe handicaps born to a couple who worked in a plant which posed clearly identified reproductive hazards?

Natural and Man-Made Disasters

In the space of only a decade, hazardous waste has become a central concern of citizens in every part of the United States

EPA journal

A **disaster** is generally defined as a "a great, sudden misfortune resulting in loss of life, serious injury, and property damage."[1] Although the loss of even one person could be considered a disaster, a more correct use of the term would refer to an occurrence that kills and injures a relatively large number of persons or damages a large amount of property.

Disasters take many forms. They may involve attack (nuclear or conventional warfare, terrorism), man-made hazards (chemical spills, major transportation accidents), and natural hazards (floods, hurricanes, tornadoes). Table 9-1 lists some of the disasters to which you may be exposed. Disasters and emergencies affecting large areas and many people can sometimes develop quickly, as in the case of a flash flood or tornado, while others are preceded by a "build-up period," which provides more time for taking protective measures. For example, the path of a hurricane may be traced for a number of days, thus allowing weather personnel to warn people who are in potential danger areas.

Some of these emergencies are more likely to occur in certain parts of the country; for example, hurricanes are more common along the Gulf and Atlantic Coast states, tornadoes are more frequent in the Midwest and southern states, and earthquakes occur more often in the western states.

Although natural disasters have not increased in frequency, a growing population and the development of areas where these disasters occur have increased public vulnerability to hazardous environmental conditions. For example, the construction of housing tracts along once uninhabited, low-lying coastal areas of the southeastern United States has increased the risk of exposure to hurricanes for thousands of

Table 9-1 Types of disasters to which one may be exposed

Attack	Man-made	Natural
Biological	Epidemic	Drought
Chemical	Fire	Extreme cold
Nuclear	Accident-rural and urban	Fire from lightning or spontaneous
Conventional war	Arson	combustion
	Hazardous material accident	Forest fire
	Fixed site	Range fire
	Transport	Other
	Nuclear and radiological	Flood and other water
	Fixed site	Landshift
	Transport	Earthquake
	Pollution	Earthslide or mudslide
	Resource and energy disruptions	Erosion
	or shortages	Snow and ice
	Reservoir or dam breaks	Tsunami and sea surge
	Major gas and water main breaks	Volcanic eruption
	Major transportation accidents	Wind
	Mine disasters	Cyclone, hurricane, and typhoon
	Pipeline explosions	Tornado
	Terrorism	Sand and dust storms
	Civil disorders and riots	Severe fog and smog
	Strikes	Agricultural blight or infestation

Courtesy: Federal Emergency Management Agency. Source: Fire and Emergency Management Project, Washington, D.C., NaCoR, Inc.

Americans who have moved to these new communities. The construction of new high-rise structures along earthquake faults on the West Coast presents similar dangers.

In recent years, the rapid development of hazardous materials has increased technological dangers and compounded the disaster problem. The U.S. Environmental Protection Agency (EPA) estimates that hazardous waste is produced in this country at the rate of 700,000 tons per day, or approximately 250 million tons per year. Hazardous waste can pollute ground water, rivers, and lakes; it can pollute the air; and it may even burn or explode. Of the more than 30,000 toxic waste sites identified by the EPA, it is estimated that as many as 3000 present an "imminent and substantial" danger to human health.[6] In the next decade, the cost of decontaminating these areas is expected to run to the billions of dollars.

The transportation of hazardous materials presents another problem. Every day planes, trains, and trucks carry hazardous and toxic materials across the United States. In a recent 7-year period, the U.S. Department of Transportation's Material Transportation Bureau received 72,000 hazardous-incident reports of accidents that caused 6729 injuries, 457 deaths, and millions of dollars in property damage.[6]

As an alternative fuel source, nuclear energy came to the forefront in the mid-1970s when there were increasing shortages of petroleum. However, in March 1979 the question of nuclear safety became a widely debated issue, following the accident at Three Mile Island, Pennsylvania. Could an accident at a nuclear power plant that released high concentrations of radiation possibly result in the deaths of hundreds of people?

DISASTER PLANNING

The time for planning is before a disaster occurs, not during or after the event. Too often, community officials find themselves responsible for emergency operations that are unfamiliar. They may preside over agencies and organizations that have conflicting interests, or they may be forced to make quick decisions that have long-range consequences. In a disaster, the responsibilities are enormous. Many lives and vast amounts of property and personal possessions (many of which are irreplaceable) are in jeopardy. People will depend on local authorities for leadership both during and after the crisis.

A system of comprehensive emergency management (CEM) is essential to ensure that everyone knows his or her role when disaster strikes. CEM means that all levels of government (local, state, and federal) and the private sector coordinate their efforts to manage a disaster. Table 9-2 lists the agencies that may become involved in an emergency.

Since most of the damage and suffering occurs at the local or community level, effective emergency management must begin here. Emergency management encompasses four phases of activity: (1) hazard reduction, (2) preparedness, (3) response, and (4) recovery. The key to developing the emergency management system is the emergency operations staff. In large metropolitan areas full-time personnel may be hired to conduct emergency and disaster programs. Disaster operations in a smaller community may be the responsibility of the mayor, his or her assistant, or perhaps the fire chief. A chain of command must be established to coordinate available emergency resources in a smooth and efficient manner.

Hazard Reduction

One of the first steps in comprehensive emergency management at the local level is to determine what hazards pose a threat to the community and the significance of the risks involved. To set some type of priority in terms of the various hazards, a probability and vulnerability analysis is often used. *Probability* refers to the chance of an event happening in a given year, based on past history [11,13]; for example, communities in Illinois, Indiana, and Michigan have a significantly greater chance of being damaged by a tornado than do communities in California. *Vulnerability* represents the number of lives and amount of property that would be in jeopardy in the event of a particular disaster. [11,13] The development of coastal areas in the southeastern United States has created a high-vulnerability situation should a hurricane strike in one of these areas. On the other hand, in undeveloped coastal areas vulnerability is very low.

By having an idea of what disasters could occur and their potential destructive power, community planners can seek ways to prevent disasters if they are avoidable,

Table 9-2   Four levels of participation in disaster activities

Private sector	Local government	State government	Federal government
Charities	Elected officials	Office of the governor	President
Volunteer groups	Police	State emergency office	Congress
Volunteers	Fire	State police	Federal Emergency
Religious organizations	Emergency medical services	National Guard	Management Agency
Service groups	Local emergency coordinator	Transportation agency	U.S. Department of
News media	Sheriff	Human resources	Agriculture
Educational	Human resources	departments	National Oceanic and
Organized labor	Educational	Natural resources	Atmospheric
Professional organizations	Agricultural extension service	departments	Administration
Business and industry	Public works	Agricultural department	Military departments
Knowledge	Public health organizations	Regulatory commissions	Transportation agencies
Equipment	Interorganizational and	Ad hoc advisory councils	Construction agencies
Financial institutions	Interjurisdictional bodies	Quasi-public utilities	Human resource agencies
Insurance companies	Ad hoc advisory councils	Planning divisions	U.S. Department of Housing
Private-nonprofit		Judiciary	and Urban Development
organizations		Legislature	Federal Bureau of
			Investigation
			Internal Revenue Service
			U.S. Department of Labor
			Veterans Administration
			Small Business
			Administration

Courtesy: Federal Emergency Management Agency. Source: Fire and Emergency Management Project, Washington D.C., NACoR, Inc.

or at least minimize their impact if they are unavoidable. Using "site zoning," a community could reduce the possibility of an explosion disaster by limiting construction of a gasoline tank farm to an uninhabited area of the county. To minimize the impact of future earthquakes, a community at risk may want to establish building codes that require structural reinforcement of multistory buildings.

Officials must have community support to be successful in the hazard-reduction phase of a comprehensive emergency management program. It is the responsibility of local citizens to become informed of potential hazards, to abide by community codes and ordinances, and to follow the procedures that have been established to protect them.

Preparedness

Preparedness activities are necessary to the extent that hazard-reduction measures have not prevented or cannot prevent disasters. These activities generally refer to identifying and organizing resources available both from inside and outside a locality.[11] Probably the two most important questions that must be asked are: (1) What will need to be done should an emergency arise? and (2) Who will be responsible for performing these tasks?

The most probable tasks are identified first, then appropriate resources are sought to accomplish them. This will help to prevent duplication of services in one area and a lack of services in another area. Using a building collapse as an example, let's see what needs to be done and who should respond. If such a situation were to occur, tasks to be considered include:

1. Evacuation of surrounding buildings.
2. Extrication and rescue of victims.
3. On-scene emergency medical treatment.
4. Security of the area from gas and electrical hazards.
5. Crowd and traffic control.

Now that we have an idea of what may need to be accomplished immediately, who will perform these tasks? Who will be responsible for evacuation of endangered areas? Police, fire fighters, ambulance personnel? Who would be best prepared to stop a gas leak in the building? Do you see the difficulties that could occur without some type of organized disaster plan?

The system will not work without a coordination of services. In the case of the building collapse it is likely that both fire and police personnel will respond immediately. If you look at their normal job descriptions, it makes sense to assign police officers to building evacuation and crowd and traffic control and fire fighters to victim extrication and rescue. Ambulance personnel (EMTs and paramedics) would be given the responsibility of treating and transporting the victims. To handle gas leaks or downed power lines, specially trained personnel from the various utility companies would be needed. As seen in our example, each of these agencies has specific responsibilities in the formulated disaster plan.

Response

In the event of a disaster, the resources that have been identified in the preparedness stage are activated to provide assistance for victims and to reduce the probability of further casualties and damage.

The most critical information in the early-response period is the extent and nature of damages and injuries. Based on this initial assessment, decisions will be made concerning requests for additional personnel and equipment, evacuation of nearby residences, and notification of hospitals. The most likely first responders, fire and police personnel, should receive training in damage assessment and triage. (Triage is a method used to determine which victims need immediate medical attention and which victims can tolerate a delay in treatment.)

A chain of command and a communications network should be implemented to limit confusion and chaos at the emergency scene. A chain of command helps to answer the question, Who's in charge? This should be established long before a disaster occurs. The command structure may vary, depending on the type of disaster. In our previous example of a building collapse, fire personnel would probably be in charge at the scene; an inner-city riot would call for police leadership; whereas a bus accident involving multiple casualties would come under the direction of ambulance and rescue personnel. By establishing a chain of command, rivalries and jealousies among agencies do not become a problem at the emergency scene.

During a major emergency, the sources and volume of information are staggering. A communications network needs to be established as soon as possible. Radio communication and telephone lines are usually connected between the command post at the disaster scene and an emergency operations center (EOC) where officials such as the mayor, city manager, and county supervisors can be kept informed. With information received from the scene, officials will make policy decisions about requests for private sector, state, or federal assistance. The EOC can also be used to provide a single, authoritative source of information for the media and the public.

With a well-organized emergency response effort, the problems of underresponse and overresponse can be avoided. Delays in calling for assistance may result in a higher number of deaths because of a lack of trained personnel at the disaster site; however, too much assistance on or near the emergency scene can create confusion and seriously hamper the efficiency of the rescue effort. Coordination of resources and program planning are essential to have a successful response.

Recovery

The final phase of comprehensive emergency management (CEM) is the "return to normal" or recovery. The main activities during this time involve the restoration of homes, businesses, and public facilities as well as the rejuvenation of the economy and social structure of the community. Insurance claims and requests for state and federal disaster assistance will be a priority. Even at this stage, planning is important, because the process for requesting assistance may be rather complicated. Specific information is necessary to expedite requests. If officials do not know the proper channels for assistance, the community's recovery will be delayed.

Reassessment is another activity of the recovery phase. Based on the type of disaster that occurred, emergency management personnel, community leaders, and citizens may need to consider changes that might prevent, or at least reduce, the chances of a recurrence of the disaster. At the same time, they will be able to review and update their comprehensive emergency management plan.

ANALYSIS OF A DISASTER: NEED FOR CHANGE

On the afternoon of January 13, 1982, in a heavy winter snowstorm, Air Florida's Flight 90 crashed shortly after taking off from Washington, D.C.'s National Airport. During its descent and eventual crash into the Potomac River, the airplane struck the northbound ramp of the 14th Street Bridge, crushing a number of vehicles that were on the heavily traveled route during the afternoon rush hour. All but 5 of the plane's 80 passengers and crew perished, and a number of persons traveling on the bridge were also killed.

In the weeks following this tragedy, government officials, emergency management personnel, and several citizens' groups began to reevaluate disaster planning in the nation's capital. Let's examine the four phases of disaster planning as they relate to the Air Florida crash.

Ultimately, the cause of the plane crash was determined to be a heavy buildup of ice on the plane's wings, which prevented it from gaining sufficient air speed to maintain flight. Hazard reduction questions that needed to be answered included: Why were planes allowed to take off during the snowstorm? What were the runway conditions at the time of take-off? What de-icing procedures had been used before take-off? Post accident analysis revealed that pilots were given a wide latitude in determining if and when their craft should take off and whether they should be de-iced. It was also found that information regarding runway and weather conditions relayed to pilots might have lacked sufficient updating. In other words, runway and weather conditions could deteriorate significantly while a plane was waiting for take-off, yet the pilot might not be notified.

Suggestions that have been made to minimize the potential for similar bad-weather crashes include requiring more frequent de-icing of planes in bad weather and improving communication between the control tower and pilots concerning weather and runway conditions. Because its runways are relatively short, National Airport is particularly hazardous for planes taking off in icy conditions. If they fail to attain the minimum take-off speed and attempt to abort a take-off, pilots may still be in jeopardy because they may not be able to stop the plane from going off the end of the runway and into the Potomac River. For this reason, a number of air safety groups have recommended that officials shut down operations at National Airport more readily during inclement weather than they have in the past.

A major hazard reduction issue concerning National Airport that is still unresolved is the high volume of air traffic at the airport, which is located in a densely populated area. Unlike nearby airports, such as Dulles International and Baltimore-Washington International (which have large open areas surrounding them), National is located in the heart of the Metropolitan Washington area near Alexandria, Virginia. Flight patterns into and out of the airport force planes to fly at low altitudes over numerous office buildings and apartment complexes. Had Air Florida's Flight 90 remained aloft a few moments longer and crashed into one of these structures, the death toll would probably have been significantly higher. Federal and private aviation agencies have requested a significant reduction in the number of flights arriving at and departing from National Airport.

The analysis of the Air Florida disaster also identified a number of shortcomings in the emergency management system for Metropolitan Washington, which includes the District of Columbia and nearby government jurisdictions in Virginia and Maryland. Although such an air crash had been discussed, no detailed rescue plan had been developed by these jurisdictions at the time of the Air Florida accident. This lack of coordination of resources led to doubt about who was in charge at the crash site. Additional problems arose when fire and rescue personnel from the various jurisdictions could not communicate with one another, since they did not operate on the same radio frequencies. There was confusion about the type of rescue apparatus and personnel that were needed at the scene. Later, the communication difficulties hampered efforts to identify survivors and the hospitals to which they had been taken. Had there been more survivors, these response problems could have been even more momentous.

Since the Air Florida crash, Metropolitan Washington emergency services planners have instituted a number of organizational changes in developing an areawide rescue plan. The various jurisdictions are establishing command structures based on the types of emergencies that may occur. They have also procured operational control vehicles equipped with multiple-channel radio receivers so that communication can be maintained with equipment from several communities, using local radio frequencies.

In April 1987, this emergency management system was again tested when a tour bus hit a roadway overpass, killing one person and injuring 28 others. Fire and rescue personnel from three communities were credited with saving the lives of many victims, the result of a rapid, coordinated response. Without an organized emergency plan, this kind of joint rescue effort would not have been as effective.

A PERSONAL APPROACH TO DISASTER PLANNING

In the first few pages of this chapter, we have discussed disaster planning from the standpoint of community responsibilities. On an individual or personal level, disaster planning is just as important. In fact, the four phases of a comprehensive emergency management program can apply as readily to an individual or family as it can to an entire community.

Hazard reduction for the individual is a process of self-awareness and education. Is the property that you are buying located in a flood plain? Do you know what types of natural disasters occur in your part of the country? Does your community have an early warning system (sirens, whistles, horns) to alert people of an impending emergency? What are the federal guidelines for anchoring house trailers in high-wind areas? To answer such questions, you may need to contact a variety of organizations; for example, the county extension service, county health department, and local or state governmental agencies. However, an awareness of possible disaster hazards where you live is not enough.

The second phase of planning requires preparation for disaster; for example, now is the time to make sure your trailer is properly anchored. After finding that you live in a frequently flooded area, it may be wise to purchase flood insurance, since your regular homeowner's policy will not cover damage from such a disaster.

A major disaster may interfere with your normal supplies of food, water, heat, and other daily necessities. You should keep on hand (in or around your home) a stock of emergency supplies sufficient to meet your family's needs for at least a few days, preferably a week. The most important items to keep on hand are:[15]

1. Water in plastic jugs or stoppered containers.
2. Canned or sealed-packaged foods that do not require refrigeration or cooking.
3. Medicines needed by family members and a first aid kit.
4. Blankets or sleeping bags.
5. Flashlights or lanterns.
6. Matches and several candles in a waterproof container.
7. Battery-powered radio.
8. Extra batteries.
9. Large plastic trash bags.
10. An extra set of clothing for each family member.

In parts of the country subject to hurricane, flood, or wind damage, preparedness may include keeping materials on hand to protect your home. Plywood sheeting or lumber could be used to board up windows and doors, while plastic sheeting or tarpaulins would provide protection for furniture, appliances, and family members.

Response activities are those things you need to do to protect yourself or your family during a disaster. We will focus on personal response in each of the disaster categories to be discussed. The type of disaster with which you are faced will determine the method of response.

Recovery after a disaster is a personal as well as a community responsibility. While local governmental agencies are attempting to clean up and reorganize public facilities, homeowners will face their own major cleanup operations.

After a disaster, especially one in which you have had to evacuate your home for any length of time, there are some special precautions that need to be taken:[15]

1. Keep your radio tuned to the designated emergency broadcast station for advice and instructions from local authorities. They will be able to provide you with information about housing, clothing, food, and medical assistance.
2. *Do not* return to your home until it has been broadcast that it is safe to do so.
3. *Do not* visit the disaster area, since onlookers often hamper rescue and emergency operations.
4. When you return home, use caution on entering the structure, since it may have been damaged or weakened by the disaster.
5. Stay away from fallen or damaged electric wires—they may still be dangerous.

6. *Do not* take torches, lighted candles, or cigarettes into the structure, since there may be a potentially dangerous gas buildup from leaking pipes. Check for leaking gas in your home by smell only. If you suspect a gas leak, notify the gas company or fire department, and don't reenter the house until you are told it is safe to do so.

7. *Do not* handle live electrical equipment in wet areas; it should be checked and dried before it is returned to service.

8. Check your food and water supplies before using them. Food that requires refrigeration may be spoiled if electric power was off. Food that has come in contact with flood waters should be discarded.

9. After the emergency, write or phone relatives to let them know that you are safe; this will alleviate their fears and reduce the workload of rescuers whose job it is to locate missing persons.

In the following sections, let's examine some of the personal responses you may need to take in situations involving natural and man-made disasters.

NATURAL DISASTERS

Tornadoes and Severe Thunderstorms

Of all the winds that sweep the earth's surface, tornadoes are the most violent. A **tornado** is a short-lived, local storm, made up of high-speed winds usually rotating in a counterclockwise direction.[34] The classic trademark of the tornado is the funnel-shaped appendage that seems to be attached to a storm cloud (Fig. 9-1).

Scientists now believe that tornadoes begin within thunderstorm clouds and gradually rotate downward to the earth's surface, where they do their damage. Although many questions remain unanswered, the most widely accepted theories of tornado development suggest that the merging of warm, moist air from the Gulf Coast and cool, dry air masses from Canada creates a rotary circulation of winds, which may spawn a violent storm and resulting tornado.

Tornadoes occur in many parts of the world and have been recorded in all 50 states; however, the areas that suffer the most damage annually are the Gulf Coast and midwestern states.[32] In February and March, states along the Gulf record the greatest number of tornadoes, since cool air from the North penetrates into the southern states. During the late spring (April, May, June), the meeting point for cool and warm air masses is over the midwestern states, which will now suffer the bulk of the damage. During the late summer, fall, and early winter there are fewer encounters between warm air and overriding cold systems; consequently, there are fewer tornadoes during this time.

Although there may be some debate about how tornadoes develop, there is no question about their destructive force. Some major tornadoes having wind speeds of up to 300 mph have caused damage in areas measuring 1½ miles wide and 200 miles long. On the average, tornado paths are only ¼ mile (400 yards) wide and 10 to 15 miles long; they rarely last more than 20 to 30 minutes. Nonetheless, during their

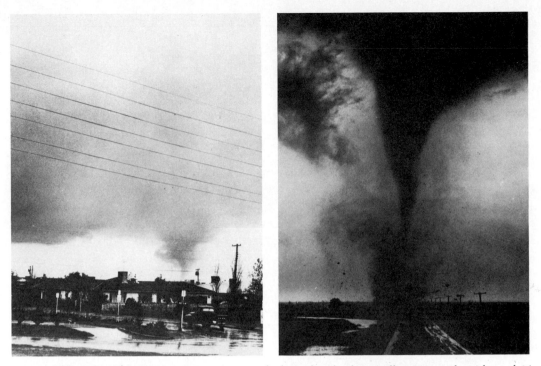

FIG. 9-1   This Texas twister cut a swath through suburban Dallas 200 yards wide and 16 miles long.

Courtesy: Federal Emergency Management Agency, National Oceanic and Atmospheric Administration.

short life span, tornadoes, with their rotating winds of 150 to 200 mph, flatten virtually everything in their paths. (Fig. 9-2 and Fig. 9-3).

Tornadoes do their destructive work through a combined action of strong rotary winds, the impact of windborne missiles, and the partial vacuum in the center of the vortex.[34] As the tornado travels along the ground, it sweeps up debris in its path (piles of wood, metal, concrete) and spins it along its outside edge, literally ripping open anything in the way. The debris is by no means small; it may include such objects as cement blocks, two-by-fours, and drainage pipes. A recent Kansas tornado carried a home freezer more than a mile from its original location.[43]

As a tornado passes over a building, its leading edge pushes nearby walls inward; however, as the spinning continues, the storm's center, with its partial vacuum, causes a pressure reduction that blows other walls of the structure outward. Each year, the approximately 650 tornadoes in the United States are responsible for 200 deaths and nearly $700 million in property damage.[11]

No one can stop a tornado, but there are precautions that can be taken to safeguard lives and property. The first line of defense against the destructive effects of tornadoes is the National Weather Service (NWS), an agency within the National Oceanic and

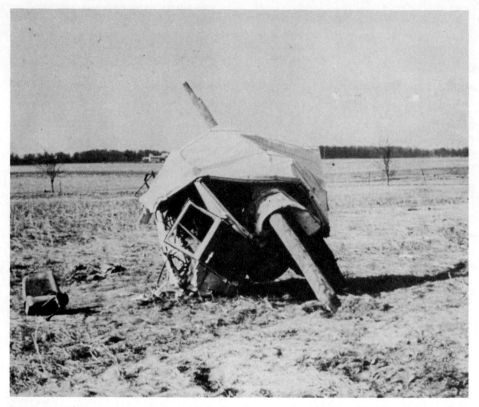

FIG. 9-2   This was someone's truck before it was twisted around a telephone pole by a tornado.

Source: Federal Emergency Management Agency, National Oceanic and Atmospheric Administration: Tornado Safety Campaign.

Atmospheric Administration. It coordinates the efforts of local officials, spotter networks, law enforcement personnel, and other emergency forces in detecting and tracking severe storms. The National Weather Service is responsible for issuing warnings and watches that alert the public to potential danger. Meteorologists at the National Severe Storms Forecast Center constantly monitor weather patterns across the country. When they spot conditions that suggest a high probability for tornadoes or severe thunderstorms in a particular area of the country, they contact local National Weather Service officials who, in turn, issue a tornado watch. A tornado **watch** means that tornadoes are possible.[32] The weather conditions that are conducive to severe thunderstorms are also the conditions that can produce a tornado, so it is not unusual to have a combined tornado and severe thunderstorm watch. The watch bulletin broadcast over local radio and television stations states approximately where and for how long the severe storm will exist.

A tornado **warning** is issued only after a tornado has been sighted in the immediate area. Any person who sees a tornado can call the nearest National Weather Service station or a local emergency agency such as the sheriff's department, state police, or

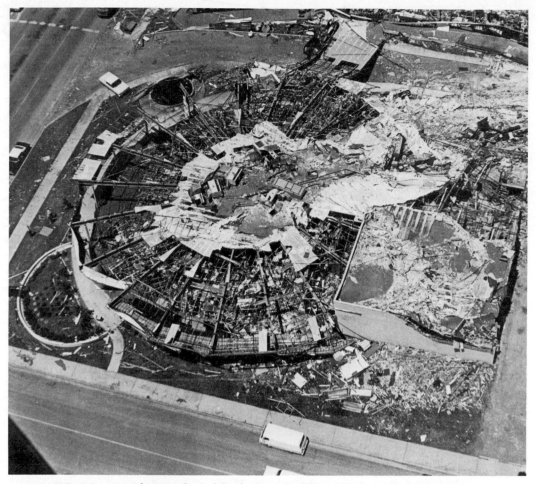

FIG. 9-3 Aerial view of a Lubbock, Texas building-supply store that was torn apart by a tornado.

Courtesy: *Avalanche—Journal*, Lubbock, Tex.

fire rescue service to report the sighting. In recent years the National Weather Service, aided by thousands of volunteers, has developed a nationwide tornado warning network known as "Skywarn."[32] Trained volunteers act as observers when a tornado watch is announced in their area. When a tornado is sighted, its location, size, direction, and speed of movement are quickly reported to the National Weather Service, which, in turn, identifies the area that is most likely to be affected. Although their direction of movement may be erratic, most tornadoes move from *southwest to northeast;* consequently, an early sighting could save countless lives. Once the sighting has been confirmed by radar, tornado warnings are broadcast on radio and TV. In many communities the local warning system includes a steady blast of sirens, horns, or whistles for approximately 5 minutes.

Tornado safety tips. When a warning is received, persons close to the storm should take cover immediately. Actions that you can take depend on your location at the time of the warning.

1. *At home.* Opening windows on the side of the house away from the approaching tornado may prevent damage from a sudden pressure drop if a tornado does hit. After this is done, quickly take cover in a sheltered area. Be sure to take along a flashlight and a battery-operated radio. The best place for shelter is underground; the basement is most often used for this purpose when a separate underground shelter is not available. The safest places to be in the basement are in a corner or under the stairway. For added protection, get under something strong, like a workbench or heavy table. A basic rule to follow is *avoid windows,* since flying debris and broken glass are the cause of death in most tornado fatalities.

If a basement is not available, move to the center of the house, to an interior closet or bathroom (be sure it has no windows). Because the walls are tied together closely in these locations. they offer better protection in high winds.

2. *Mobile homes.* Because it is particularly vulnerable to strong winds and windborne missiles, a mobile home is among the least desirable places to be in a tornado or high-wind situation. Its relatively large surface area and thin protective coating make the mobile home susceptible to being rolled over or penetrated by large pieces of debris. This danger was sadly illustrated on April 26, 1991, when a tornado with 250 mph winds hit Andover, Kansas, killing 14 people. In Andover's trailer park, 220 of the 240 trailers were completely destroyed; all 14 of the town's fatalities lived in the trailer park.[43] If you live in a tornado-prone area, your mobile home park should have an underground shelter for its residents. If it does not, you had better make arrangements with neighbors who have basements.

3. *Offices and apartments.* Safety rules for offices and apartment dwellers are basically the same as those for the homeowner. Go to the basement, if one is available, or to the innermost portions of the structure, such as a hallway, on the lowest floor.

4. *Schools, shopping centers, and factories.* These structures should have designated shelter areas, such as strengthened interior hallways that offer protection from the strong winds and airborne debris. During the tornado season, schools and industrial plants should hold regular drills for students and workers, whereas shopping centers should clearly display directions to shelter locations. A problem with many large open structures, such as gymnasiums, supermarkets, and shopping centers, is that their roofs are supported solely by the outside walls. The partial destruction of the outside supporting walls may lead to the sudden collapse of the entire roof.

5. *Motor vehicles and outdoors.* Two other highly undesirable locations during a tornado are outdoors and in motor vehicles. If you are trapped outside and there is no underground protection or building available, seek shelter in the nearest depression of land; for example, a ditch, gully, or roadside culvert. Lie down flat and remember to cover your head as much as possible.

Against the 150 to 200 mph winds of a tornado, a car or truck offers little protection. Debris carried by a tornado can quickly shatter windows, and the high winds can transform a 4000 pound vehicle into a flying missile. Never try to outrun the tornado in your car; it is estimated that nearly half of those killed or injured in tornadoes were attempting to flee in their cars. If you spot a tornado, stop your vehicle, get out, and seek shelter nearby. Do not get under or next to the vehicle—it may roll over on you.

Although there is no guaranteed safe place during a tornado, these suggestions can increase your chances of survival if they are practiced.

Severe thunderstorms and lightning. Tornadoes are only one of a thunderstorm's killer elements. Heavy rains, high winds, hail, and lightning can also pose a threat. Heavy, sudden rainfall from these storms may cause small streams and sewer lines to overflow. Become familiar with areas of your community that may be prone to flash flooding and avoid them after a heavy rain. If you must be outside, never try to cross stretches of fast-moving water that are more than knee deep. Do not let children play near drainage ditches and roadside culverts, since they are likely to contain the fast-flowing runoff from the storm.

Although they are rarely killers, strong winds in excess of 60 mph and hail (three-quarters of an inch in diameter or larger) often accompany severe thunderstorms, causing millions of dollars in damages to crops and property. The opposite holds true for lightning, which may also occur during this violent weather. Lightning kills more than 50 persons each year; however, it does little in terms of annual property damage.[22]

At the first signs of nearby lightning, get inside a building or an automobile. If you are caught outside, avoid tall, isolated trees; they tend to act as lightning rods. If you can, seek shelter in a ravine or valley; this will prevent you from projecting above the surrounding landscape and becoming a likely target. Finally, avoid contact with metal objects such as bicycles and the metal parts of cars, golf clubs, clotheslines, and fences. Also, avoid using the telephone and appliances.

Hurricanes

No atmospheric disturbance combines duration, size, and violence more destructively than a hurricane. With its elements of driving winds, torrential rain, and storm surge, a hurricane has the potential to kill great numbers of people and destroy vast amounts of property. It is, by far, the most dangerous of all storms.

A **hurricane** is a violent tropical storm in which winds reach constant speeds of 74 mph or more and blow in a large spiral around a relatively calm center—the "eye" of the hurricane.[16] This circular band of heavy rains and strong winds may have a diameter of nearly 300 miles; gusting winds near its center may exceed 200 mph.

Although hurricanes occasionally develop along the southern California coast, they are generally much weaker than their Atlantic counterparts. (Hurricanes occurring in the Far East are called "Typhoons.") States along the Eastern Seaboard and the Gulf of Mexico are the most frequent targets of hurricanes. Most of the damage occurs in August, September, and October; however, the hurricane season lasts from June 1 to November 30. Luckily, major hurricanes are relatively rare events. The most recent hurricane to cause significant loss of life and property damage in the United States was Hurricane Hugo. Hugo, the 10th most intense hurricane since 1900, hit the

South Carolina coast on September 21, 1989, leaving 20 dead and $6 billion in damages. The storm cut a 150 mile-wide swath from Charleston, South Carolina, to Charlotte, North Carolina.

In recent years, a major concern of officials at the National Hurricane Center in Miami has been the rapid development and expansion of coastal communities throughout the Sunbelt. As major industries have relocated in the South, there has been a significant population increase in these states. Millions of these new coastal residents have never experienced a major hurricane and may hesitate to evacuate their homes should a storm emergency occur. The popularity of the Barrier Islands off the coasts of Florida, Georgia, North and South Carolina, and Texas especially concerns hurricane safety personnel. These low-lying islands offer little protection against heavy seas in a major storm. It is likely that a number of them would be under as much as 20 feet of water should a hurricane hit.[9] In the past, many of these islands were sparsely populated and evacuation was not a serious problem; however, today, over-development and outdated evacuation plans have created a situation that could result in the deaths of thousands of residents. The National Hurricane Center can give about 12 hours of warning for an approaching hurricane, but it is estimated that adequate evacuation of many of these communities would take 20 to 30 hours.

In the case of Hurricane Hugo, the Barrier Islands of South Carolina, which lie north and east of Charleston, took the brunt of the storm's winds. More than 300

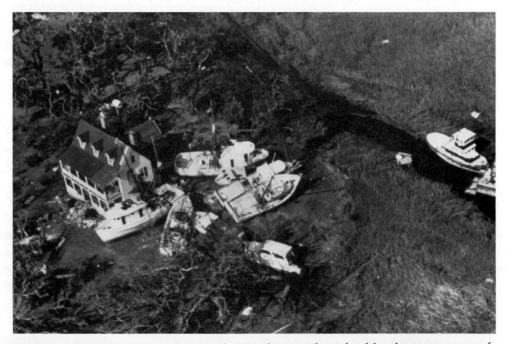

FIG. 9-4 These boats were deposited more than 3 miles inland by the storm surge of Hurricane Hugo.
Courtesy: Federal Emergency Management Agency.

oceanfront homes were destroyed along with several hundred sailboats and yachts. Because of the impending severity of the storm, most of the islands' 5000 inhabitants had been evacuated under police order the day before Hugo arrived.

Elements of destruction. While a hurricane's strong winds and heavy rain threaten life and property, its most dangerous element is the accompanying high tides and rough seas known as a "storm surge."[33] The storm surge, which accounts for approximately 90% of hurricane-related deaths, is a great dome of water caused by a combination of low pressure and high winds around the eye of the storm. It can stretch as much as 50 miles across and rise 20 feet or more above sea level. It does not slam into shore like a tidal wave; rather, it rises like a quick tide to flood low-lying areas (Fig. 9-4). Add to this wind-driven waves of 5 feet or more which ride along the top of the storm surge, and the effects are devastating. Breakers coming ashore on top of the storm surge travel about half the speed of winds in the storm and act like a battering ram, smashing into buildings, while the high tides erode long stretches of beach, undermining support for these structures. (See Fig. 9-5.) Hurricane Hugo's storm surge was measured at 17 feet.

For some structures, the force of high winds is sufficient to cause destruction. In this regard, mobile homes are particularly vulnerable. Another threat from a hurricane's winds is flying debris; lawn furniture, signs, roofing materials, and lumber are only a few of the objects that may become deadly missiles. Wind speeds vary greatly from storm to storm, but hurricanes having sustained wind speeds of 100 to 150 mph and gusts of 175 to 200 mph are not uncommon.[16] The sustained wind speeds of Hurricane Hugo measured 135 miles per hour. To put this into perspective, think about those days when you have been outside with winds gusting at 30 to 40 mph. Now, multiply that 4 or 5 times! (See Fig. 9-6.)

As a hurricane moves inland, its winds diminish; however, it still has the potential to do harm with its torrential rains and subsequent flooding. On the average it takes 24 hours for one of these tropical storms to move through a community; in that time as much as 30 inches of rainfall might occur. Part of the massive damage caused by Hurricane Hugo in 1989 was the result of severe flooding in South Carolina and North Carolina. In some areas more than a foot of rain fell in less than 12 hours.

When a hurricane threatens. The best time for preparation is before the hurricane season. Become familiar with the area in which you live: How far from the beach is your home? What is the elevation above sea level? Is it built on pilings or on a cement slab? A storm surge from a major hurricane can damage residential areas on low ground as far as 10 miles inland. Homes built on wood pilings driven deeply into the sand offer more protection, since there is no way to anchor a building adequately to a smooth cement surface.

Review your insurance policy to make sure that you are adequately covered. A homeowner's policy covers damage from wind and rain, but it does not cover flood damages. A separate flood insurance policy is required.

Also before the hurricane season, it would be wise to review the best routes for evacuating the area, locations of the nearest community shelters, and your inventory

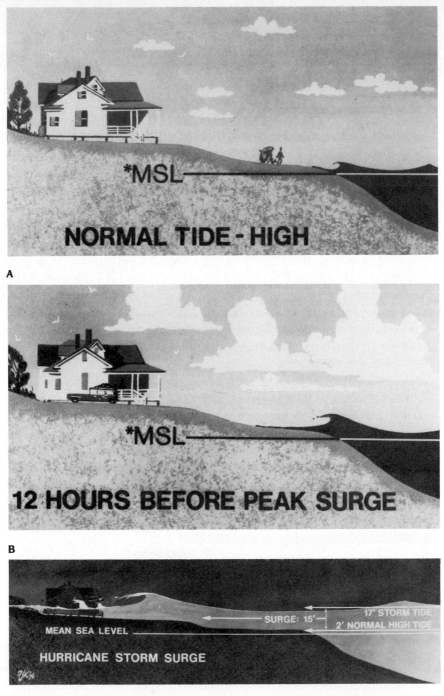

A

B

C

FIG. 9-5 Three illustrations on this page show the formation and effects of the hurricane storm surge. **A,** Sea rises and falls predictably with astronomical tidal action; however, a hurricane has developed, and a hurricane watch is in effect. **B,** With the hurricane 12 hours away, the watch has been upgraded to a warning. The tide is somewhat above normal as water moves up the beach and the size of the waves increases. **C,** As the hurricane moves to shore, it brings with it a 15-foot storm surge topped by battering waves.

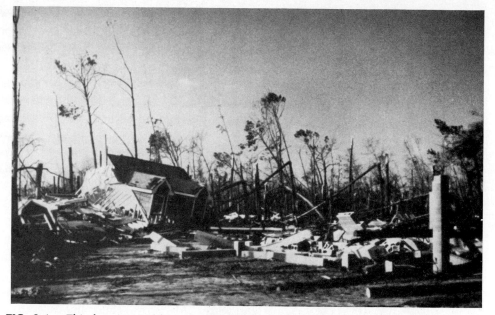

FIG. 9-6   This home was blown from its cement block foundation by Hurricane Hugo's winds. Notice the trees in the background which have been sheared off.
Courtesy: Federal Emergency Management Agency.

of emergency supplies. This inventory may include plywood to cover windows and entrances, batteries for flashlights and radios, plastic sheeting for waterproofing, canned goods and nonperishable foods, a first aid kit, and any special medications.[15] Do not wait until a storm is heading toward shore; supplies will be difficult to locate, so purchase them ahead of time.

With the aid of modern detection and tracking devices, the National Weather Service's Hurricane Center in Miami can usually give 12 to 24 hours' warning to coastal residents about an approaching hurricane. A hurricane watch is issued whenever there is a threat of hurricane conditions developing in the next 24 to 36 hours. Persons in the watch area should listen for further advisories, check supplies and equipment, and fuel their cars.

A hurricane warning is issued when winds of 74 mph or higher or a combination of dangerously high water and very rough seas are expected in a specific coastal area within 24 hours.[16] When a warning is issued, it's time for immediate action:
1. Continue to listen to the radio or TV.
2. Prepare for high winds by anchoring objects outside or bringing them indoors; for example, toys, bicycles, garden tools, lawn furniture.
3. Protect windows and glass with plywood coverings or shutters. To reduce the danger of shattering glass, put tape across windows and close drapes over them.
4. Move valuables to upper floors if possible.
5. Store drinking water in jugs, bottles, cooking utensils, sinks, and the bathtub.

Perhaps the biggest decision that you will have to make is whether or not to evacuate your home. If you live on the beach, on a offshore island, near a river, or in a flood plain, *plan to leave*. These areas are likely to be damaged by the storm surge and torrential rains. If you live in a mobile home, *plan to leave*, since it offers little or no protection against high winds.

If you live on high ground, away from the coastal beaches, you may want to consider staying. If you decide to stay, remain indoors on the downwind side of the house, away from windows until the all clear signal is broadcast by emergency personnel. Regardless of your location, if local authorities recommend evacuation, do so; their advice will be based on information concerning the strength and destructive power of the hurricane. If you must leave, post a note in a conspicuous place including: time you left, destination, and condition of family members.

Floods

If you had been an early settler in this country, where would you have made your home? Chances are you would have located near the sea or near a river. Actually, our forefathers had little choice; it was a necessity, since these bodies of water provided drinking water, food, transportation, and power. Towns sprang up along river banks, on fertile deltas, and on low coastal plains. When these communities were small, high water and flood damage was minimal; however, as cities became more densely populated, flood hazards became more serious. Since 1900, more than 10,000 people have died in the United States as a result of floods and flood-related accidents. It is estimated that annual property losses from floods now total more than $1 billion each year.[11]

A **flood** is a river flow or ocean elevation that threatens or causes damage. The most common are the rainstorm or river flood and the coastal flood (resulting from an unexpected increase in sea level). Other, less-common floods result from the melting of ice and snow, ice jams and river blockages, and dam or levee failures. In some communities, inadequate storm-sewer drainage after a heavy rainfall may result in the flooding of neighborhood streets and homes. This is known as ''sheet flooding''; it seldom threatens lives, but it can cause major property damage on a regular basis.

Normally, flooding will be a relatively slow process, allowing for adequate warning. The buildup to flood conditions will take several days and can be monitored closely by the local office of the National Weather Service. A storm's magnitude and duration are important factors in flood-flow calculations and are the subject of detailed study and evaluation by meteorologists. For persons working in flood control, warning of approaching storms allows for more efficient preparation, especially when predictions are made for amounts of precipitation. However, a warning of impending high-water conditions is not always possible.

Intense localized storms can produce heavy runoff into nearby streams. In Texas, areas as small as 10 to 50 square miles have been inundated with as much as 4 inches of rain in 1 hour. The soil quickly becomes saturated and the excess rainwater or runoff causes small streams and drainage ditches to overflow their banks; this situation is known as a **flash flood.** In mountainous portions of New Mexico and California, heavy rains in the higher elevations can produce deadly flash flooding. The runoff from steep slopes can create a raging torrent at lower elevations (foothills and valleys) in just a few hours. Often, unsuspecting campers in the path of the flash flood become the victims.

Through its River Forecast Centers and River District Offices, the National Weather Service issues flood forecasts and warnings when rainfall is significant enough to cause rivers to overflow their banks and when melting snow combines with rainfall to produce similar effects.[17] Flood warnings are forecasts of impending high water conditions, the expected severity of the flooding, and when and where it will begin. They give people in the affected areas a chance for prompt response and careful preparation to reduce property loss and to ensure personal safety. Flash flood warnings are the most urgent type of flood warning issued; they are concerned with ensuring personal safety, since there may be little time to respond before flood waters arrive.

As with any disaster situation, preparation is of the essence. Do you live on a "flood plain" (an area that is subject to flooding; under certain conditions it is likely to be inundated)? If so, you may want to consider flood insurance. A homeowners' policy does not cover flood damage, but flood insurance may be purchased at reasonable rates from the National Flood Insurance Program (NFIP). The NFIP is a federal program established by Congress in 1968 to assist persons living in flood-prone areas. In return for this federal assistance, communities carry out local flood-plain management to protect property from future flooding. To find out more about flood insurance eligibility and your property's risk of exposure to flood, contact your local insurance agent. Persons living in areas that are likely to be flooded should keep on hand materials such as plastic sheeting, plywood, and sand bags, which can be used to protect property. Also, a flashlight and portable radio are two pieces of emergency equipment that every household should maintain. Learn the safest and quickest route from your home to the designated emergency shelter in your area.

In the event of a flood warning, your personal safety is the most important consideration. Since flood waters can rise very rapidly, be prepared to evacuate should emergency personnel make that request. If time permits, a number of steps may be taken to lessen flood damage:[17]

1. Turn off all electrical circuits at the fuse or breaker panel. If this cannot be done, unplug all electrical appliances.
2. Fill the bathtub, sinks, and plastic jugs with fresh water, since supplies may later become contaminated. Once this is done, shut off water service to the home.
3. If there are gas appliances in the home, shut off the main gas line.
4. Move all valuables to upper floors if possible.
5. Open basement windows to equalize water pressure on the walls of the foundation. If sandbags are used as a barrier against the rising waters, do not place them against the walls of the house. When wet, they may create an added pressure on the structure.

If the plan is to evacuate, stock the car with nonperishable foods, several jugs of water, blankets, dry clothing, a first aid kit, flashlight, and portable radio.[15] Drive to the home of friends or relatives who live outside the danger area or head to the nearest emergency shelter. Do not drive where water is over the roads—sections may be

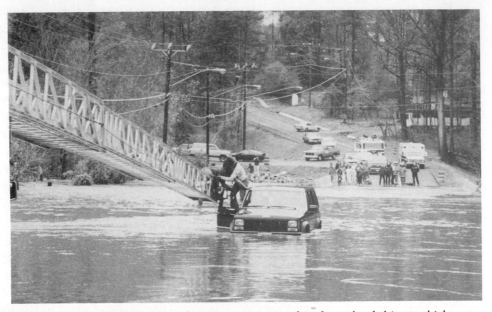

FIG. 9-7 A short time after the passengers in this four-wheel-drive vehicle were rescued, rising flood waters swept it away.

Courtesy: Fairfax County Fire and Rescue Department, Fairfax, Va. (photo by Paul Torpey).

washed out or missing. Also, cars that stall in the floodwaters should be abandoned; rising waters can quickly sweep a car and its occupants away (Fig. 9-7).

Floods are deceptive. People do not realize the force and power exerted by floodwaters. Be sure to avoid all areas that are more than knee-deep. If the water exceeds that depth around your home, stay put and move to the second floor or the roof if necessary, then wait for rescue personnel.

Winter Storms

Winter can be an enjoyable time of the year, providing conditions for recreational activities such as skiing, ice skating, sledding, snowmobiling, and tobogganing; nonetheless, you must also be aware of its hazards. Having a comfortable and safe winter is a matter of planning. If you do not plan, winter can be a killing season.

It is estimated that nearly 500 Americans die from cold-related causes each winter.[35] Winter storms cause death in a number of ways, including auto accidents, home fires, exposure and freezing, carbon monoxide poisoning, overexertion, and falls. Such winter tragedies could be prevented by taking some basic precautions. Let's examine them.

One of the most important safety measures during winter is to keep posted on weather conditions. Even a few hours' warning can help you to better cope with severe weather. The National Weather Service issues watches and warnings concerning winter storms. A winter storm watch is issued when atmospheric conditions might produce severe winter weather conditions (ice, snow, heavy winds) in a particular area. Winter storm warnings are issued when the weather conditions are imminent and will specify the type of weather to occur:[35]

1. Ice storm warning: significant, possibly damaging ice accumulation; precipitation is expected to freeze when it hits exposed surfaces

2. Heavy snow warning: A snowfall of at least 4 inches in 12 hours or 6 inches in 24 hours is expected

3. **Blizzard** warning: Considerable falling and/or blowing snow with winds of at least 35 milers per hour are expected; a Severe Blizzard Warning is issued when winds are at least 45 miles per hour and the temperature is 10° F or lower

4. High wind warning: Winds of at least 40 miles per hour are expected for at least 1 hour.

Severe winter weather can present hazards both in the home and on the road. A heavy snowfall accompanied by bitterly cold temperatures may isolate people in their homes for several days. During this forced isolation, residents will have two primary needs for survival: food and heat. With a little preparation, these hardships can be eased significantly. Before winter weather arrives, stock up on foods that require no cooking or refrigeration. A variety of precooked, canned items (meats, vegetables, and fruits) can be purchased. *Be sure to have a nonelectric can opener available in case of power outages.* Easily stored, quick-energy foods, such as raisins, nuts, and dried fruits, are excellent in an emergency situation. All of these supplies do not have to be purchased at once. Purchase just one or two extra items with each visit to the grocery over a period of months, so it won't affect your budget. Persons who wait until a snow emergency hits often find store shelves bare, since delivery trucks are unable to reach their destinations.

Regular supplies of fuel may also be limited by storm conditions or extremely low temperatures. Homes using heating oil may not be resupplied for several days if fuel trucks cannot make their rounds. In extremely cold weather, an excessive demand for electricity can lead to power shortages; a similar demand for natural gas can also create problems for homeowners heating with gas. In an emergency, an alternative heating source could keep at least one room warm enough to live in. Three of the more popular methods of heating are fireplaces, wood-burning stoves, and kerosene heaters. However, these must be used with care; proper ventilation is necessary and extra caution is needed to reduce potential fire hazards. For directions concerning the proper use of these alternative heat sources see Chapter 5.

Not every home has an alternative heat source if a blizzard should knock out power; for example, people who live in an all-electric apartment or home. The alternative in this case is to dress warmly.

Dress in thin layers, preferably using wool clothing. The layers entrap insulating air, which is warmed by the body; and wool, with its loosely woven fabric, allows moisture to evaporate from the skin. If you get too warm, a layer of clothing can be peeled off.

The body can lose as much as 50% of its heat through the head and neck;

therefore, whether you are outdoors or in an unheated home, wearing a knit cap can keep you much warmer.[7] This applies whether a person is in bed at night or up and around during the day. Mittens should be used instead of gloves to keep the hands warm, since they allow the fingers to touch (which uses body heat more efficiently). If you have no mittens, a pair of wool socks covering your hands will be as effective.

If you have elderly persons living in your household, special care must be taken to ensure their safety. Older people are especially susceptible to a condition known as **hypothermia** (a significant drop in body temperature—below 95° F). Often an elderly person's body temperature regulating mechanisms do not function well; they may not have the sensation of being cold, even though their body temperature is dropping. Other problems that contribute to hypothermia difficulties in the elderly are reduced physical activity, decreased body fat, and poor circulation. If the body temperature continues to drop, cardiovascular and respiratory distress are likely. As many as 50,000 Americans over 65 years of age and who suffer from hypothermia are admitted to hospitals each year. A significant number of them die.

What can be done to protect the elderly? Unless there is a problem, such as a power outage, the elderly should never be in a room in which the temperature is below 65° F—regardless of the savings on fuel costs. Dressing warmly is also extremely important. Besides the layered clothing, mittens, and headgear, thermal underwear should be a regular part of an elderly person's winter wardrobe. This ventilating net underwear provides an important added layer of warmth without restricting the evaporation of perspiration from the skin. A final precaution to ensure sufficient warmth for the elderly is to take a daily body temperature reading; if it is lower than normal, steps should be taken to provide additional warmth for them.

With a stock of quick-energy foods and a supply of warm clothing a family should be able to survive a winter emergency with little difficulty. Don't wait until the snow or winter emergency hits—plan early for a cold winter.

On the road. No one should drive in bad winter weather unless he or she absolutely must; however, it is not surprising to find that many people do not heed this advice. Business obligations and holiday plans usually win out when a travel decision must be made. People often underestimate the force of a winter storm; in some cases, they pay with their lives.

If you must travel during the winter, some special planning is in order. Whether your trip is 60 miles or 600 miles, plan it carefully:[23]

1. Be sure the car or truck is in good condition and properly serviced. Check the battery, radiator, hoses, fan belts, brake fluid, engine and transmission oil levels, lights, and tires. Snow tires or chains are a must. In many states you may get fined if you get stuck during a snow emergency without snow tires or chains.

2. Determine your route of travel. Try to stay on major highways and drive during daylight hours.

3. Let a friend or relative know when you are leaving home, when you expect to arrive, and the route you are taking.

Even with these precautions, people can still get stranded during a sudden winter storm. If you have ever traveled on an interstate highway during the Christmas season, you may be familiar with the following list of circumstances: It is snowing heavily; the wind is blowing; and visibility is poor. Suddenly,

1. The car in front of you stops.
2. The car in front of you goes into a slide.
3. Wind and turbulence from a passing tractor-trailer obstruct your vision.
4. A vehicle attempting to pass you goes out of control.
5. You hit a patch of ice.

You attempt to avoid a collision and end up in a ditch!

Depending on the amount of traffic and the severity of the storm, it may be some time before you and your vehicle can be rescued. This is why it is wise to carry an emergency car kit during your winter travels. Essential elements of this kit include the following:[11]

1. Several blankets or sleeping bags.
2. A stack of newspapers (for extra insulation).
3. Extra winter clothing (wool caps, mittens, and boots).
4. Flashlight with extra batteries and a portable radio, if your car does not have one.
5. A first aid kit.
6. A supply of quick-energy foods (nuts, dried fruit, and candy).
7. A small sack of sand and a shovel; if your car is not mired too deeply in the snow, you may be able to dig yourself out and use the sand for added traction.
8. A set of booster cables.

Most deaths in winter storms occur in and around automobiles in noncollision situations, as described in the following case studies:

> *A number of motorists who did not have adequate warm clothing left their cars to seek other shelter. They quickly became disoriented in the blizzard conditions and could neither find shelter nor return to their cars. The combination of exposure to the elements and a lack of physical conditioning led to hypothermia and death.*

Persons who are found alive often lose extremities (hands or feet) to frostbite. Unprotected hands and feet freeze; oxygenated blood flow to them stops and tissues begin to die. If circulation cannot be restored quickly after rescue, the extremities must be removed surgically to prevent infection from damaging additional tissue.

> *In a recent winter, blizzard conditions over a 3-day period in northwestern and north central Indiana claimed five lives and seriously injured 20 other persons. The majority of the victims had been stranded in vehicles along a 150-mile stretch of Interstate 65 from Chicago to Indianapolis. Most of them had failed to follow the first rule of winter survival: when trapped in a car, stay in the car and don't panic.*
>
> *Many of the victims were businessmen who were not dressed for the weather; with winds exceeding 40 mph during the storm and temperatures hovering around 0°F, the resulting wind chill index (the actual cooling effect on the skin) was -54°F.[32] At this temperature, tissues can freeze in a matter of minutes. In addition, much of Interstate 65 cuts through flat or gently rolling farmland, which offered no protection from the arctic*

winds of the blizzard. Consequently, without the protection of their vehicles or proper winter attire, these motorists paid a dear price for their lack of knowledge and preparation.

Although they do not guarantee total protection, if you are trapped in a car during a blizzard, the following safety tips give you the best chance of survival:[12]

1. Do not attempt to leave your car to seek shelter, unless you can answer yes to all of the following:
   a. Can you clearly see the structure?
   b. Do you have warm clothing?
   c. Are you in good physical condition?
   If you cannot answer yes to all three questions, stay in your car because you are more likely to be found here than if you are out wandering aimlessly in the snow.
2. If you stay in the car, give some indication that you are in trouble:
   a. Turn on your flashers.
   b. Tie a cloth from the antenna or door handle.
   c. At night, turn on your dome light to make the vehicle visible to search crews.
3. To stay warm, run the engine and heater for short periods of time. To reduce the danger of carbon monoxide poisoning, open the windows slightly to allow for adequate ventilation. Be sure to check that snow does not block the exhaust pipe and increase the risk of carbon monoxide poisoning. If the car's engine will not start or you run out of fuel, mild exercises involving arm and leg movement will help to warm you. Now is the time to use those blankets and sleeping bags you have stored in the trunk. If you have failed to prepare an emergency kit, rubber floor mats and the car's floor carpeting can be used as a blanket to conserve body heat.
4. If someone is with you, take turns sleeping in 1- or 2-hour shifts; if you are alone, try to stay awake. Your top priority is to be rescued, so someone needs to be awake to alert rescuers. At the same time, the potential for hypothermia and its fatal consequences increases the longer you sleep and are inactive in an unheated vehicle. Remember, the key to your survival in this winter storm emergency is to maintain adequate body warmth.

Earthquakes and Tsunamis

One of the most destructive phenomena in nature is the earthquake. An **earthquake** is characterized by vibrating movements of the earth's surface known as ''seismic waves.''[14] These vibrations result from the sudden dislocation and shifting of the underlying plates that make up the earth's crust. Extreme pressures deep within our planet's core cause the solid rock crust to break in certain areas. In the breaking process, energy is released and seismic waves are generated outward from the break.

It is estimated that perceptible shocks (2.5 or higher on the Richter Scale) number about 150,000 annually worldwide. However, the number of reported earthquakes that are associated with extensive damage or loss of life (6.0 or higher on the Richter Scale) is approximately 140 per year.[27]

Throughout history, major earthquakes have caused catastrophic damage and extensive loss of life. It is estimated that in the past 4000 years, over 13 million deaths have been caused by these violent disturbances. One of the most devastating earthquakes was recorded in the province of Tangshan, China in 1976; the death toll exceeded 600,000.[27]

In contrast to these figures, the death toll and property damage caused by earthquakes in the United States has been comparatively small. There have been approximately 1300 deaths and $14 billion in property damage since the first earthquake was recorded in the colonial town of Plymouth, Massachusetts in 1638. More than half of the U.S. deaths (700) occurred in the 1906 San Francisco earthquake. The most recent major earthquake was located in the San Francisco Bay area in 1989. To date, it was the most expensive earthquake on the North American continent, causing $7 to $10 billion in damages.[28]

Do the above figures indicate that the United States is relatively free from a serious earthquake threat? Not really—about 33% of the people in the United States (80 million), living in areas west of the Rocky Mountains, are under a significant risk from earthquakes. Another 160 million Americans who live east of the Rockies have at least a moderate chance of suffering injury or property damage from an earthquake in their lifetime. The only places in the United States that seem to be free from earthquake hazards are parts of southern Florida, Alabama, Mississippi, and Texas. Fig. 9-8 is a seismic risk map of the 48 continental states. Alaska and Hawaii are also at risk for major destructive earthquakes.

Although the magnitude of strength of the seismic waves plays an important role in determining an earthquake's destructive potential, other factors are more important. These include the size of the population involved, the time of day the quake

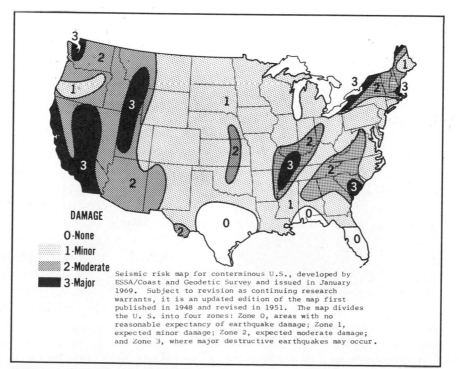

DAMAGE

0 - None
1 - Minor
2 - Moderate
3 - Major

Seismic risk map for conterminous U.S., developed by ESSA/Coast and Geodetic Survey and issued in January 1969. Subject to revision as continuing research warrants, it is an updated edition of the map first published in 1948 and revised in 1951. The map divides the U. S. into four zones: Zone 0, areas with no reasonable expectancy of earthquake damage; Zone 1, expected minor damage; Zone 2, expected moderate damage; and Zone 3, where major destructive earthquakes may occur.

FIG. 9-8   Seismic risk map.

Courtesy: U.S. Geological Survey.

occurs, the type of housing in the area, and the geographic location of the affected area. The most important of these factors is population.

A major earthquake in a metropolitan area will do far more damage than an earthquake of even greater magnitude in a sparsely populated location. The Good Friday earthquake of 1964, which severely damaged a number of Alaskan communities and claimed 300 lives, measured 8.6 on the Richter Scale, whereas a 1985 earthquake in Mexico City that killed over 10,000 registered 7.3 on the same scale, and an earthquake in Soviet Armenia in 1988 that claimed nearly 40,000 lives measured 6.9. The great loss of life associated with earthquakes is often a result of the poor design and construction of buildings.

In the United States, unreinforced masonry buildings constitute the greatest seismic hazard. In the event of an earthquake these structures are more likely to collapse or partially break apart, sending down debris such as bricks and glass. Although California has had earthquake-resistant building codes since the 1930s, it is estimated that as many as 40,000 buildings, housing 15% to 20% of the total population of Los Angeles County, offer little or no earthquake resistance (Fig. 9-9).[28]

To alleviate some of the danger, engineers have designed ways to retrofit these older buildings; for example, anchoring adjoining walls to floor and roof structures with steel cables and bolts increases their stiffness and strength. Additional support can be provided by installing steel and rubber shock-absorbing devices at the base of the building's foundation.

Building collapse and falling debris are not the only hazards in an earthquake.

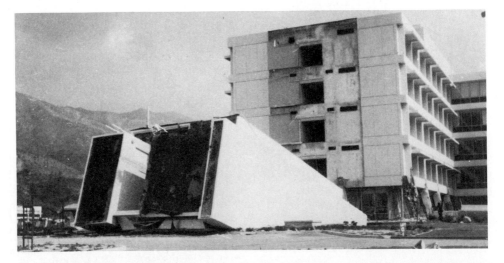

FIG. 9-9   Fallen section of Olive View County Hospital, Los Angeles, Calif. Note the wheelchair dangling from the roof of the fallen section.
Courtesy: Federal Emergency Management Agency.

Earthquakes that occur near coastal areas may be accompanied by destructive sea waves, which can quickly flood an entire community. Known as **tsunamis** or **tidal waves,** they are generated by the sudden displacement of the sea bottom.[4] When the ocean floor moves vertically, it forces water before it like the paddle of a boat. In deep water the tsunami is usually less than 3 feet in height and moves very quickly; it would not generally be noticed by large vessels. As the wave moves into shallow water, it slows down and begins to increase in height to as much as 60 feet above sea level. Such a massive wave may run inland for nearly half a mile, inundating and smashing anything in its way. Often more than one sea wave is generated by the earthquake; they may be separated by several minutes or nearly an hour. People are lulled into a sense of security after the first wave passes and prematurely return to their homes to clean up. During the 1964 Alaskan earthquake, a tsunami generated in Alaskan waters hit the northern California town of Crescent City, killing 119 persons and causing $104 million in damage. It consisted of a series of four waves. The first two caused only minor flooding, and many people returned to their homes; however, two more waves of much greater magnitude hit sometime later, causing death and destruction.

Secondary hazards that may compound the damage from an earthquake include fires, floods (resulting from dam failures), and landslides. The San Francisco earthquake of 1906 and its ground tremors caused approximately 20% of the damage to the city, while devastating fires, which occurred after the earthquake, did the rest of the damage. Over 7 square miles of the downtown area were destroyed by fire. A more recent example of fire hazards associated with an earthquake is the Managua, Nicaragua, disaster of 1972, which killed 5000 people. The initial earthquake destroyed most of the fire apparatus in this city of almost 2 million residents. In addition, the local water system was devastated by a number of pipeline breaks. It took more than 7 days before fires burning in the city could be controlled.

In hilly and mountainous regions that are seismically active, earthquake tremors can set in motion large amounts of loosely packed soil and rock; this phenomenon is known as a **landslide.** Tremors in southern California have set off thousands of landslides over the years, which have killed many residents and caused millions of dollars in property damage.

The most tragic quake-related landslide in recent years occurred in the Peruvian Andes in May 1970. A wall of earth, snow, and rock approximately 200 feet high and traveling at speeds in excess of 150 mph buried the villages of Ranrahirca and Yungay and killed 20,000 people. Ironically, the same villages had been damaged 8 years earlier by a similar landslide that claimed 4000 lives.

The lessons of Loma Prieta. On Tuesday, October 17, 1989, at approximately 5:04 P.M., an earthquake (measuring 7.1 on the Richter Scale) struck the Oakland-San Francisco Bay area. Its epicenter or starting point was an area along the San Andreas fault 50 miles southeast of San Francisco in the Santa Cruz Mountains known as Loma Prieta (Black Hill). Shock waves traveling from the shifting plates in the earth's

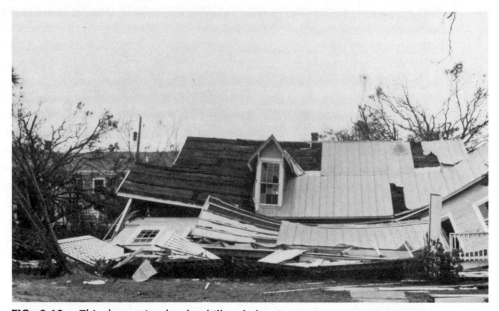

FIG. 9-10   This home in the foothills of the Santa Cruz Mountains was one of the casualties of the Loma Prieta earthquake.
Courtesy: Federal Emergency Management Agency.

surface damaged communities both north and south of the epicenter (Fig. 9-10). The communities of Santa Cruz, Watsonville, Hollister, Los Gatos, San Jose, Redwood City, and San Mateo suffered significant damage and a number of fatalities. However the bulk of the damage occurred in the densely populated and developed Oakland-San Francisco area (Fig. 9-11).

In the aftermath of the quake, approximately 70 people had been killed and damage was estimated to be between $7 billion to $10 billion. Why so few deaths from a relatively strong and destructive earthquake? The answer is threefold:

1. Major high-rise structures extensively use steel which is strong enough to support a building, yet is flexible enough to bend under seismic stress without breaking. Older low-rise structures which used brick and masonry for support could not withstand the lateral movement caused by the seismic waves.

Nearly 50 of the 70 deaths were the result of the structural collapse of a mile-long section of the double-decked Nimitz Freeway in Oakland. Built in the 1950s before there was an emphasis on earthquake-resistant construction, the freeway's concrete support columns had minimal steel reinforcement.

2. Building codes requiring the retrofitting of older structures with earthquake-resistant designs led to the reinforcement of buildings which normally would not have tolerated the forces of the earthquake. One technique that has been used on older concrete and masonry structures is known as "base isolation." Engineers insert reinforced rubber stilts between the building's walls and its foundation; thus, the

rubber absorbs most of the shock from an earthquake and little vibration is transferred to the building.

3. The emergency medical, fire, and rescue systems in the various communities hit by the Loma Prieta earthquake provided a rapid response for the extrication and rescue of victims, on-scene emergency treatment, and security of damaged areas. These coordinated efforts not only reduced the severity of injuries and property damage, they enabled their communities to quickly return to normal.

Earthquake hazards: some preventive measures. Unlike disasters such as storms, tornadoes, and floods, earthquakes are not easily predicted. Although some advances have been made in determining the probability of occurrence of small earth tremors, the principal concern for seismologists (earthquake researchers) is the determination of disturbances that are a threat to life and property. These larger earthquakes are believed to develop over long periods of time; consequently, it will take a number of years of close and detailed observation of quake-prone areas before accurate prediction techniques can be developed.

In the meantime, a number of preventive measures can be taken by high-risk communities to substantially lessen the damage of future earthquakes. A first step in this direction is land-use planning and management. Facilities such as hospitals,

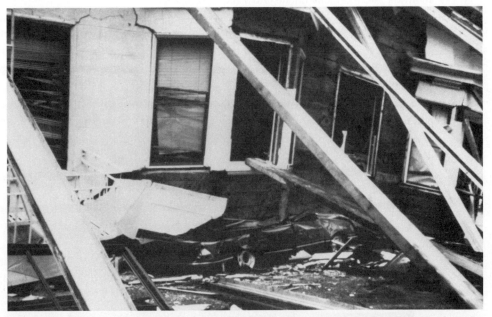

FIG. 9-11   This is the third floor of an older apartment building that collapsed in the Marina District of San Francisco. Notice the crushed vehicle under the windows of the structure.
Courtesy: Federal Emergency Management Agency.

schools, fuel storage tanks, and high-rise apartments should be constructed in areas that have a higher degree of earthquake protection. These structures should never be developed over fault lines or areas that have exhibited significant seismic activity. A concern for southern Californians is where nuclear power plants can be safely located. Can one of these plants withstand a major earthquake?

Once a site has been determined to be a safe place to build, the next step is the design and construction phase. Earthquake-resistant buildings are a key element in protecting high-risk areas. Although it may not be feasible to have every structure follow special building codes and ordinances, facilities that house large numbers of people or that may affect a populated area must be structurally sound. Older structures that are not earthquake resistant may need to be phased out and replaced with new structures or refitted to comply with updated building codes.

The third phase of this community action program involves public information and education. Since major earthquakes occur infrequently in the United States, it is important for people to understand the need to take preventive steps that may be costly and inconvenient at times. Also, knowledge of procedures that provide protection both during and after an earthquake will be invaluable should such an emergency occur.

Some personal tips for earthquake safety. As in the case of homeowners living in floodplains who purchase special flood insurance, owners of homes in earthquake hazard areas would be wise to invest in earthquake insurance. Along the West Coast, such an endorsement can usually be added to an existing homeowners' policy. In some cases, the coverage will also provide protection against damage from landslides and tsunamis. However, coverage for older, unreinforced dwellings is generally not available, since they are likely to be a total loss in an earthquake-related disaster.

Preventive measures that can reduce earthquake hazards in and around the home include:[11]

1. Checking for potential fire risks. Are electrical wiring and gas connections in good condition? Gas appliances should be bolted down or firmly anchored; flexible hosing and connections should be used wherever possible for both gas and water connections.

2. Knowing where and how to shut off electricity, water, and gas at main switches and valves.

3. Securing shelves to walls and bracing top-heavy objects, such as china cabinets. Be sure to place breakable items, such as bottles, dishes, and glasses, on lower shelves.

4. Reinforcing and anchoring overhead light fixtures. Deep cracks in ceiling plaster should be investigated, since this may result in large pieces of plaster falling during a seismic disturbance.

Should an earthquake occur, remember these basic rules:

1. Many injuries occur when people are struck by debris while entering or leaving buildings. If you're outdoors, stay outdoors and move away from buildings and utility

wires. If you're indoors, stay indoors and take cover under a heavy desk or table. Also, stay away from glass doors and windows.

2. If you're in a car, proceed to an open area away from buildings, overpasses, and power lines. Stop the car and stay in the vehicle—it's a relatively safe place to be. When the tremors stop, proceed cautiously, watching for falling objects and damaged roadways.

After the initial earthquake vibrations there may be a series of weaker tremors called "aftershocks." These may last several hours or several days. If your home has been severely damaged, take care when entering because the continued aftershocks may put further stress on the building.

Check utilities. Earth movement may have broken gas, electric, or water lines in your house. Be especially careful if you smell gas; open windows and shut off the main gas valve. Report the leak to emergency personnel, since a ruptured gas line can endanger an entire neighborhood. Damage to electrical wiring in the house can also present a substantial fire hazard, so shut off power if any wiring is shorting out.

Damage to water mains in the community may create a water shortage for a period of time. Remember, emergency water supplies may be obtained from hot water tanks and toilet tanks. During this disaster emergency continue to listen to the radio for the latest bulletins and instructions from local authorities.

MAN-MADE DISASTERS

As humans have progressed into the twentieth century, the changes in society have been fantastic. Many of the diseases that claimed thousands of lives in the early part of this century have become medical rarities. Food production has continued to increase to accommodate a growing population. Even persons living in the northern parts of the country can have fresh fruits and vegetables all year long. Easy-to-care-for fabrics have taken at least some of the drudgery out of housework as have new and better cleaning agents, waxes and polishes. The list of labor- and time-saving innovations that have been introduced just since World War II is immense.

During this era of advancing technology, America's chemical industry has been at the forefront. More than 40% of all goods and services rely in some way on chemicals; and nearly 75% of all fibers used in clothing and home furnishings are chemically based.[41]

Nevertheless, everything has its price. With the benefits of new and exotic chemical compounds come certain hazards. Many chemicals used in industrial and manufacturing processes can pose a significant threat not only to plant workers, but also to the public. In December 1984, more than 2000 people died and 40,000 were injured as a result of an accidental release of methyl isocyanate (MIC) into the atmosphere in Bhopal, India.[1]

A November 1986 fire in a Basel, Switzerland chemical warehouse resulted in the emission of large amounts of nitrogen oxide and sulfur dioxide over the countries of

Switzerland, West Germany, and France, causing respiratory problems for thousands of residents. Further problems resulted when 66,000 pounds of mercury compounds and a variety of pesticides were washed into the Rhine River as fire fighters attempted to control the fire.[29]

This contamination of mercury compounds caused massive fish kills and damage to the marine ecosystem, which has yet to be determined; it is expected to take a number of years for the river's aquatic life to make a comeback.

In our chemically-oriented society, hazardous materials not only present problems during the manufacturing process, but they also must be handled appropriately during transport and disposal. A hazardous material is identified by any of the following four characteristics:[37]

1. Ignitability: These wastes pose a fire hazard during routine management. Fires not only present immediate dangers from heat and smoke, but they can also spread harmful particles over wide areas.

2. Corrosiveness: Corrosive wastes require special containers because they can destroy most standard packaging materials. Corrosives can also dissolve and carry other toxic contaminants in solution.

3. Reactiveness or explosiveness: These hazardous wastes tend to react violently with air or water. When containers carrying these wastes are heated or suddenly jolted, there is a chance for explosion and generation of toxic gases.

4. Toxicity: Toxic wastes pose a substantial biological threat to all living organisms—humans, animals, or plants. Certainly, chemicals that can burn, explode, or corrode tissue can be classified as toxic; however, the definition of toxicity is broader. Many toxic chemicals are not corrosive or explosive; they will do their harm internally and, perhaps, over a period of time. Toxins in this category are also known as "pollutants."

Hazardous Materials Transport

Every day, products that have the potential to burn, explode, or produce highly toxic vapors are shipped from coast to coast. They travel by train and truck through densely populated areas and over heavily traveled thoroughfares. How many times have you seen a tank truck marked *flammable, corrosive,* or *poison* traveling on the interstate, or a railroad tank car with similar markings moving through a busy commercial area? Is there a need for concern? In an average year 1 of every 3 trains and 1 of every 10 trucks is carrying hazardous materials.[11]

On the evening of November 10, 1979, a number of tankers on a 106-car Canadian Pacific freight train derailed in the city of Mississauga, Ontario (population 276,000). Three of the cars, carrying liquefied propane gas (LPG), broke open and exploded, rattling windows as far as 30 miles away. When fire fighters arrived, they found a nearby tank car leaking deadly chlorine gas vapors. If that car exploded, it could have spread a deadly fog of chlorine gas over much of the city. That evening the largest evacuation in Canadian history took place, with most of the city's inhabitants moving to temporary emergency quarters in nearby Toronto. After several days of painstaking, hazardous work, emergency crews were able to patch the damaged tanker and residents were able to return to their homes.

As many as 1000 rail mishaps a year involve hazardous cargoes. An estimated 100,000 people are evacuated from towns and cities annually. An even larger number of hazardous-cargo accidents involve motor vehicles. In a country like the United States, which uses massive amounts of energy, the demand for fuel transportation is quite large. These trucks carry gasoline, diesel fuel, home-heating oils, and a variety of liquified gases (for example, natural gas, propane, butane). Add to this trucks that transport corrosives, explosives, and radioactive materials, and you may begin to get an idea of the scope of the problem (Fig. 9-12). The Chemical Manufacturers Association of America estimates that 90 million shipments of hazardous materials are made each year in the United States.

Realizing the potential for disaster, both private industry and government agencies have become actively involved in efforts to prevent such an occurrence. New chemical tank cars have a double-walled design—actually a tank within a tank. If the outer wall is damaged, there is an inner wall to retain the contents. Since the ends of railroad tank cars are more prone to damage in an accident, these areas have been

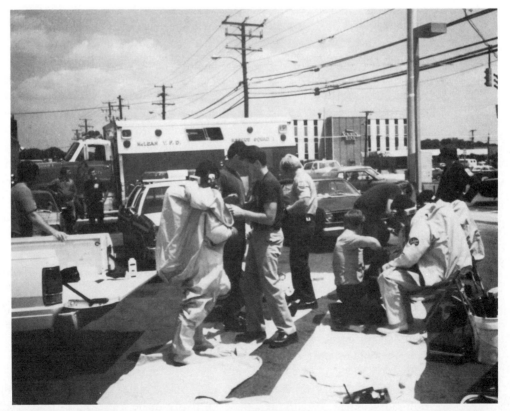

FIG. 9-12 Hazardous-materials response team members don protective gear before entering an overturned tractor-trailer to remove unmarked, leaking chemical drums.
Courtesy: Fairfax County Fire and Rescue Department, Fairfax, Va.

reinforced. To further reduce the possibility of container puncture, special coupling devices have also been installed. Similar structural designs have been incorporated in the manufacture of tractor-trailer tanks as well.

In spite of its design, no chemical tank is unbreakable or puncture-proof. With this in mind, many states and local jurisdictions have enacted legislation that limits shippers of hazardous material to specific routes of travel. In Ohio, legislation has been enacted that requires shippers of nuclear materials to notify the Ohio Disaster Services Agency at least 48 hours before the material reaches the Ohio border. In addition, the scheduled route of the shipment must be designated. Ohio authorities feel that such information would allow emergency personnel to respond in a quicker, more efficient manner, if an accident were to occur.

Recognizing the wide array of hazardous materials that are being shipped nationwide and the need for special handling of these products, many communities are developing **hazardous materials response teams.** These teams usually consist of fire fighters who have received training in the identification, containment, and cleanup of hazardous materials spills (Fig. 9-13).

To assist these units in identifying and controlling hazardous materials, the Chemical Manufacturers Association in conjunction with the U.S. Department of Transportation has developed the Chemical Transportation Emergency Center (CHEMTREC) located in Washington, D.C. CHEMTREC provides immediate advice for persons at the scene of an emergency, then promptly contacts the shipper of the hazardous materials involved for more detailed assistance. Operating around the clock, 7 days a week, CHEMTREC can usually provide hazard information warnings and guidance when given the identification number or name of the product and the nature of the problem. Identification of hazardous materials through the use of I.D. numbers on shipping papers or placards attached to tanks and trailers has been standardized by the Department of Transportation. All hazardous materials transported in the United States have been assigned a specific four-digit code. Using this coding system, the Department of Transportation developed an emergency response handbook for fire fighters, police, and other emergency services. The guide lists initial actions to be taken by emergency personnel to protect themselves and the public during a hazardous materials incident. More specific information can be obtained from CHEMTREC.

Recently, the Environmental Protection Agency (EPA) and the U.S. Coast Guard have developed hazardous material data bases that can be used with portable computers installed on emergency response vehicles. Information from these programs, which can be provided immediately at the emergency scene, includes personal safety precautions, disposal information, handling and storage procedures, hazard levels, effects on humans, air, soil, and water, and procedures for notifying the proper authorities.

The public also has a role to play in a hazardous materials incident. In a highway or railroad accident, the first responder is likely to be a private citizen. When approaching the scene of an accident involving any cargo, especially tank trucks or rail

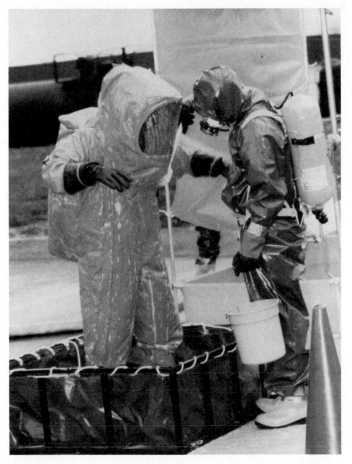

FIG. 9-13 This HAZMAT team member is going through the process of decontamination after repairing a leak in a railroad tank car.

Courtesy: Fairfax County Fire and Rescue Department, Fairfax, Va. (photo by Paul Torpey).

tank cars, never get closer than several hundred yards. If someone is with you, have him or her call the local fire or police service to report the accident while you attempt to warn and keep others away from the scene. Avoid inhaling gases and fumes. If you see smoke or a vapor cloud, quickly move away from it. Even if there is no smell, gases can still be highly toxic. Above all, never walk into or touch any spilled material. By protecting yourself and others, you can play an important role in preventing a hazardous spill from becoming a disaster.

Hazardous Wastes: What Can Be Done?

Waste disposal mismanagement has the potential to affect a significant portion of the U.S. population. Improperly disposed wastes can pollute ground water, rivers, and lakes (Fig. 9-14). In the 1980s, cities in Michigan, Minnesota, Massachusetts, and Tennessee were forced to use bottled water after it was found that local wells had become contaminated with pesticides and suspected carcinogenic compounds from local landfills and manufacturing firms.

In 1982, the small town of Times Beach, Missouri, was abandoned when it was discovered that much of the surrounding soil had been contaminated with highly toxic dioxin. (In the 1970s an oil truck that was used to spray unpaved roads had also been used to haul waste sludge from a number of chemical plants.) Purchased by the EPA, the empty community is now used as a research plot by companies working on methods of detoxifying the land.

Either directly or indirectly each of us will pay if uncontrolled and improper disposal of toxic waste is allowed to continue. People living in areas like Times Beach, Missouri, and the Love Canal (a neighborhood in Niagara, New York, that had to be abandoned in the late 1970s after hazardous waste contaminated ground water) have been directly affected. However, all taxpayers have been indirectly affected, since federal and state governments have been forced to pay for the majority of cleanup operations.

Recognizing the potential for repeated hazardous waste disasters, Congress enacted major legislation. Passage of the Toxic Substances Control Act (TSCA) and the Resource Conservation and Recovery Act (RCRA) brought important changes to the day-to-day operations of the U.S. chemical industry. With TSCA the Environmental Protection Agency was given the task of identifying and controlling chemical products that pose an unreasonable risk to human health or the environment through their manufacture, distribution, use, or disposal.

Under RCRA a multistep regulatory program has been developed. The first and most important step has been the implementation of a "cradle-to-grave" control system for hazardous wastes. The keystone of this system is the monitoring of hazardous waste from point of generation through treatment, storage, and ultimate disposal. All companies involved in handling these wastes (generators, transporters, and disposal facilities) must have EPA identification numbers that are used in filing reports. EPA standards have been established for the proper packaging, transportation, and disposal of wastes.

Ultimately, the company that produces the hazardous waste (the generator) is responsible for its safe disposal. No longer can companies use the cheap alternative of the "midnight dumper" or "gypsy hauler" to dispose of their hazardous materials. With only a truck and a total disregard for public safety, midnight dumpers would take hazardous wastes off generators' hands for relatively modest fees and then dispose of them by dumping the materials into city sewers, rivers, lakes, or onto county roads or private property (such as farmland). If EPA investigators find that generators have not properly disposed of their wastes, they are likely to be responsible for an expensive cleanup bill.

In 1980, a third phase of this national hazardous waste management program was established with the enactment of the Comprehensive Environmental Response, Compensation, and Liability Act (CERCLA). Popularly known as "Superfund," this

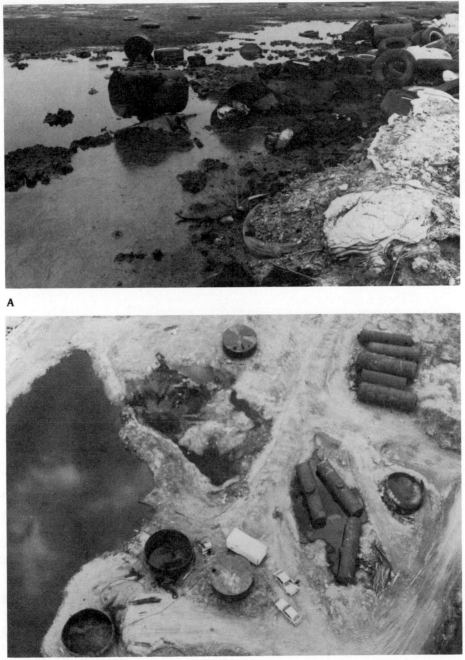

A

B

FIG. 9-14   A, This is one of a number of open pits near La Marque, Texas that were used by independent haulers of hazardous liquid waste. **B,** Known as Bruin Lagoon, this hazardous-waste dump site is adjacent to Bear Creek, a stream that empties into the Allegheny River. The Allegheny is an important water supply for many Pennsylvania communities, including Pittsburgh.

Courtesy: U.S. Environmental Protection Agency.

legislation provided $1.6 billion for the identification and cleanup of abandoned or uncontrolled toxic waste sites.

What has happened since the passage of this legislation? Waste management personnel have found that the dimensions of the toxic and hazardous materials problem are staggering. During the first 6 years of the Superfund more than 30,000 potentially dangerous hazardous waste sites were reported to the EPA. Of these sites, it is estimated that more than 3000 present a substantial danger to human health and the environment. Completion of cleanups has proved more difficult and time consuming than expected; from start to finish the average time for completing decontamination of top priority sites has been 5 years.[6]

The EPA has indicated that cleaning up abandoned hazardous-waste sites and those operating under environmentally unsound conditions could eventually cost as much as $44 billion—only part of which is likely to be paid for by the owners of the sites. With the enactment of the Superfund Amendments and Reauthorization Act in October 1986, Congress mandated an additional $8.5 billion for correcting the toxic waste problem as we move into the 1990s.[6] As more companies follow the guidelines for prudent waste management that have been designed by TSCA and RCRA, the need for a Superfund may someday be eliminated.

Hazardous waste control: some new technologies. The technologies available for processing hazardous wastes present a variety of possibilities. Using physical, chemical, thermal, and biological processes, scientists and engineers can extract useful materials from many hazardous wastes and put them back into production. Some wastes can be changed into harmless materials while other waste can be totally destroyed.

Waste exchange enables one factory's hazardous residues to become another factory's raw material supply. Acid and solvent wastes from some industries can be used by others without processing. Heavy metals such as arsenic, cadmium, and mercury can be extracted from waste solutions and recycled.

Biological processes, such as activated sludge treatment to destroy organic compounds, composting of organically rich wastes, trickling filters to promote decomposition, and controlled application of these chemicals on land to degrade organic compounds, can reduce the amount of hazardous waste that must be disposed of directly on land. This is crucial, since land available for disposal is decreasing while waste tonnages are increasing.

For wastes that can't be handled in any other way, special high temperature incinerators, equipped with pollution control and monitoring systems, have been highly successful in destroying organic wastes without posing a threat to the environment. They have been especially successful in destroying bromine and chlorine-containing wastes, which are very toxic because they resist degradation and can accumulate in living tissues. These incinerators have a combustion efficiency of over 99%; only traces of the wastes are discharged unburned into the atmosphere. A number of hard-to-handle pesticides, including DDT, were almost totally detoxified in tests of these incinerators. Incinerators have also been used to destroy stockpiles of the defoliant Agent Orange (which was used in Vietnam and later banned because of fears that it caused cancer and birth defects) and the controversial polychlorinated biphenyls (PCBs) (which were used in transformer oils and were also found to be carcinogenic).

Because of limited space for landfill operations and strict government regulations, a practice of incineration at sea developed in Europe in the late 1960s. The combustion products of water, carbon dioxide, and a variety of acids drop into the sea. The acids do not present a problem at sea, since they are quickly neutralized by sea salts. A land-based incinerator would have to have special pollution devices to trap escaping acid gases. Another advantage of sea-based incineration is that one incineration ship can handle 10 times the amount of a land-based incinerator.

An incineration device that shows promise for the future is a portable unit dubbed the "blue monster" by EPA researchers. It can be moved from site to site, thus enabling a number of different hazardous waste generators to use it.

Although many of these environmentally sound technologies for waste disposal have existed for some time, they have not been widely used because of their high cost. In the past, the predominant practice for generators of hazardous waste was to store the materials on their property in unlined ponds or landfills. Now, with the stricter EPA controls and regulations that limit the amount of liquid waste that can be placed in landfills and that also require new landfills to install special synthetic leakproof liners, the old methods of hazardous waste disposal aren't as cheap anymore. The rising costs of landfill disposal will make the environmentally sound technologies more practical and appealing.

Citizens' role in hazardous waste management. Successful development and implementation of the EPA's national hazardous waste regulatory program depend on public support. However, before this can happen, citizens need to understand the complex political, social, and economic issues involved. Since 1979, the EPA has funded groups such as the American Public Health Association, the Environmental Action Foundation, and the National Wildlife Federation to assist in keeping the public informed about significant issues. Through this program, known as "Waste Alert," a number of informative booklets concerning hazardous wastes and their management have been produced. Information on these programs is available from the technical information staff of the Office of Solid Waste Management Programs, EPA, Washington, DC 20460.

Events such as the Bhopal, India, tragedy and the Chernobyl nuclear accident have made people more concerned than ever about the need to be aware of chemicals and the hazards they pose. Recognizing this need, Congress established the Emergency Planning and Community Right-to-Know Act in its 1986 Superfund legislation. This act requires federal, state, and local governments and industry to develop emergency response plans as well as provide the public with information about the presence of hazardous chemicals in their communities. For specific details about hazardous materials in your community, contact your Local Emergency Planning Committee (LEPC) or your local fire department.

Citizens can be most effective by working close to home on the local or state level. Become aware of the possible chemical problems to which you and your family might be exposed. If you work with chemicals, find out what they are and what procedures are used to dispose of them. If you find what appears to be a hazardous chemical problem, contact county or state agencies for assistance. The proper authorities include departments of environmental protection, public health, and water resource management.

It is often more productive to make an impact on the planning process than to fight a situation that's already bad. Be aware of new development projects in your community. Will the new county landfill be located over the community's groundwater supply? Will the new industrial park be located near a stream that feeds the county's reservoir and supply of drinking water? Informed citizens can play an important role in seeing that new facilities are located in secure areas, and that they will operate in an environmentally sound manner.

Protection in the Nuclear Age: From Three Mile Island to Chernobyl

Probably one of the least understood, yet most feared, forms of energy is nuclear power. The devastating force of the explosions at Hiroshima and Nagasaki at the end of World War II have made a lasting impression—as they should; however, comparing the destructive potential of an atomic bomb to energy production in a nuclear reactor is invalid. That is not to say that a mishap at a nuclear plant would not present some danger, but the probability of physical harm to the general public from a nuclear accident in the United States is low. How low? The risk of death from a nuclear accident for a person living less than 1 mile from a nuclear plant is approximately 1 in 100 million per year, whereas the chances of dying in a motor vehicle accident is 1 in 4000 per year.

The public misconception of nuclear power has continued to grow since the incidents at the Three Mile Island (TMI) nuclear plant (near Middletown, Pennsylvania) on March 28, 1979, and at the Chernobyl nuclear plant in the USSR on April 26, 1986.

Let's take a look at what actually happened at TMI and Chernobyl. A nuclear power plant's function is to generate electricity. It does this by heating water that, in turn, produces steam that drives a turbine that turns a generator, thus producing an electrical current. The heart of the nuclear plant is its reactor, which heats water. It accomplishes this through the process of nuclear fission—the splitting apart of atoms.

The reactor contains fuel assemblies (which consist of uranium fuel rods, control rods, and small spaces between the rods for the flow of water). These fuel assemblies make up the reactor's core. The core fits into a steel tank known as the ''reactor vessel.''

To initiate a nuclear reaction, the control rods (which block nuclear activity) are withdrawn from the core and uranium atoms begin to split. One of the products of this splitting or fission is heat. Water that surrounds and covers the fuel rods in the core is heated through this process. This super-hot water is then pumped through steam generators that contain a separate supply of cooler water. Water in the steam generators absorbs heat from the reactor water and changes to steam, which is used to generate electricity. In the meantime, reactor water returns to cool the fuel rods. It will absorb more heat from the fuel and repeat the cycle. As long as there is adequate water to cover and cool the fuel rods, the reactor will operate safely.

Although they are of different technical designs, the nuclear reactors at both Three Mile Island and Chernobyl suffered what is known as a "severe loss-of-coolant" accident. Without adequate water flow to cool the reactor's core, steam can build up to explosive levels within the reactor vessel or fuel rods can melt; this is called "meltdown." If either of these occurrences goes unchecked, the surrounding population may become exposed to high levels of radiation.

At Three Mile Island (TMI), a malfunction in the cooling system and a number of human errors caused 30,000 gallons of radioactive water to boil out of the reactor and uncover 30% to 40% of the fuel rods. When this happened, temperatures in the reactor's core exceeded 5000° F, and portions of the uranium fuel reached melting point and allowed highly radioactive gases to escape from the reactor to the surrounding containment building (Fig. 9-15).

Although there was serious damage to the internal equipment of the plant, all but a negligible amount of radiation remained isolated in the containment structure; a small amount of radioactive water was pumped into an auxiliary storage building during the first few minutes of the accident. It was from this building that some radioactive gas escaped into the atmosphere. During the emergency at TMI, the maximum amount of radiation received by local residents was 70 millirems; this is equal to the quantity of radiation you receive from an x-ray (Fig. 9-16).

As with all nuclear power plants built in the United States, TMI had a number of backup systems and protective mechanisms to provide maximum safety to the public. Early in the accident, as temperatures in the reactor's core escalated, control rods automatically dropped into place, shutting off the process of fission and heat production. Backup systems initiated the high pressure injection of water into the reactor vessel to stabilize and cool the fuel rods. Probably the most significant protection was provided by the overall design of the plant. The reactor vessel in which the nuclear fuel is housed is a 40-foot high steel tank with walls 8 ½ inches thick. It is further surrounded by concrete and steel shields, which measure an additional 9 ½ feet in thickness; they absorb radiation from the reactor's core. Finally, all this equipment is located in a containment building, a 193-foot-high, reinforced concrete structure with walls 4 feet thick.

Although the emergency at TMI was officially declared "over" on April 9, 1979, the accident will continue until the long cleanup is completed. Waste disposal and the cost of replacement power for the utility company will be nearly $2 billion; if the plant cannot be put back into operation, the costs will be significantly higher.

Unlike the incident at TMI, which released minimal amounts of radiation, a steam explosion at a reactor in the Soviet city of Chernobyl on April 26, 1986, became the

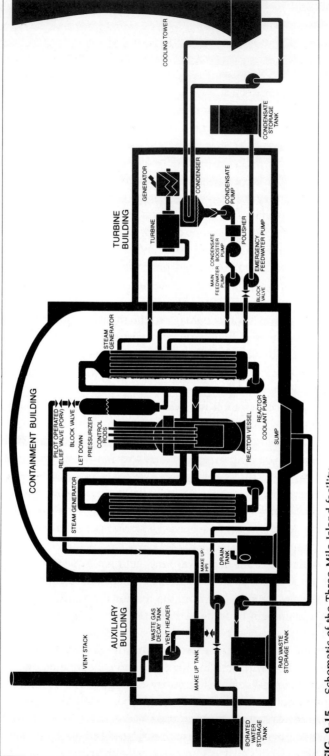

FIG. 9-15 Schematic of the Three Mile Island facility.

Courtesy: Nuclear Regulatory Commission.

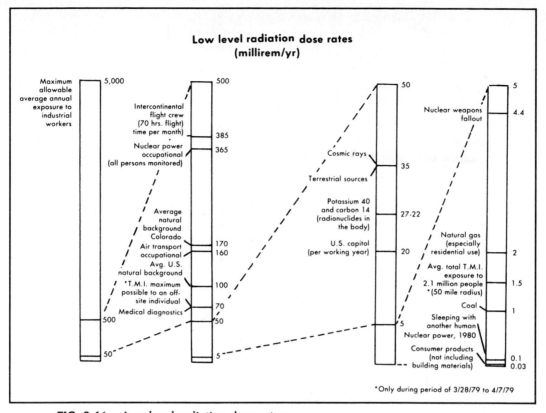

FIG. 9-16   Low-level radiation dose rates.

Source: U.S. Congress, House Committee on Science and Technology.

worst nuclear power accident in history. Thirty-one persons were killed, more than 200 persons were hospitalized with acute radiation syndrome, and an estimated 24,000 residents living near the plant received serious radiation doses of about 50 rem.

Although they had proved to be relatively safe and effective, Russian nuclear reactors could become unstable at low power levels. During the testing of an electrical generator at the Chernobyl plant (which required a power reduction), operators allowed the power to drop to dangerously low levels, breaching a number of safety standards. While operators tried to correct this situation, a rapid increase of thermal energy caused water in the reactor to change to steam and blow it apart.

The explosion and ensuing fire sent up a plume of contaminants 15,000 feet in the air. Ultimately, more than 116,000 people in an 18-mile radius of the plant were evacuated. Since the accident, an additional 90,000 people have been evacuated from surrounding regions because of continuing high-level background radiation and contamination of farmland and water supplies.[8]

The remains of the nuclear plant have been encased in a concrete and steel containment structure. The building will be monitored closely to ensure that no radioactive material can leak into the surrounding groundwater. Although there is some debate, many nuclear safety personnel feel that stronger shielding around the reactor and a containment building similar to those used in the United States could have prevented much of the radiation from escaping into the atmosphere.

Many changes have been made to prevent a recurrence. Technicians, engineers, and managers at all Soviet nuclear plants have received detailed retraining, and new safety features have been added at the remaining nuclear facilities. It is also likely that significant design changes will be seen in future nuclear facilities in the Soviet Union.

Radiation exposure. Since they cannot be seen, tasted, or smelled, radioactive particles have a certain "mystique" about them. Exposure to radiation terrifies many people because they have no idea about what could happen. Every day we're exposed to a certain amount of radiation from the atmosphere. The average annual U.S. exposure is 100 millirems; if you live in Colorado, it is about 200 millirems; and if you fly on a regular basis, you may receive about 400 millirems of radiation each year. Add to this diagnostic x-rays that you may receive in a given year, and you get an idea of how small the amounts of radiation were at TMI (70 millirems; see Fig. 9-16).

What does radiation do, and how can it affect you? It is generally accepted that radiation affects the cell's ability to divide normally; it may cause affected cells to die or reproduce in an abnormal manner, as in the case of cancer.[19] One of the long-term effects of exposure to high doses of radiation is an increased incidence of leukemia. This is not surprising, since it is known that blood-forming cells in the bone marrow are especially sensitive to radiation.

Tissues whose cells normally divide at a rapid pace are most susceptible to radiation injury. A growing child or a developing fetus, with their rapid cellular activity, would be more prone to radiation injury than an adult. This is what prompted the recommendation that pregnant women and young children leave the vicinity of Three Mile Island as a precautionary measure.

Two factors that affect the extent of damage to the body from radiation exposure are the amount received and the period of time in which it is received. The higher the dosage and the shorter the period of time in which it is received, the greater the damage to tissues;[11] that is, if a high radiation dosage is received in a very short period of time, such as 24 hours, the damage to tissues will be much more severe, than if the same dosage were received during a 1- or 2-week period.

Radiation exposures are of two types: short-term, high-level; or long-term, low-level. In a nuclear facility accident we are essentially concerned with short-term, high-level exposures; that is, receiving a large dosage in less than 24 hours. Long-term, low-level exposure would be a concern for people who work with radioactive materials over a period of years.

To put things in perspective, remember that the largest dose that anyone received from the TMI incident was 70 millirems, or 0.07 rem in a 24-hour period; while more than 200 victims of the Chernobyl disaster received between 200 and 600 rems, and an additional 24,000 received 50 rems or more.[10] Table 9-3 compares dosages and their effects.

Table 9-3 Short-term effects of acute radiation exposure

Dose (rems)	Effect
0 to 50	No visible effects.
50 to 200	Some will suffer nausea; about 5% will require medical attention.
200 to 400	Most will require medical attention and about 50% of the persons who receive doses around 400 rems will die in 2 to 4 weeks.
400 to 600	Serious radiation sickness; all require medical attention. Most of the persons who receive doses around 600 rems will die in 1 or 2 weeks.
600 +	Nearly 100% of the victims will die within 2 weeks.

Courtesy: Nuclear Regulatory Commission.

It is important to note that exposure to radiation, even in high doses, is not necessarily fatal. In most cases, if death does not occur within about 6 weeks, recovery from high, but nonlethal, radiation exposure eventually occurs. A factor that complicates studies of radiation effects is that some people are less sensitive to radiation than others; consequently, most tables have a range of exposure, rather than being more precise.

Injury to the bone marrow (blood-forming tissues) is probably the most significant effect of radiation exposure and is the most common cause of death. Another problem is that radiation destroys large numbers of white blood cells, thus greatly reducing the body's ability to fight infection for several months.

Certain characteristic signs follow exposure to high levels of radiation: nausea, fatigue, vomiting, and fever will appear during the first days after exposure. Reddening of the skin similar to a sunburn may also occur. The occurrence of these symptoms does *not* mean that a person will die from the exposure; these are simply signs that the person has received a high dosage of radiation.

Are there long-term effects after the initial recovery? The answer to this question is highly controversial. Researchers who have followed the survivors of the Hiroshima and Nagasaki atomic bombings found that there was a slight increase in the incidence of leukemia over a 15-year period; however, keep in mind that persons in the study had received exposure of 100 rems or more in a very short period of time. In the next 30 years, scientists will be able to observe thousands of Soviet citizens who received varying levels of radiation exposure. Such research is likely to yield valuable information about the relationship between radiation and cancer.

Radiation protection. We must expect and be prepared for nuclear accidents. As with a variety of disasters, a nuclear power plant accident would normally allow time for warning residents in the area. An important step for local emergency management agencies would be the development of crisis relocation or evacuation plans for residents within a 5 to 10-mile radius of the facility. This needs to be done ahead of time, because such an evacuation may include the removal of patients from hospitals and nursing homes.[11]

Even if there was little warning about a nuclear power plant accident, people could reduce their exposure to radioactive fallout by staying in their homes. Materials such as concrete, brick, and lumber can absorb significant amounts of radiation; thus the basement of a home or the inner hallways of an apartment building could offer quite a bit of protection.

Since radiation passing through food does not contaminate it, food in the home would not present a hazard. The same holds true for water supplies in the home. Water in hot water heaters and toilet flush tanks would not be contaminated. Underground water supplies, such as wells, would also be protected from radioactive fallout. Communities whose water is supplied by open reservoirs, lakes, and streams might have a problem for several weeks with radioactive material that has been dissolved in the water.

In some cases, state or federal authorities might distribute small doses of potassium iodide to local residents 1 or 2 days before exposure to radiation. This is done to protect the thyroid gland from the effects of iodine-131, a radioactive substance likely to be released in a nuclear accident. The nonradioactive potassium iodide saturates the thyroid, thus preventing the absorption of the harmful iodine-131.[19]

After several weeks, much of the radioactivity will have dissipated; it is likely that people would be able to go outside to begin the cleanup process. Since fetuses and young children are most susceptible to radiation, pregnant women and small children may need to stay indoors longer. Before you attempt to go outside or return to your community (if you are evacuated), make sure that emergency personnel have declared the area "safe."

SUMMARY

The time for preparation is before a disaster occurs. In every community a system of comprehensive emergency management involves both public and private sectors. It involves four phases of activity: hazard reduction, preparedness, response, and recovery. Disaster planning even involves preparation on a personal level.

Although we have been able to control the environment a little more with each succeeding generation, certain natural phenomena cannot be controlled. Tornadoes, severe thunderstorms, hurricanes, floods, winter storms, and earthquakes present a variety of dangers.

Tornadoes appear in the late spring when warm, moist air masses meet cooler, dry air. Their funnel-shaped, rotating winds can generate speeds of 200-300 mph.

Occurring mostly along the eastern seaboard and the Gulf of Mexico, hurricanes do most of their damage in the late summer and early fall. A secondary danger often associated with hurricanes is flooding, as heavy rains move inland.

Normally flooding is a relatively slow process, giving adequate warning; however, in some regions of the country heavy rains can produce dramatic stream elevations known as flash floods.

Although winter can provide conditions for a variety of recreational activities, it can also bring hazardous winter storms. The hazards may be both at home and on the road. Heavy snows and bitterly cold temperatures may isolate people for days. During this forced isolation, people must be concerned with survival: food and heat. A variety of methods can be used to provide temporary heat for a family, but some of these methods are extremely dangerous. A well-stocked supply of quick-energy foods are excellent in an emergency situation.

Although no one should drive in a winter storm unless it is essential, if you must, preparation for possible driving emergencies is absolutely necessary. An emergency kit for the car should include warm clothing, blankets, and quick-energy foods.

The earthquake is one of the least understood natural disasters. The seismic waves produced by breaks in the earth's crust can put a tremendous stress on buildings miles away from the actual break. Areas around the world that lie near cracks in the earth's crust, known as "faults," are more likely to suffer earthquake damage. For high-risk communities, the design and construction of earthquake-resistant structures can lessen the damage should a quake occur.

Twentieth-century technology has brought a number of risks. The wide variety of chemicals used in the production of plastics, synthetic fibers, pesticides, and a variety of other materials has created problems involving handling, transportation, and storage of these highly toxic substances. Also, the improper disposal of hazardous wastes imperils both human health and the environment.

To handle problems such as chemical spills during transport, the Chemical Manufacturers Association developed an emergency center known as CHEMTREC. It provides immediate advice to local emergency personnel around the country who are faced with a hazardous materials accident. Many communities are developing their own specialized emergency groups known as "hazardous materials response teams."

Recognizing the potential for repeated hazardous waste disasters, Congress enacted the Resource Conservation and Recovery Act. Under this act, a cradle-to-grave control system has been developed to ensure the proper disposal of these wastes. With these new, strict regulations forcing waste generators to be more careful, a number of technologies which were once considered too expensive may be the answer to waste disposal in the future.

Certainly, one of the most feared and least understood forms of energy production is nuclear power. With the accidents at Three Mile Island and Chernobyl, public misconceptions have increased. A close analysis of the operation of a nuclear facility and the many precautions that are designed in the system demonstrates the degree of safety of nuclear power. The public must be better informed about how nuclear power plants work, what the real hazards are, and how it can protect itself against these hazards.

Key Terms

Blizzard   Considerable falling or blowing snow accompanied by winds of at least 35 miles per hour.

Disaster   A great, sudden misfortune resulting in loss of life, serious injury, or property damage.

Earthquake   Vibrating movements of the earth's surface caused by the sudden dislocation of its underlying crust.

Flash flood   Heavy water runoff produced by intense localized storms.

Flood   A river flow or ocean elevation that threatens or causes damage.

Hazardous materials response teams   Emergency personnel trained in the identification, containment, and cleanup of hazardous materials spills.

Hurricane   A violent tropical storm in which winds reach constant speeds of 74 miles per hour or more.

Hypothermia   A drop in one's body temperature below 95° F.

Landslide   The rapid movement, down a slope, of large amounts of loosely packed soil and rock.

Meltdown   The destruction of radioactive fuel in a nuclear reactor, resulting from the loss of coolant.

Tornado   A short-lived, local storm, containing high-speed winds usually rotating in a counterclockwise direction.

Tsunami or **tidal wave**   A destructive wall of water generated by the sudden displacement of the sea bottom.

Warning (flood, hurricane, storm, tornado)   Means that such an event is impending or has occurred nearby.

Watch (flood, hurricane, storm, tornado)   Means that conditions are possible for such an event to occur.

References

1. Baker, D. P.: Deadly chemical returns by convoy: MIC, cause of India disaster, is hauled to Georgia, The Washington Post, Dec. 30, 1984, p. A-4.
2. Benjamin, M. R.: Top of A-plant reactor core is found reduced to rubble, The Washington Post, Sept. 7, 1984, p. A-8.
3. Bohlen, C., and Pincus, W: Anatomy of an accident: a logistical nightmare, The Washington Post, Oct. 26, 1986, p. A-1.
4. Bolt, B. A. and others: Geological hazards, New York, 1975, Springer-Verlag New York, Inc.
5. Brownlee, S. H.: Waiting for the big one, Discover, July 1986, p. 52.
6. Coco, M.. Pollution doesn't pay: a landmark case, EPA Journal 13(2):6, 1987.
7. Department of Energy: Winter survival: a consumer's guide to winter preparedness, No. DOE/OPA 0019R(9-80), Washington, D.C., Sept. 1980.
8. Dobbs, M.: A radioactive visit to the killing zone, The Washington Post, April 26, 1991, p. A-38.
9. Dvorchak, R.: Storm brews over beachfront building, The Washington Post, Oct. 14, 1989, pp. F-31, 32.
10. Edwards, M.: Chernobyl—one year after, National Geographic 171(5):632, 1987.
11. Federal Emergency Management Agency: Are you ready?: your guide to disaster preparedness, H-34, Washington, D.C., Sept. 1990.
12. Federal Emergency Management Agency: Disaster driving: safety tips for motorists in emergencies, No. L-1 16, Washington, D.C., June 1981.
13. Federal Emergency Management Agency: Disaster operations. a handbook for local governments, CPG 1-6, Washington, D.C., July 1981.
14. Federal Emergency Management Agency: Earthquakes: safety tips, No. L-111, Washington, D.C., 1980.
15. Federal Emergency Management Agency: Family emergency preparedness: disaster supplies kit, Washington, D.C. Jan. 17, 1991.
16. Federal Emergency Management Agency: Hurricanes: safety tips, No. L-105, Washington, D.C., April 1980.
17. Federal Emergency Management Agency: In the event of a flood, No 593-237, Washington, D.C., Aug. 1981.

18. Federal Emergency Management Agency: In time of emergency: a citizen's handbook on emergency management, No. H-14, Washington, D.C., 1980.
19. Federal Emergency Management Agency: Planning for survival, H-20, Washington, D.C., July 1988.
20. Federal Emergency Management Agency: Shelter management handbook, No. P & P-8, Washington, D.C., Sept. 1981.
21. Federal Emergency Management Agency: Standards for local civil preparedness, No. CPG 1-5, Washington, D.C., Nov. 1980.
22. Federal Emergency Management Agency: Thunderstorms and Lightning, L-139, Washington, D.C., June 1984.
23. Federal Emergency Management Agency: Winter survival resource kit, Washington, D.C., May 1982.
24. Horan, M.: Tornadoes: winds of destruction, Family Safety and Health 45(2):28, 1986.
25. Lafferty, L.: Earthquake threat shakes fire department into action, Firechief 28(8):48, 1984.
26. Lippman, T. W.: Reactor plays out worrisome scenario, The Washington Post, March 22, 1990, p. A-40.
27. Liu, B.-C.: Earthquake risk and damage functions: application to New Madrid, Boulder, Colo., 1981, Westview Press, Inc.
28. Mathews, J.: Final quake toll estimated below 80, The Washington Post, Oct. 25, 1989, pp. A-1, A-20-23.
29. McCartney, R. J.: Europe tries to cope with poisoned Rhine, The Washington Post, Nov. 14, 1986, p. A-29.
30. National Fire Protection Association: The hazards of some hazardous materials, Fire Journal, Jan. 1979, p. 53.
31. National Governor's Association: Comprehensive emergency management, 008-040-0079-6, Washington, D.C., March 1979, U.S. Government Printing Office.
32. National Oceanic and Atmospheric Administration. Severe local storm warning service, NOAA/ PA 77018, Washington, D.C., Oct. 1981.
33. National Oceanic and Atmospheric Administration: Storm surge and hurricane safety, NOAA/ PA 78019, Washington, D.C., 1981.
34. National Oceanic and Atmospheric Administration: Tornado, NOAA/ PA 77027, Washington, D.C., 1980.
35. National Oceanic and Atmospheric Administration: Winter storms: terms to know/how to survive, NOAA/PA 78022, Washington, D.C., 1979.
36. Parker, L.: Carolinas bear brunt of Hugo's devastation, The Washington Post, Sept. 23, 1989, pp. A-1, A-14, 15.
37. Segel, E. and others: The toxic substances dilemma, Washington, D.C., 1980, The National Wildlife Federation.
38. United States Congress, House Committee on Science and Technology: Nuclear powerplant safety after Three Mile Island, Washington, D.C., 1980, U.S. Government Printing Office.
39. United States Environmental Protection Agency: Administration of the Toxic Substances Control Act (1980), OPA 100/ 10, Washington, D.C., April 1981.
40. United States Environmental Protection Agency, Office of Water and Waste Management: Everybody's problem: hazardous waste, SW-826, Washington, D.C., 1980.
41. United States Environmental Protection Agency: Toxic substances control act. report to congress for fiscal year 1981, Washington, D.C., Jan. 1982.
42. United States President's Commission on the Accident at Three Mile Island: Report of the President's Commission on the Accident at Three Mile Island. The need for change: the legacy of TMI, Washington, D.C., 1979, U.S. Government Printing Office.
43. Walsh, E.: Spring terror in tornado alley, The Washington Post, April 26, 1991, p. A-38.

Resource Organizations

American National Red Cross
17th and D Streets N.W.
Washington, DC 20006

American Nuclear Society
555 North Kensington Avenue
LaGrange Park, IL 60525

Armed Forces Radiobiology Research
Institute
8901 Wisconsin Avenue
Bethesda, MD 20814

Aviation Safety Institute
Box 304
Worthington, OH 43085

Bureau of Explosives
50 F Street N.W.
Washington, DC 20001

Environmental Action Foundation
1525 New Hampshire Avenue N.W.
Washington, DC 20036

Environmental Action, Inc.
1525 New Hampshire Avenue N.W.
Washington, DC 20036

Environmental Protection Agency
Radiation Programs
Washington, DC 20460

Environmental Protection Agency
Toxic Substances
401 M Street S.W.
Washington, DC 20460

Federal Aviation Administration
Aviation Safety
800 Independence Avenue S.W.
Washington, DC 20591

Federal Emergency Management Agency
500 C Street S.W.
Washington, DC 20472

Federal Insurance Administration
500 C Street S.W.
Washington, DC 20472

Geological Survey
National Earthquake Prediction Evaluation
Council
National Center
Reston, VA 22092

Hazardous Materials Advisory Council
1110 Vermont Ave., N.W., Suite 250
Washington, DC 20005

National Council on Radiation
Protection and Measurements
7910 Woodmont Avenue, Suite 1016
Bethesda, MD 20814

National Oceanic and Atmospheric
Administration
Environmental Science Information Center
11400 Rockville Pike
Rockville, MD 20852

National Transportation Safety Board
Bureau of Accident Investigation
800 Independence Avenue S.W.
Washington, DC 20594

National Weather Service
8060 13th Street
Silver Spring, MD 20910

Nuclear Information and Resource Service
1616 P Street N.W., Suite 160
Washington, DC 20036

Nuclear Regulatory Commission
Nuclear Material Safety and Safeguards
Washington, DC 20555

U.S. Council for Energy Awareness
1776 I Street N.W., Suite 400
Washington, DC 20006

U.S. Department of Transportation
Research and Special Programs
Administration
400 7th Street S.W.
Washington, DC 20590

CHAPTER 9

Applying What You Have Learned

1. Utilizing the following checklist, develop an all-weather emergency car kit for your travels:

a) Blanket/sleeping bag ☐
b) Set of clothing (cap, gloves, boots, pants, shirt, sweater or jacket) ☐
c) Flashlight with extra set of batteries ☐
d) First aid kit ☐
e) Supply of quick-energy foods ☐
f) Small shovel, screwdriver, pliers, and adjustable wrench ☐
g) Set of booster cables ☐
h) Additional items _____

2. Contact a local industrial plant, your community's fire/police department, or your university's safety and security personnel to find out what type of comprehensive emergency management program they have. Base your discussions with them on the following four management phases.

a) Hazard reduction:

b) Preparedness:

c) Response:

d) Recovery:

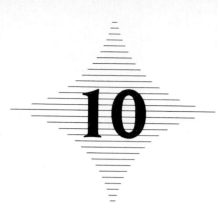

10 Recreational Safety

Approximately 9% of all injuries occur in places of recreation and sport.

National Center for Health Statistics

During the 1970s Americans began to switch from watching to participating. The physiological and psychological benefits of exercise as well as the importance of fitness throughout the life cycle have been well documented. In the 1990s there has been a growing trend toward the development of lifetime activities. These leisure pursuits are geared toward the individual; that is, to be active and enjoy success, one does not have to depend on others, nor does the individual have to compete against someone else. The activity can be as demanding as the person chooses.

However, a corollary trend that seems to be evolving has some disturbing implications: taking maximum risks in activities. A phrase that describes this approach to recreation is "taking it to the limit." In a society that continues to offer the worker more comfort and fewer challenges, people find it necessary to fulfill themselves in other ways. A person whose job is to input data into a computer 8 hours a day, 5 days a week, 50 weeks a year can get rather bored. So where is the challenge? It's on Saturday and Sunday, flying an ultralight (a hang glider with a motor). But it's not just flying; instead, the person "takes it to the max" by flying higher and faster than the manufacturer recommends.

Another example is the all-terrain vehicle (ATV) rider who pushes to the limit. Have you ever seen an ATV rider go up a sand dune and become briefly airborne? Of course the individual was wearing no protective gear because that would lessen the challenge. It's not that risks should never be taken; but, as mentioned in Chapter 1, the idea is to minimize the risks so that we can maximize success. There will still be plenty of risk, but it will be a more controlled risk.

In this chapter we will investigate a number of activities that offer both challenge and enjoyment. Our emphasis will be how to receive the maximum challenge and enjoyment with a minimum of risk. As you cover each of these activities, keep in mind the four factors that one must consider in attaining a safe level of performance: (1) knowledge and understanding of the risks involved, (2) skill development, (3) the state of the performer, and (4) the condition of the environment.

361

A SAFE APPROACH TO FITNESS FOR THE 1990s

During the late 1960s and early 1970s, the concept of fitness, as we know it today, had its beginnings. As much as anyone else, Dr. Kenneth Cooper, an Air Force physician, was responsible for demonstrating the importance of regular exercise in one's daily life. He popularized the term *aerobics,* which involves a variety of activities that stimulate heart, lung, and blood-vessel function. These include jogging, cycling, swimming, and racquetball.

This concept of fitness in the 1990s involves not only development of muscular and cardiorespiratory health, but also enhancement of the capacity to enjoy life fully. With this in mind, it is not surprising to find that more than 55 million American men and women jog, 70 million own bicycles, and over 18 million play racquetball. There were no commercial racquetball facilities in the United States in 1970; now there are over 2500. Another 20 million Americans work out at over 8000 health clubs and spas. Most of these clubs have appeared only in the last 10 to 15 years.

Although the benefits of participation far outweigh any detrimental factors associated with these activities, there are risks involved, and they must be addressed.

JOGGING

On any given day nearly 20 million Americans run for their health.[42] They can be found on jogging paths, bike trails, sidewalks, and city streets. As with any activity, there are going to be injuries—blisters, muscle pulls, backache, runner's nipple (from the repeated rubbing of one's shirt), and runner's toe (from the jamming effect of shoes that are too short) are just a few of the problems that may occur.

For the runner who takes to the streets, there is an added danger—being hit by a car—and, in these man-versus-machine collisions, the machine always wins. Fewer than 100 runners are hit by vehicles each year; however, nearly half of them die and the remainder of the victims receive serious or critical injuries.[34] While this is a relatively small number, the problem should not be downplayed or ignored. As the running population continues to increase, these injuries and deaths will increase unless runners take measures to reduce their risks. Runner-vehicle collisions involve the more experienced individual as well as the beginner. And as more people in this country make running a way of life, their experience on the road could become a detriment if they develop an attitude of invincibility, as many runners do. No matter who is at fault in a collision, the runner will pay the price.

Just as sports medicine specialists can give runners advice about training injuries, there is a need for the safety specialist to advise runners about precautions to take when training on public roadways[16,42,43]:

1. If you must use the roads, select areas with little traffic. Preferably, the roadway should be wide or at least have a wide shoulder on which to run. The roadway surface may be more level and firm than the shoulder, but running on this surface puts both you and an oncoming driver in danger, especially if he has to swerve to avoid hitting you. Whatever you do, don't challenge a car!
2. Always run against, rather than with, traffic. In the typical runner-motor vehicle collision,

the runner is moving with traffic and is hit from behind. You can better anticipate vehicle movement when running against the traffic flow (Fig. 10-1).
3. When running with others along the roadside, run single file. In cases investigated where runners were proceeding side by side, the one nearest the traffic flow was injured.
4. When crossing an intersection where a car is stopped, make sure the driver sees you before you proceed. Often drivers stopped at stop signs will be looking to their left and will then proceed once traffic is clear. They will not see a runner approaching from the right. Also, yield to vehicles turning into an intersection that you are crossing. It is likely that these motorists are thinking only about vehicular traffic, not runners in the crosswalk.

Here is where the experienced runners get into trouble. They challenge an oncoming car by yelling, screaming, and swearing as they proceed into the right of way. Yes, the pedestrian has the right of way, but it does you no good if the driver doesn't see you. Don't take the chance; wait until they pass by.

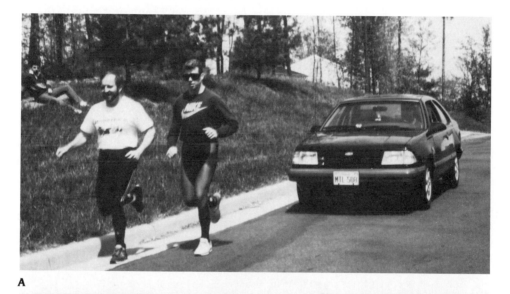

A

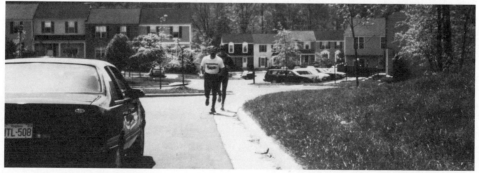

B

FIG. 10-1   A, If the driver lost control of this vehicle, these runners would have little or no warning. **B,** By running single file and against traffic, these runners have significantly reduced the possibility of a pedestrian vehicle collision.

5. Avoid running on roads during non-daylight hours. Over 50% of runner-vehicle collisions happen after dark, with another 10% to 15% occurring at dawn or dusk. This can be an especially serious problem during the winter, when it gets dark around 5:30 P.M. and doesn't get light until around 7:30 or 8 A.M. If you have no choice, then run wearing light-colored clothing with reflective materials; however, what might be better is to go to a school, library, or shopping center that is well lighted in the evening. The scenery may be boring, but you'll be much safer.

6. A new trend that has the potential for creating problems for the runner is that of wearing the lightweight stereo headset. It can certainly make a run more pleasant, but it also blocks out all sounds such as honking horns and screeching tires. This may be especially detrimental to your health if those honking horns or screeching tires are meant for you (Fig. 10-2).

Summertime Running

Summertime—and the living isn't necessarily easy for the runner, especially during those really hot midsummer days. When training or racing in this weather, a person may fall victim to a number of heat-related difficulties (heat cramps, heat exhaustion, and heat stroke) if precautionary measures have not been taken.

Although we will direct our comments to the runner, the guidelines apply to a

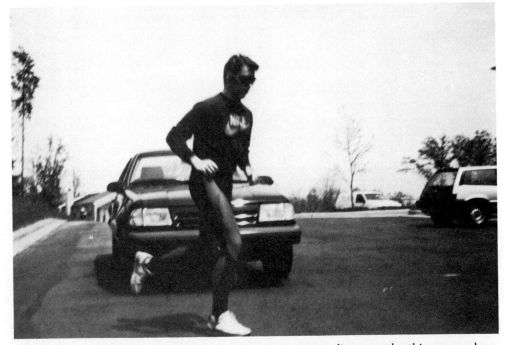

FIG. 10-2 With his stereo headset blocking out surrounding sounds, this runner has not heard the approaching vehicle as he darts into the street.

number of groups that are particularly susceptible to exposure to high temperatures. These include the elderly, the chronically ill, the overweight, children under 2 years of age, construction and factory workers, and persons participating in a variety of summertime sports (for example, tennis, football, and golf).

Heat cramps. The person who is unaccustomed to vigorous exercise in warm weather is a prime candidate for **heat cramps**—a very painful, yet not particularly dangerous, condition.

> *Allan had been running somewhat irregularly during the spring, but now on his 2-week vacation he was going to do some serious training. On Monday morning he ran 4 miles instead of his usual 2 ½; that afternoon he played tennis for 2 hours. He worked up a good sweat during his two workouts and other than a little stiffness that evening felt fine. On Tuesday he repeated his running and tennis, but as he was sitting on the side of the court drinking a beer, he screamed, fell out of his chair, and grabbed the backs of his legs. Allan was suffering from heat cramps. After the application of ice to the backs of his legs for 15 to 20 minutes and some mild massaging, the cramping subsided. However, that night at home he had several more bouts of cramping. His problem was twofold: (1) During his 2 days of heavy exercise, Allan did not replenish lost salt (sodium-potassium) and water, and (2) his muscles were not accustomed to that much activity.*

Let's look more closely at this problem. Perspiration is nature's way of cooling the body. Evaporation of sweat from the skin helps to maintain a steady internal temperature, regardless of the temperature outside the body. Sweat is basically a salt-water solution; so when you perspire you lose not only water but also the salts, sodium and potassium. Sodium and potassium (known as electrolytes), play an important role in muscle contraction as well as the retention of fluids in the system. If one does not adequately replace the lost water and salts, heat cramps may occur. However, this is not the only reason for the muscle cramping. Another factor that seems to be of equal importance is conditioning. Muscles must be acclimated to additional stress on a gradual basis. This is why people who suffer from heat cramps are usually just beginning a program of heavy exercising, or they are suddenly increasing their amount of training. Football players, basketball players, and wrestlers, during their preseason workouts, are likely to suffer from heat cramping because they are losing large quantities of salt and water and are stressing muscle groups that haven't been used for some time. The most effective way to deal with heat cramps is to prevent their occurrence. During the warm summer months, put a little extra salt on your food at mealtimes. This will help to maintain sodium levels and decrease fluid loss. At the same time, bananas, cantaloupe, apricots, and tomato or orange juice can help to maintain adequate levels of potassium.

Before exercising vigorously in hot weather, acclimate yourself to the higher temperatures. Take a week or two and gradually build up to the level of activity at which you want to participate.

Heat exhaustion. Another heat-related problem involving salt and fluid loss is **heat exhaustion.** Not everyone who loses large amounts of salt and water will suffer from heat cramps, especially those who have been training prior to warm weather.

These people are used to heavy exercise, but they misjudge the amount of fluid they lose with each workout. It is likely to take several days of training or working in hot weather before heat exhaustion becomes a problem.

Carla Roseanne ran 4 miles five times per week religiously, rain or shine. She was also conscious of her weight and diet, so she limited her salt intake and watched her fluid intake. Carla generally ran in the early morning; however, a change in her work schedule forced her to train in the early afternoon when the temperatures were much higher. After her first three afternoon workouts, Carla noticed that she had lost 4 pounds and she felt sluggish and tired. On the fifth day of training, in the middle of her run, she became very weak and dizzy. She was sweating profusely and certainly didn't feel hot, but the longer she stood the worse she felt, until she fainted in a neighbor's yard. Carla had suffered a classic case of heat exhaustion.

Again, prevention of heat exhaustion is much simpler than treating its occurrence. In hot weather a person's body weight is a good way to judge fluid balance. A sudden drop of 1 or 2 pounds the day after a workout means that you are not adequately replenishing lost fluids, and with the loss of water comes a loss of sodium and potassium. A simple rule of thumb is that each pound of weight loss is the equivalent of losing 1 pint of water. If you lose 2 pounds during your run, you will need to drink about a quart of fluid to replace it. The extra salt at mealtimes and the addition of potassium-rich foods to the diet will adequately maintain electrolyte balance.

The individual suffering from heat exhaustion is basically suffering from a mild form of shock. When a person sweats profusely and the fluid loss is not replaced, there is a drop in blood volume. This in turn reduces blood flow to major organs, especially the brain; thus the runner becomes weak and dizzy and is likely to faint. Treatment consists of replenishing the fluid loss and seeing that the victim has 2 or 3 days of rest before resuming activity. Drinking fresh fruit juices will help to replace lost electrolytes as well as the lost fluids.

A word to the wise about salt intake to prevent heat cramping or heat exhaustion—do not take salt tablets. This concentrated form of sodium not only irritates the stomach lining, but it also can have a dehydrating effect on the body. Two or three salt tablets in the stomach will affect water balance by drawing fluid out of the cells and into the stomach cavity. At the same time, as the person exercises, he or she will lose further bodily fluids through perspiration. Blood volume will drop rapidly, increasing the individual's chances of heat exhaustion.

If you are concerned about fluid loss during workouts, take a break about each half hour to replace lost fluids. The amount depends on the size of the individual, how vigorous the exercise is, and how much he or she perspires. Thirst is not necessarily a good way to judge fluid loss; many people will not feel a strong urge to drink during exercise, even though they may be losing anywhere from a pint (16 ounces) to a quart (32 ounces) per hour. Another suggestion for runners is to drink about 16 ounces of fluid 10 to 15 minutes before exercising.[42, 43] This will afford added protection during exercise.

Many people wonder what drink is best to replace fluid loss from the body. Advertisers of drinks such as Gatorade, which contain added sodium and potassium salts, claim that these drinks are rapidly absorbed into the system; however, studies have indicated that their sugar content actually slows down water absorption. The best and most economical fluid replacement is just plain water.

Heat stroke. By far the most dangerous heat-related problem is **heat stroke.** Also known as sunstroke, this condition results when the body's heat-regulating mechanism fails and a person's temperature reaches 105°F or higher.[22] Although heat stroke occurs most often among the elderly and those whose bodies cannot adequately regulate temperature, it may occur in healthy individuals performing work at such intensity that heat produced from muscle contraction cannot be adequately dissipated (for example, runners). It usually occurs during heat waves, especially if the humidity is high.

Normally a person loses about 60% of body heat production through the process of radiation—the transfer of heat from the body into the surrounding air. However, at temperatures above 90°F there is very little heat loss from the body through radiation. A second important means of temperature control, especially in warm weather, is evaporation of perspiration from the skin. However, this process does not work well if the humidity is more than 80%.

In August of 1980, a 10-mile race through one northern Virginia community resulted in the deaths of two of the participants and the hospitalization of a number of others. At the start of the race the temperature was 88°F; and by the time the last of the 600 participants had finished, temperatures were in the mid-90s.[15] If one considers the number of distance races held throughout the United States each summer, it is easy to see the potential for serious injury or death for a significant number of people. Studies have indicated that during races of as few as 6 miles, a runner's body temperature can rise to more than 105°F during hot, humid weather.[15]

Whether you are racing or doing your regular training during the summer months, there are preventive measures that can be taken to reduce the chance of heat stroke:

1. During those times of the year when temperatures are regularly exceeding 80°F, running should be completed before 9 A.M. or after 4 P.M.[15]
2. Since sweating and fluid loss play an important role in cooling the body, fluids should be consumed frequently during races or training runs (about every 2 ½ to 3 miles). As with prevention of heat exhaustion, drinking a glass or two of water 10 to 15 minutes before you run will provide extra fluid for cooling the body during exercise.

Runners should be aware of the early warning signs of impending heat stroke: erection of hair on the arms or chest, chilling, throbbing headache, dizziness, and hot, dry, flushed skin. If you notice these signs or you see another person exhibiting these signs, immediate action is essential. Often a person suffering from heat stroke will be mentally confused; and unless someone recognizes the difficulty, the person's temperature will continue to escalate until he or she collapses. The greatest danger from high internal body temperature is brain damage and subsequent cardiac arrest. Another serious consequence of elevated blood temperature is liver and kidney failure. Because of delays in the recognition and treatment of heat stroke victims, approximately 80% of them die.

On determining that a person may be suffering from heat stroke, the rescuer's priority is to cool the victim's body as quickly as possible. The first choice would be to immerse the person in a tub of cold water; if this is not available, get them into a cold shower or wrap them in sheets soaked in cold water. To speed up the cooling process, place ice packs along the sides of the neck, under the arms, and in the groin area; in each of these locations large blood vessels pass close to the skin surface. Application of cold packs across the forehead will also help in the cooling process. Other methods of cooling that can be improvised include the use of a garden hose as a makeshift shower and cold cans of soda or beer as a modified form of ice pack.

Any combination of these treatments should be used until the victim's temperature drops below 102°F. If the cooling measures are stopped too soon, the patient's temperature will quickly start to elevate. Using the methods described, a rescuer can lower body temperature by as much as 4° in 30 minutes. If the victim has been incoherent or has lapsed into unconsciousness, seek emergency medical support immediately as you continue cooling the body. If the victim has remained alert and you have reduced the body temperature below 102°F, watch the person closely for at least an hour to make sure that the body temperature has stabilized.

If there is one piece of advice to give anyone who exercises vigorously during the summer, that would be to consistently drink plenty of fluids before, during, and after exercising. A person with a good fluid balance is far less likely to suffer heat-related problems than a person who takes in only small amounts of fluid.

WALKING/VOLKSMARCHING

A less strenuous, low-impact exercise that produces many of the benefits associated with jogging is that of walking. Weight loss, improved cardiovascular health, stress reduction, increased lean body mass, and strengthening of the skeletal structure are benefits that can be accrued from walking as well as jogging. It is estimated that more than 20 million Americans walk at least twice a week.[2] An additional 3 million people participate each weekend in a walking activity known as Volksmarching.

Volksmarching (a German word for peoples' walking) is a non-timed, non-competitive walk of a least 10 kilometers (6.2 miles) over a marked course.[2] Many volksmarching clubs provide additional trails for those who want to walk greater distances during these weekend events.

In terms of safety, walkers/volksmarchers need to take the same precautions as runners. Walking on or near public roadways presents the same hazards as those for joggers. Also the warm-weather walker is just as likely to suffer the same heat-related problems if hc or she does not maintain adequate fluid balance.

RACQUETBALL

Probably the fastest growing competitive recreational activity in the country today is racquetball. With over 18 million active participants, the sport has had a phenomenal growth since the early 1970s. Unlike tennis, handball, and squash, which take considerable practice before one can actively participate, racquetball offers even the beginner a moderate amount of success and an excellent opportunity for developing cardiovascular fitness. The compact size of the court, the softer, larger rubber ball, and the smaller racquet, which make the activity easier to play, at the same time increase one's chance of injury. Let's look at each of these factors to see what might be done to lessen the potential for injury.

Although they are seldom serious, wall-related injuries are a common problem for novice racquetballers. In their zest to cover the 40-foot by 20-foot playing surface, beginners tend to misjudge distances and inadequately control their momentum. As a consequence, a new player will lunge for a shot, miss it, and crash into a wall. Contusions of the shoulder, elbow, and forearm commonly result as a person falls into the wall and tries to control the impact with the arms. In rare instances a player may suffer a shoulder separation if the impact has been severe. With experience one learns to better control body movement. Wearing good shoes that prevent slipping can also provide more body control.

More serious racquetball injuries involve contact with the ball or racquet. Surprisingly, experience does not seem to reduce one's chance of injury in these cases. It has been suggested that as one becomes more experienced, there is a greater tendency to become more aggressive when playing.

Racquet-related injuries usually result from carelessness or overenthusiasm as players get in the way of the swinging racquet. The majority of wounds involve facial lacerations. As a player is hitting a shot, his opponent will crowd next to him to get into position for a return. However, as the first player follows through, he may hit his opponent in the face with the racquet. This is more likely to occur on backhand returns.

Following the basic rules of court etiquette could eliminate many of these injuries[15,17]:

1. Always give your opponent plenty of room to swing and follow through.
2. Toward the end of a close game, do not crowd your opponent; when he is hitting a shot, it is safer to stand diagonally to his rear than directly at his side.
3. If a player gets in your way on a shot, call a "hinder" rather than attempt to hit the ball and possibly injure someone.
4. All players should have racquets with a thong that must be securely wrapped around the wrist when playing.

Although it is relatively soft and easily compressible, the racquetball presents the greatest danger to a player. The ball cannot only attain a high velocity when it is hit (in excess of 100 mph), but upon contact it will conform to the surface it strikes. In other words, if the racquetball hits the wall, it will momentarily flatten out before it regains its shape and bounces back; however, if it hits near a person's eye, it will conform to the shape of the bony orbit surrounding the eye and penetrate inward, damaging tissues.[5,17]

Because of its compressible nature, a racquetball can injure players wearing some eye guards. A popular model that is stocked in most sporting goods stores is the open eye guard. It works well in preventing slashing injuries about the eyes from racquets, but since it offers no protection between the upper and lower rims, this device cannot prevent direct shots from penetrating into the eye[5] (Fig. 10-3). It is the direct shot that has the greatest potential for permanent visual impairment.

Likewise, regular prescription eyeglasses consisting of hardened glass or plastic lenses do not provide adequate protection from high-velocity direct shots. Near-sighted players are at greatest risk, since their eyeglass lenses are thinnest at the center. Prescription eyeglasses also offer little protection from racquet injuries.

Because of the racquetball's potential for serious eye injury, special precautions are needed for adequate player safety. The most significant measure would be the mandatory use of goggles. They consist of special polycarbonate lenses mounted in a wraparound, impact-resistant plastic frame[5] (Fig. 10-4). An additional suggestion, especially for novice players, is never to turn around to view the opponent's return. Keep your eyes on the front wall until you are ready to make a shot (Fig. 10-5).

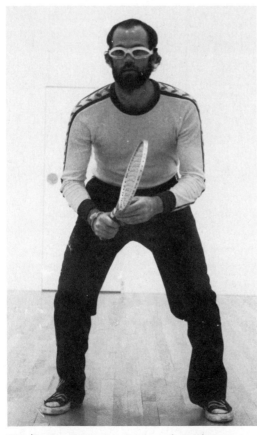

FIG. 10-3   An open eye guard. (Did you notice that his racquet is firmly anchored by the strap around his wrist?)

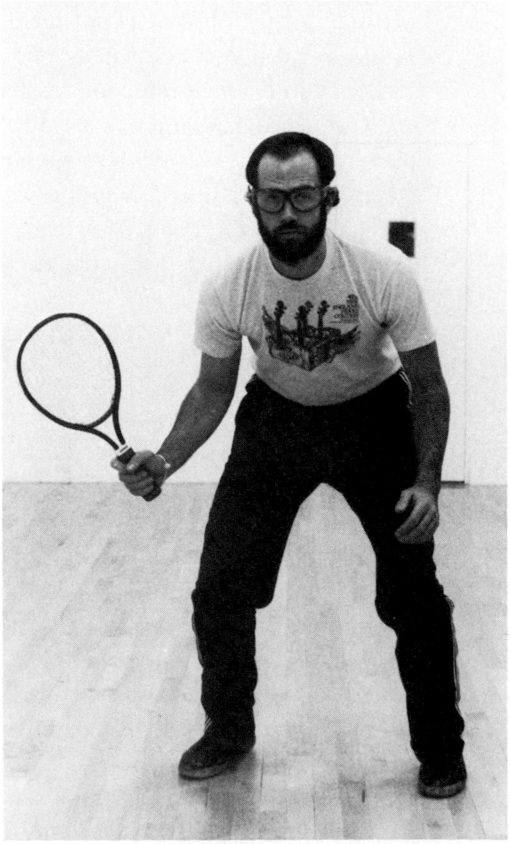

FIG. 10-4   These wrap-around goggles have both impact-resistant lenses and frames.

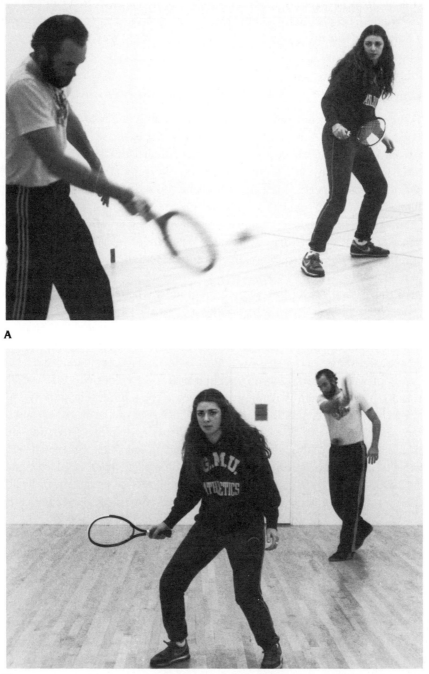

A

B

FIG. 10-5   A, Never turn around to view an opponent's return; this is the way ball-related eye injuries occur. **B,** By keeping her eyes on the front wall, this player significantly reduces her chance of being hit in the eye by the high-velocity shot of her partner. (However, if they want maximum protection, both should be wearing safety goggles.)

Racquetball is excellent for conditioning and it is a sport that can be played by a wide range of people, but it is not without its hazards. Using the proper equipment and following the rules of the court will go a long way in making this a safe recreational activity.

AEROBIC DANCE

While it is not a competitive activity like running and racquetball, aerobic dance has become a widely popular form of cardiovascular exercise. By bringing music into the workout, aerobic dance offers a somewhat artistic outlet, while meeting the criteria for improving heart, lung, and blood-vessel function in participants. In a study of aerobic dancers, Metcalf and others[32] found that heart rates of participants remained between 150 and 190 beats per minute for a considerable portion of each 30-minute training session. This meets or exceeds the criterion for aerobic training, which is 75% of the maximal heart rate. When these sessions are repeated three or four times per week, the training effect is similar to that received by a person running an equal amount of time.

For this reason, a word of warning is in order. A man or woman who begins an aerobic dance program should be aware that this activity can put a significant stress on the heart. An additional finding of the Metcalf study indicated that aerobic dancing can disturb the cardiac rhythm of certain susceptible individuals. A person's age, current health status, and fitness level must be taken into consideration. For those over 35 years of age or for those who have not exercised vigorously for several years, a check-up by a physician is recommended before beginning this activity.

The aerobic dancer should be aware of the need for proper warm-up and stretching before and after the activity. Using routines involving explosive twisting and turning movements as well as high kicks, aerobic dancing has been associated with muscle damage to the trunk, lower back, and legs of some participants. Before signing up for that 12-week program at your local Y, community recreation center, or health spa, be aware that aerobic dancing is not the benign form of exercise that many consider it to be.

In recent years a variation of traditional aerobic training which tends to be less stressful on the feet and legs of participants is "low-impact aerobics." With low-impact aerobics (LIA) there is more stepping, scooting, and walking than in classic aerobic routines, which require strenuous kicking, bouncing, and jumping. Additionally, LIA uses more upper-body movement and stretching than regular aerobic training. Although both of these forms of aerobic training improve cardiorespiratory function of participants, LIA reduces those wear-and-tear injuries to the lower extremities.[1]

WEIGHT TRAINING

Whether you water ski, hang glide, or play tennis or golf, almost every recreational activity requires some muscular strength. Depending on the activity, the amount of strength desired varies greatly; consequently, most people will want to adopt a weight-training program suited to their particular needs and interests. The beauty of this particular recreational activity is that it can be geared to the ability level of the performer, it can be continued throughout one's lifetime, and it may be performed competitively or noncompetitively. Couples find weight training an excellent recreational activity, since it allows them to work out together without necessarily competing against one another.

But weight lifting, like any other fitness activity, has certain hazards. The U.S. Consumer Product Safety Commission estimates that over 43,000 weight-training injuries requiring hospital emergency-room treatment occur each year. Most of the injuries are contusions, sprains, and strains; however, at least 5000 of them involve a bone fracture, and an additional 1000 injuries involve crushing or amputation of tissues.[59] The lower back and shoulder are prone to muscle strain, whereas the hands and feet are where fractures and crushing injuries are likely to occur.

Most of these injuries can be blamed on a lack of knowledge about the use of weight-training equipment and a lack of skill development in performing the various lifts. Weight-training equipment design and development has become a big business in the last 10 years. Today almost every high school in the country has some type of weight-lifting equipment. Universal Gym, Nautilus, and York are just a few of the well-known weight-lifting equipment companies. Each of these companies offers a wide assortment of apparatus that, when used correctly, enable an individual to make significant gains in strength and muscle tone.

Whether a person trains on a weight machine or uses free weights (bar and removable plates), there are a number of safety precautions to be taken if that individual is to have a positive and relatively injury-free experience.

Technique

For every muscle group that one wants to develop or strengthen, there are specific lifts or exercises; and for each of these lifts, there is a proper way to perform it. One of the quickest ways a beginning lifter can get hurt is to have poor technique in executing these lifts.

Before starting a weight-training program, do some reading. There are a number of excellent texts that outline correct lifting technique. Talk to people who have been actively involved in the sport for a number of years. Many colleges and universities have full-time strength coaches who could offer valuable assistance. Such faculty departments as physical education, exercise physiology, and kinesiolgocial sciences will have personnel with the expertise to assist you.

What about your local health spa? Too often these establishments do not have people who are adequately trained. What about your coach? Coaches have experience and training in the performance of skills for a particular sport; however, they generally have little knowledge when it comes to developing muscular strength and endurance in athletes. Basketball coaches know the intricacies of the sport; they don't necessarily know how to increase the strength of their players.

The lower back is most often injured when a person uses poor technique. A common fault of the novice lifter is attempting to lift weights from the floor by bending at the waist and keeping the knees straight. As the person attempts to bring the weights up in this manner, extreme stress is placed on the lower back muscles (erector spinae), and this commonly results in a slight tear known as a muscle strain. Although it usually heals with no problem, the lower back muscle strain can be a very painful injury. When one lifts weights from the floor, the knees should be bent before the lift is made and the back should be kept in a vertical position. In this way the stress will be placed on the large muscles of the upper legs, not on the smaller and weaker muscles of the lower back.

Another technique error made by many lifters that usually affects the lower back is known as "cheating." This consists of hyperextending the lower back and exaggerating the normal curvature of the spine. By doing this the lifter can exert more force on the weight he or she is attempting to move, but at the expense of the spinal column. Three exercises that commonly involve the "cheating" technique are the military (overhead) press, bench press, and curls. The inherent danger of this activity is that extreme hyperextension of the vertebrae causes them to exert pressure on the spinal disks. The spinal or intervertebral disks act as protective cushions between the vertebrae. If the pressure on the disks is severe enough or they have been weakened from a prior injury, one or more of them may herniate, or rupture. When this occurs the damaged disk may exert pressure on the spinal cord and peripheral nerves. It is likely that surgery will be required to repair the damage.

When lifting, protect the normal curvature of the back. If you cannot lift the weight without hyperextending the back, then you are probably attempting to lift too much weight. Drop the resistance by 5 to 10 pounds and perform the lift properly (Fig. 10-6).

The correct technique for proper breathing when executing any lift is to exhale during muscle contraction. When you are pushing or pulling the weight, you should be exhaling. As you let the weight return to the starting position, you should be inhaling.

During extreme effort novice lifters often hold their breath and experience what is known as the **Valsalva maneuver.** The combination of holding one's breath and straining against a heavy weight increases pressure in the chest and abdominal cavity. Initially, large amounts of blood will be pumped quickly from the heart, elevating blood pressure, but as the lifter continues to strain, returning blood flow to the heart decreases and blood pressure starts to drop. As the lifter finishes the lift and starts to breathe, the blood pressure will drop for several more seconds, then suddenly rebound to an extreme level, since blood flow into the chest cavity has returned to normal. While this doesn't seem to present a problem for the healthy individual, the two sudden elevations in blood pressure at the beginning of the lift and after the lift could be dangerous for the person who has a cerebrovascular weakness, because this sudden pressure increase could cause a blood vessel hemorrhage.

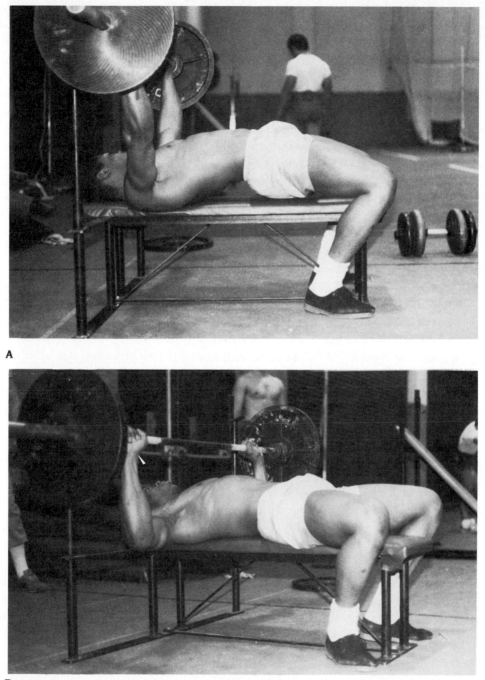

FIG. 10-6   A, This photograph illustrates how many novice weight lifters hurt their backs while performing the bench press exercise. (Notice the extreme curvature and hyperextension of the lower spine.) **B,** In this photograph we can see that the lower back and pelvic region are well supported by the bench when the man performs the exercise correctly.

The first time a weight lifter experiences this phenomenon, it may be somewhat frightening. It frequently occurs when a person is doing the bench press (a lift performed while lying on a bench). Immediately after completing this lift, most people quickly sit up or stand. Just after pressure on the chest cavity is released, the blood pressure drops to its lowest point; this usually coincides with the lifter's sitting up. Momentarily, blood flow to the brain is greatly reduced and the person gets extremely dizzy or may faint. The dizzy period induced by the low blood pressure is quickly replaced by a sudden throbbing sensation resulting from the rebounding high blood pressure. In seconds the blood pressure levels off and returns to normal. Although it is a rather complex physiological occurrence, the whole process (blood pressure increase/decrease/increase/and return to normal) usually takes less than a minute. If you breathe properly during training, you don't have to worry about this problem.

Aids to safe performance. Although they are not always necessary when a person weight trains, the following suggestions can provide an extra margin of safety as well as enhance performance (Fig. 10-7):

1. Use spotters: Spotters are individuals who help the lifter who cannot handle the weight he or she is attempting. They should always be present when one is performing heavy squats or bench presses. Depending on the amount of weight that's being handled, one or two people may be needed.

2. Use collars: These detachable locking devices which hold plates in position on the bar should always be used. If the bar is tilted while a person is lifting, the weights will be prevented from falling on the floor and injuring the lifter or someone standing nearby.

3. Work in a hazard-free area: Before performing a particular exercise, make sure the area in which you are working is free of hazards. Don't be like the lifter who was stepping back with 500 pounds and tripped over a collar that was lying on the floor. After you use the weights, put them away so that no one gets injured because of your actions.

4. Wear weight belts and wraps: To provide added support when lifting, especially when the exercise involves the low back, a 4-inch-wide leather lifting belt is recommended. For exercises in which there may be added stress on the knees (squat, deadlift), wraps will provide added support for the knee joint.

5. Use chalk: To provide a better grip of the bar, especially when hands are wet from perspiration, magnesium carbonate should be placed on the lifter's hands and/or the bar. Blocks of magnesium carbonate can be purchased in any gymnastics store, since this is the same material used by gymnasts.

6. Wear leather gloves: After lifting for a number of weeks, most individuals develop thick calluses across the hands. The tissue underlying these calluses tends to get very sore when one attempts to hold the bar firmly. To slow down the development of calluses, many individuals wear weight-lifting gloves. Some sensation or feel for the bar may be lost, but these gloves significantly reduce wear and tear on the hands.

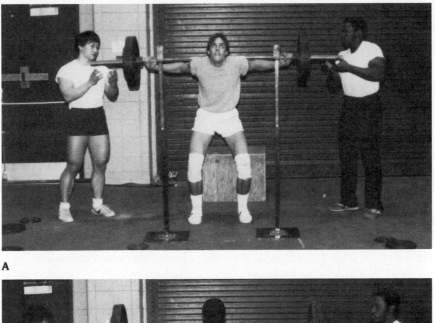

A

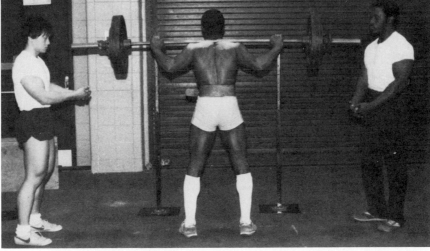

B

FIG. 10-7 **A,** If the lifter performing this squat has trouble handling the weight, spotters will assist him in the completion of the lift. The wraps that he wears provide support for the knees. **B,** Collars on the ends of the bar will keep the weights from shifting during the exercise; the chalk on the lifter's shoulders prevents the bar from slipping; and the belt will give added support to the musculature of the lower back.

BICYCLING

A recreational activity that not only provides elements of cardiovascular and strength fitness, but also provides an economical means of transportation is cycling. From the early 1900s to the early 1970s, the bicycle industry grew slowly and steadily. The major recipients of both the pleasures and dangers of bicycling were children; the cycling population consisted mainly of children under 15 years of age, with a few older adult riding enthusiasts.

However, all of that changed with the "bike revolution" of the 1970s. Research studies that demonstrated the importance of aerobic exercise in reducing heart disease indicated cycling as one of the best methods for improving heart-lung function. Escalating gasoline prices and shortages forced many to consider alternative means of traveling, especially to and from work. At the same time more and more people were becoming aware of pollution problems created by motor vehicles. Cycling provided a quiet, nonpolluting form of transportation. Today there are over 70 million bicycles on the road, with an additional 10 million being purchased annually.[4]

With this sudden increase in bicycle traffic over the last 15 years, one might think that an equally sudden increase in the number of traffic-related deaths would have occurred. Surprisingly, the death rate for bicyclists has decreased since 1970; however, there have been some significant changes in the ages of persons dying or being injured. The proportion of persons 15 years of age and older who die in cycling accidents has steadily increased. In 1970 persons 15 and older accounted for about 30% of all cycling deaths; now they account for approximately two thirds of the fatalities.[34] And don't think that the majority of these deaths involve 15- to 19-year-olds or 15- to 24-year-olds; cyclists 25 years of age and older are injured or killed almost as often as the younger groups. Bicycling and bicycle safety aren't just for kids anymore.

Your Bike and Your Body

The foremost consideration for the beginning bicyclist is to select a bike that fits your body[9, 12, 23]:

1. The rider should be able to straddle the top bar of the bike with both feet flat on the ground. Preferably there should be about a 1-inch clearance between your crotch and the top bar. Do this in stockinged feet. Preferably, a woman should purchase the same type of bike as a man, since this top bar provides additional structural support for the frame.

2. Saddle height plays an important role in riding efficiency. While you are seated on the bicycle, completely extend the leg in a downward position. The heel of the foot should be in contact with the pedal in its lowest position. Since a rider pedals with the ball of the foot, this method of measurement will allow some slight flexion in the leg throughout the revolution of the pedal. If you must completely extend your leg during pedaling, the bicycle seat is too high, and you will have to expend more effort to keep the bike moving.

3. To prevent placing excessive weight on your hands while riding, handlebar height

and stem length must also be adjusted. The top of the handle bar should be level with the top of the saddle. Stem length is the distance from the front of the seat to the point where the handlebar attaches to the stem. This distance should be equal to the length of the rider's arm from the tip of the elbow to the tips of the fingers.

Incorrect handlebar height or stem length has been associated with a condition known as ulnar neuropathy or **handlebar palsy.** After an extended period of riding, the cyclist may notice a loss of sensation in the hands and an inability to coordinate finger movement, generally in the ring and little fingers of both hands. A combination of road vibration and the extra pressure placed on the hands caused by inadequate handlebar placement causes irritation of the ulnar nerves. Once the condition develops, it may take several weeks before it clears up. Besides correct bicycle adjustment, the wearing of padded cycling gloves and the application of padded tape to handlebars can help to eliminate this problem.

Almost every part of the bicycle can be adjusted for safer and more efficient riding. The staff of a reputable bike shop can fit your bicycle to you and your needs.

Equipment Needs

The bicycle will be only part of your purchase. A number of accessories are suggested for maximum protection. Because nearly 75% of serious or fatal bicycle accidents involve head injuries, a sturdy helmet is first on the list.[35] It provides protection against falls and collisions and offers the additional protection of making cyclists more visible.

Over the past 5 years the design and function of bicycle helmets have improved greatly. Made of polystyrene foam, today's helmet crushes, absorbing energy and slowing the rate at which your head comes to a stop.[30] To give added protection from penetration by sharp objects, newer models have a thin hard plastic shell. Before you purchase a helmet, make sure that it meets the protection standards of the Snell Memorial Foundation or the American National Standards Institute (ANSI).

With recent studies indicating that a helmet can reduce a cyclist's risk of head injury by 85%, state legislatures are taking a close look at mandatory bicycle helmet laws, especially since 50,000 bicyclists suffer serious head injuries each year.[4] Currently, California, New York, and Massachusetts have mandatory helmet laws for children under 5 years of age, while two counties in the state of Maryland require anyone under age 16 to wear a helmet when bicycling. Don't be fooled by the age limits on these laws; anyone who rides a bike is at risk. Wear a helmet!

Danger for the cyclist may come from the front or the rear. To know what's going on behind you, a small rear-view mirror that clips onto eyeglasses or helmets is highly recommended. While it takes a little practice to get used to this type of mirror, it does not require a person to look down and away from the roadway, as does a mirror attached to the handlebars.

As with motorcyclists, bicycle riders' greatest problems arise because people fail to see them. Conspicuity (the ability to be seen) can be achieved in a number of ways. Brightly colored safety vests provide a certain amount of contrast during daylight

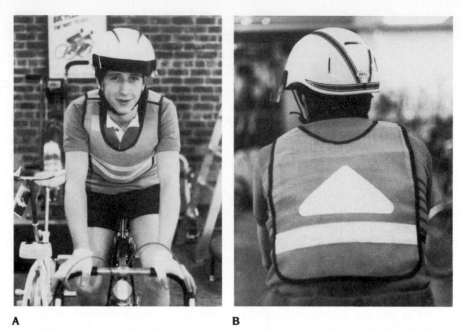

A   B

FIG. 10-8 **A,** This cyclist has taken a number of steps to protect himself by using a helmet, a rear-view mirror clipped to the helmet, padded gloves, and a safety vest. **B,** Both the helmet and vest have reflective tape, which increases his ability to be seen at night.
Courtesy: The Bicycle Exchange, Fairfax, Va.

hours. Reflective tape can be attached to jackets, vests, helmets, and gloves for riding after dusk or before sunrise. For night riding, a headlight and rear red light are essential. A portable leg-or arm light will provide additional protection (Fig. 10-8 and Fig. 10-9,A).

In heavy traffic, visual cues may not be enough to get a driver's attention if he or she is pulling in front of you or opening a car door. Miniature freon-powered horns can be attached to bicycle handlebars. They are similar to air horns found on tractor-trailers and just about as loud. They will definitely get a person's attention.

To keep pants cuffs clean and clear of the chain and sprocket, purchase a pair of trouser clips. Getting one's pants caught between the chain and sprocket is a sure way to bring on a spill. Also, getting grease out of a pair of dress slacks may be costly or impossible.

Two other accessories that will provide both comfort and protection for riders are padded gloves and toe clips. Gloves reduce much of the vibration that would normally be transferred to a person's hands and arms from the handlebars, which may lead to ''handlebar palsy.'' They also will protect one's hands if a spill occurs. Toe clips contribute greatly to cycling efficiency; they permit a combined pushing and pulling motion, whereas without the clips to hold the feet in place, there will be a transfer of power only during the downward push on the pedal. These clips will also keep the feet from sliding off the pedals, causing the cyclist to lose control of the bicycle.

Straps attached to the toe clips to hold the foot in place should be loosened slightly in city traffic so that feet can be withdrawn quickly from the pedals during a sudden stop (Fig. 10-9, B).

A variation of the toe clip and strap assembly which is being introduced on new all-terrain and mountain bikes is a device called a power grip. Power grips are laminated polyurethane straps that run diagonally across the top of the pedals.[14] After sliding one's feet into the straps, only a slight inward force with the heels will cause the straps to stay tight on the feet. When a quick stop or dismount is needed, outward movement of the heels will release the feet from the straps and the cyclist can get a foot on the ground quickly to maintain balance.

Ready to Ride

Like beginning motorcyclists or automobile drivers, beginning bicyclists must practice before they can become proficient in handling their machines. Take your new bicycle to an empty parking lot or playground and practice a variety of maneuvers. Make sure that you can ride in a straight line while giving hand signals, looking over

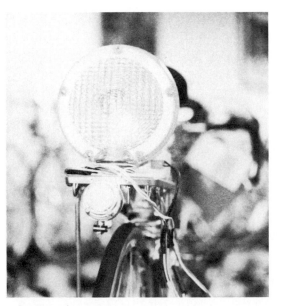

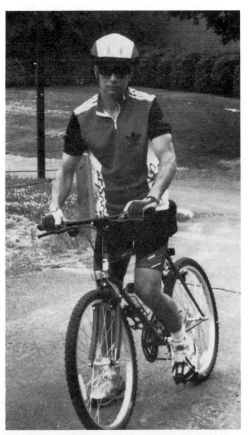

A

FIG. 10-9 **A,** An innovation that provides the night rider with a significant increase in conspicuity is the development of a dual rear-lighting system. The small light at the bottom is a red brake and tail light, while the large light above it is a flashing yellow construction marker. **B,** Notice the toe clips that hold this mountain-bike rider's feet in place on the pedals.

Courtesy: The Bicycle Exchange, Fairfax, Va.

B

your shoulder, or braking. If you have a small helmet-attached, rear-view mirror, now is the time to get used to using it. If you have front and rear caliper brakes, practice the coordinated hand movements necessary for smoothly stopping the bike. Brake pressure should be applied equally to the front and rear brakes so that the bicycle will stop in a relatively straight line. Sudden excessive pressure on the front brake may throw you over the handlebars, while too much pressure on the rear brake may send the bike into an uncontrolled slide. Take the bicycle out in wet weather also to practice braking. Remember the brakes will not stop you as well when they are wet. It takes some practicing to adjust for the variation in stopping distances during wet weather.

Check the turning radius of the bike to find out when the pedals may drag the pavement. Practice turns to the left and right using proper hand signals. Once you have developed the basic riding skills and feel confident about your abilities, the transition to riding in traffic will be a safer experience.

Safety in traffic involves three basic elements[7,8]: (1) Be visible, (2) be predictable, and (3) know the rules of the road. Clothing, lights, and helmets can provide a certain amount of visibility, but position in the lane of traffic is also important. Bicyclists must ride where drivers are expecting traffic, preferably in the right lane, riding along the line made by the right wheel of the car. If riders get too close to the edge of the lane, they blend into pedestrian traffic or parked cars, and motor vehicle drivers are not as likely to notice them. Parked cars present their own special dangers for the cyclist who is riding too close to the side of the road. A suddenly opened car door puts the cyclist in jeopardy in two ways—if he goes straight, he crashes into the car door; if he attempts to swerve, he is likely to travel into the path of a car approaching from the rear. Thus by riding further away from the edge of the road, one can avoid opening car doors and, at the same time, be seen more easily by approaching traffic.

Ride your bike as you would handle any other vehicle; in other words, be predictable. Don't ride on the left-hand side of the road and don't ride the wrong way on a one-way street. Motor vehicle drivers will not be expecting to see a bicycle rider under these circumstances. Don't suddenly turn without having given the proper hand signals to indicate your intentions.

Know the rules of the road as they pertain to your jurisdiction. Some communities may not allow bicycle traffic on certain streets, or they may restrict times of the day when bicyclists can use these thoroughfares, such as during the rush hour. Some counties require all bicycles to be registered and to carry bike tags similar to motor vehicle license plates.

The essential rule for the bicyclist is always to use good judgment and keep a cool head. Depending on traffic flow and road conditions, it may be necessary to ride somewhat closer to the edge of the road than normal, but be careful of sewer grates that run parallel to the roadway. The narrow tires of a 10-speed bike can drop through the grating easily and bring your bike to a sudden halt—while you continue over the top of the handlebars. If you are holding up a line of traffic, such as on a long hill, have the courtesy to pull off to the side to let other vehicles pass. Finally, always assume that you haven't been seen, keep an eye on developing traffic patterns ahead and behind you, and be prepared to take evasive action.

Bicycle Paths and Routes

With over 1 million people commuting on bicycles each day, cycling has become more than a recreational activity. It has become an important mode of transportation for a larger number of people.

Recognizing the potential dangers for bicycle commuters, cities throughout the country are looking for alternative ways to handle increased bike traffic and to provide cyclists with a maximum of protection. Bicycle paths probably offer the greatest protection. The typical bike path is a smooth asphalt surface that is physically separated from the road by trees or grass. It may wind along the highway or it may be constructed through a more scenic area. A variation of the bike path uses existing lanes of some city streets. One lane or a portion of a multilane street may be designated for bicycle traffic only, safely separating bicycle commuters from motor vehicle traffic flow, while the city does not have to pay for the construction of a totally new road surface.

An alternative used by other communities is the **bicycle route.** Streets on which traffic flow is not as heavy are marked with signs to inform bicycle riders that these routes are safer for traveling. At the same time the signs will indicate to motor vehicle drivers that they are likely to meet cyclists on the road. Some localities have taken this one step further by providing maps to bicycle commuters that show the safest, most direct routes through various parts of the city.

SWIMMING AND WATER-RELATED ACTIVITIES

Each year nearly 5000 people drown in the United States. Drowning is the second leading cause of death for persons 5 to 44 years of age; only motor vehicle accidents claim more lives in these age groups.[34] The deaths occur in a variety of situations, the majority of which involve swimming or playing in or falling into water at work, at home, or at a public facility such as a beach, lake, river, or pool. Additional drownings result from boating accidents. With over 100 million Americans involved in water-related activities annually, public awareness as to how these factors play a role in drownings and how they can be handled is essential.

Concerns for the Swimmer and the Boater

Many people mistakenly believe that drowning occurs primarily among the young and that once a person reaches high school age there is some built-in protection against the possibility of drowning. This is not the case. Although approximately 1200 children under age 15 died from drowning in 1989, more than 900 15- to 24-year-olds, 1300 25- to 44-year-olds, and nearly 700 persons 45 to 64 died in this manner.[34]

Almost every day from late spring until early fall, headlines report drownings:

"Three Die in Fraternity Boating Accident," "Youth Drowns in Stone Quarry Diving Accident," "Anglers Die in Lake Creely's Cold Waters." If the pertinent facts were tabulated for these various incidents, three factors would repeatedly appear: (1) The victims could not swim or were poor swimmers, (2) the water temperature at the time of the drowning was cold (below 70°F), and (3) the victims had been drinking before the accident. Very often the deaths result from a combination of these factors.

Poor swimmers generally will not risk their lives trying to swim across a lake, but poor swimmers who have had four or five beers may take the chance. On the other hand, nonswimmers will be careful about not going too far into the water at the beach, but they won't think anything of taking a canoe ride over a deep-water lake. The fisherman who is testing out a new boat and motor during the first nice weather in March may not realize that the water he could fall into after he drinks a pint of bourbon is just above freezing.

What every swimmer should know. Regardless of the recreational activity, participants must use good judgment and follow basic rules of safety. For swimming, the same rules apply to the strong and well-trained individual and the novice. In fact, good swimmers may need to follow these tenets more closely, since their example will be followed by many beginners.

1. Never swim alone or unobserved, even in a backyard pool.
2. Carefully follow the rules at the beach, lake, or pool where you swim.
3. Never dive into unfamiliar water; always go in feet first to inspect the area.
4. At beaches check with lifeguards and other swimmers about the surf and tides. Avoid swimming where rip tides and strong undertows are known to occur.
5. Keep a careful eye on family and friends; do not depend entirely on lifeguards who must watch over hundreds of swimmers.
6. If you're going to drink and swim, follow the rules just as you would if you were going to drink and drive. That means you could drink approximately one beer an hour without its inhibiting your swimming ability.
7. Do not attempt to swim long distances far from shore. Stay in close enough so that if you become fatigued, you will be able to touch bottom and take a breather.
8. Early in the swimming season watch out for cold water. Water temperatures below 70°F can quickly reduce body temperatures and lead to fatigue and muscle impairment.

Swimming safety involves more than helping oneself, it involves helping others in times of distress. Whether it's at a beach or pool, lifeguards have a major responsibility in watching over hundreds of swimmers every day. Without the help of other swimmers, guards could easily miss a great number of the people who are saved annually.

What are the signs of distress that signify "swimmer in trouble?" There seem to be three signs that universally indicate problems[46]:

1. Involuntary arm movements that result in a rapid, above-water breaststroke.
2. An open but nonvocalizing mouth.
3. A rolling back of the head.

It should be noted that these signals given by distressed swimmers usually last about 40 seconds before they slip under the surface of the water and drown. The exhaustion from overexertion and the person's inability to make the necessary movements to keep afloat result in this sequence of events. If you notice a person exhibiting these signs of distress, call for help at once.

Swimming education. There is absolutely no excuse in this country for people not to know how to swim. Mandatory education has given almost everyone rudimentary reading, writing, and arithmetic skills. A similar form of rudimentary swimming skill could easily become a part of every state's core curriculum for schools. Some states now require students to achieve a specific level of competency in reading and mathematics before they can graduate; why not require them to learn to swim before they can graduate? It would not be necessary to teach students how to become champion swimmers, but they should have the opportunity to learn basic strokes and survival skills in the water.

Drownproofing. While it cannot replace knowing how to swim as the essential component of water survival, a technique taught to swimmers and nonswimmers alike that can greatly increase their chances of rescue in a water emergency is drownproofing. Many drownings occur within as little as 10 feet of safety when people fall from boats, piers, and river banks. Had they been able to keep afloat for just a few minutes, they could have been rescued.

Drownproofing is a technique of water survival that uses a person's buoyancy and the principle that water will create an upward thrust equal to the downward pressure of the body mass. Developed during World War II to reduce the incidence of drowning in military personnel, the technique is much less physically demanding than trying to tread water or float on one's back. This five-step process is as follows[3] (see Fig. 10-10):

1. Vertical rest:
   a. Take a deep breath and sink vertically.
   b. Relax the body; let the chin drop to the chest with the arms hanging at your sides.
2. Ready position:
   a. Cross arms in front of forehead with forearms together.
   b. Raise one knee to the chest and extend the other leg behind in a striding position.
3. Exhale:
   a. Gently raise the head and breathe out; the chin should still be in the water.
4. Inhale:
   a. Gently sweep arms out and down while pushing down with the feet.
   b. Breathe in normally.
5. Return to vertical rest:
   a. As you sink back into the water, let the arms drop to the sides with the feet coming together.
   b. Drop the chin to the chest.

This method will allow the person in the water to breathe five or six times a minute while conserving much-needed energy. Although it is a simple and effective maneu-

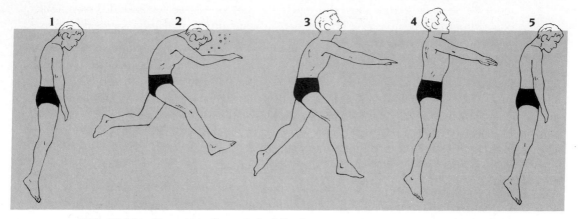

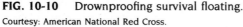

FIG. 10-10 Drownproofing survival floating.
Courtesy: American National Red Cross.

ver, beginners will have to overcome their fear of putting the face into the water, and they will need to learn that the body has a significant amount of natural buoyancy that they must use to their advantage. Once the technique of drownproofing is mastered, there is an additional maneuver known as the ''travel stroke'' that can be added, thus allowing an energy-conserving means of propulsion through the water.

PFDs (personal flotation devices). Although it is by no means an adequate substitute for knowing how to swim, a personal flotation device is a must for any nonswimmer who may be in areas where there is a strong water current, deep water, or water of unknown depth. Nonswimmers often think nothing of standing or sitting on the edge of a dock or wading in a river of unknown depth, wearing absolutely no protection. The same holds true for nonswimming fishermen who put their lives in danger when they fail to wear anything to protect them. Personal flotation devices or PFDs are made from several types of buoyant material and come in a variety of designs[51] (see Fig. 10-11).

Type I: Designed for offshore cruising, this PFD is designed to turn an unconscious person from a face-downward to a vertical or slightly backward position and provides more than 20 pounds of buoyancy.

Type II: Similar to the Type I PFD, this device also will turn an unconscious victim to a face-up position; however, its buoyancy rating is not as high at 15.5 pounds.

Type III: Designed to provide a maximum of comfort and freedom of movement during water activities, this PFD provides at least 15.5 pounds of buoyancy for its wearer, but it does not have the turning ability of the Type I and II PFDs. Most water skiers wear the Type III PFD.

Type IV: This device is designed to be thrown to a person in the water; it is not worn. The typical Type IV PFDs are the buoyant cushions found in boats and the ring buoys that are seen at most pools. While they provide adequate buoyancy, they provide no protection if the victims cannot hold onto them.

Type V: These devices are designed specifically for activities that require a max-

TYPE I - *"Offshore Life Jacket"*

- Recommended Uses: Offshore Cruising, Racing and Fishing
- Minimum Buoyancy: 22 lbs. (11 lbs. for child size)
- Best for open, rough or remote water where rescue may be slow to arrive
- Will turn most unconscious wearers face-up in water
- Offers the best protection, but bulky and uncomfortable

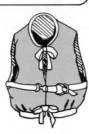

TYPE II - *"Near-Shore Buoyant Vest"*

- Recommended Uses: Inland Cruising, Dinghy Sailing and Dinghy Racing
- Minimum Buoyancy: 15.5 lbs.
- Good for protected, inland water near shore, where chance of immediate rescue is good. Not suitable for extended survival in rough water
- Will turn most unconscious wearers face-up in water
- More comfortable, but less buoyant than Type I

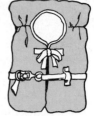

TYPE III - *"Flotation Aid"*

- Recommended Uses: Supervised activities, such as sailing regattas, dinghy races, water skiing, canoeing, kayaking and for personal watercraft
- Minimum buoyancy: 15.5 lbs.
- Good for protected, inland water near shore, where chance of immediate rescue is good. Not suitable for extended survival in rough water
- Most comfortable to wear; less buoyant than Type I
- Wearer must tilt head back to avoid face-down position in water

TYPE IV - *"Throwable Device"*

- Recommended Uses: Throw to overboard victim, or to supplement the buoyancy of a person overboard. **It is not to be worn.**
- Minimum buoyancy: 16.5 lbs. for ring buoy, 18.0 lbs. for boat cushion
- Can be a cushion, ring or horseshoe mounted on deck
- For calm, inland water with heavy boat traffic, where help is always nearby
- Not for unconscious persons, nonswimmers or children

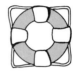

TYPE V - *"Special Use Device"*

- Recommended Uses: Restricted to the special use for which each is designed; ex., sailboard harness, deck suit, commercial white water vest, float coats. Must be worn when underway to meet minimum Coast Guard requirements.
- Minimum Buoyancy: 15.5 to 22 lbs.

Type V Hybrids - "Hybrids" have 7.5 lbs. of built-in foam buoyancy, and can be inflated to 22 lbs. by activating a CO_2 cartridge. Hybrids perform like Type I, II or III PFDs, as specified on the label. They are more comfortable than Type I or Type II, but are inadequate for unconscious overboard victims. Hybrids are recommended for boating activites where rescue is nearby. They are popular among fishermen and hunters for their stylish comfort, pockets and added warmth in cold water boating. Like other Type Vs, hybrids must be worn when underway.

FIG. 10-11   Personal flatation devices.
Courtesy: U.S. Coast Guard.

imum of movement; for example, Type V PFDs have been designed for white-water kayakers and construction workers.

Since 1973 federal regulations have required boats 16 feet or longer to carry one Type I, II or III wearable PFD for each person on board and at least one Type IV throwable PFD. Boats less than 16 feet in length and all canoes and kayaks must carry one Type I, II, III, or IV PFD for each person on board. Although the law requires that PFDs be carried on boats, it does not stipulate that they be worn. Of the nearly 900 boating fatalities in 1989, 753 (84%) were drownings; the majority of these deaths involved nonswimmers or very poor swimmers.[50] Most of the victims were not wearing PFDs when they were forced into the water. In most boating accidents there is no time to get a flotation device and put it on; the incident occurs and boaters find themselves in the water. Capsizing and falls overboard, both sudden occurrences, accounted for 547 (61%) of the fatalities.

It may not be a legal obligation that passengers (especially nonswimmers) in your boat wear PFDs; however, there would seem to be a strong moral implication that would require skippers to protect their friends and maximize their safety.

Cold water drowning. In recent years a factor that has become prominent in the investigations of numerous drownings is that of exposure to cold water, especially in boating accidents. Most swimming-related fatalities occur from mid-May to mid-September, when the water is relatively warm; however, the same does not hold true for boating fatalities. Fishermen, hunters, and canoeing and kayaking enthusiasts may be on the water from early March until late October—frequently in waters that are just above freezing. In some of the best fishing areas, water temperatures may never become much warmer than 50°F during the year. These are the people who are most likely to be faced with the dangers of cold-water immersion. The temperature of the water, the time a person stays in the water, one's body size, fat composition, and activity level in the water play a role in determining one's chances for survival.

Cold water is generally considered to have a temperature of less than 70°F, and it can affect an individual in a number of ways. The immediate effects of sudden exposure to cold water include torso reflex, muscle impairment, and possible cardiac arrest. Torso reflex is a sudden, involuntary gasping for air upon initial impact with the water. If a person's face is in the water, it can mean the inhalation of a large amount of water; this, coupled with the sudden disorientation of capsizing or falling overboard, can quickly lead to unconsciousness and death by drowning.[45] Cold water can quickly numb the extremities, making simple tasks such as holding onto a line nearly impossible; it can also reduce the ability to hold your breath. In an older, less-fit individual, the extreme shock from hitting the icy cold waters of a river or lake can affect cardiac rhythm and lead to sudden cardiac arrest.[52] The sudden immersion in cold water of a poor swimmer who is not wearing a personal flotation device may be fatal.

Even strong swimmers or people wearing PFDs can be in grave danger when they are immersed in cold water. After the initial shock and panic, there is the danger of hypothermia (loss of body temperature). If this condition goes unchecked, while victims may not drown, they will die from respiratory arrest induced by lowered body temperature. Obviously, the colder the water, the quicker the heat loss; however, a larger person will lose body heat more slowly than a smaller one. A fat person, because of the insulating qualities of adipose tissue, will lose heat more slowly than a thinner, more muscular individual.

Besides the water temperature, probably the most critical factor associated with cold-water immersion and survival is activity in the water; the more active a person is in the water, the greater will be the heat loss and the shorter will be the survival time.

What should people do if they find themselves in this dilemma? Most experts agree that getting back into the boat, if possible, is the best alternative. Owners of small boats should learn the proper procedures for righting them. If this cannot be done, try to get on top of the boat or at least as far out of the water as possible. The air may feel chilly, but cold water will rob the body of its heat more rapidly.

Shouldn't a good swimmer head for shore to get help? That depends on how far away the shoreline is. Studies indicate that some good swimmers may be able to swim as much as eight tenths of a mile in 50°F water before being overcome by hypothermia, whereas others may not be able to travel more than 100 yards.[52] Distances on the water are often very deceptive, and if you add to this unfavorable wind or water currents, your chances of safely swimming for help are rather slim. By staying with the boat, even one that has capsized, people are more likely to be spotted and rescued. However, if there is absolutely no chance of immediate rescue (for example, at a lake in an unpopulated wilderness location) or if you are a short distance from the shoreline and sure you can make it, then attempt to swim for help.

Heat-escape lessening position (HELP). In many cases the alternatives of swimming for shore or getting back into the boat are impossible. Survival in the water becomes dependent on two factors: one's ability to float and the reduction of heat loss from the body.

If you are wearing a PFD, the major concern is retention of body heat. Areas of major heat loss are the head, neck, armpits, and groin. At each of these sites large blood vessels lie close to the skin surface and will give up large amounts of heat to the water.

To reduce heat loss from these susceptible areas, you should get into the **heat-escape lessening position (HELP).**[46,52] Cross the arms over the chest; cross the ankles; draw knees to the chest and lean back. This will keep the head out of the water and protect the other heat-loss areas. If there are a number of people in the water, a huddle position is advised. Each huddle should consist of three or four people, with arms around each other's waists and chest touching chest. Small children should be placed in the middle to give them added protection. Leave on heavy clothing because it can entrap air, which provides added buoyancy and also provides insulation against the cold water (Fig. 10-12).

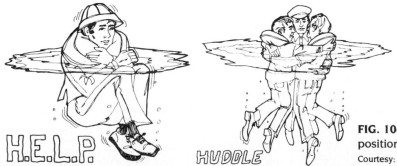

FIG. 10-12   HELP and HUDDLE positions for cold-water survival. Courtesy: U.S. Coast Guard.

What about the person who goes into the water without a PFD? This person is in double jeopardy. First he must be concerned about flotation, and subsequently there is the temperature-loss problem. Although most of us have been taught to shed heavy clothing in a water accident, this does not seem to be the best advice. As mentioned above, heavy clothing can work to one's advantage. By quickly getting into the HELP position, a person can use air trapped in water-tight boots and shoes - the bigger the boot, the more air there will be to provide buoyancy. Clothing provides the same buoyancy benefits, especially if a person is wearing several layers of clothing. A snowmobile suit will give a person a surprising amount of protection in the water. The bottom line here is that most people will need to practice before they become comfortable with this method of flotation.

In recent years a phenomenon known as the **mammalian diving reflex (MDR)** has significantly changed the approach of water-rescue personnel. MDR is a complex series of body responses that shut off circulation of oxygenated blood to most parts of the body except the heart, lungs, and brain.[22] At the same time, the body's demand for oxygenated blood is drastically reduced. What sets off this response mechanism? Sudden submersion in cold water (below 70°F) of the face and head, as in the case of drowning, activates the process.

People who have been in the water for as long as 1 hour have been successfully resuscitated with no permanent damage. MDR is stronger in young children (under age 4) and in colder water. However, new evidence has shown that even in warmer water, adults who were submerged for 15 or 20 minutes have been revived.

Most rescue personnel are taught that the cessation of breathing and circulation for more than 6 minutes results in permanent brain damage and death; however, in drowning this rule does not seem to apply. If the victim can be located within a relatively short time in warmer water (under 30 minutes), resuscitative efforts, including CPR and advanced life-support measures, should be initiated. In the case of a cold-water drowning, especially if a young person is involved, rescue within an hour may still offer the victim a chance for survival.

Boating safety tips. Since we have mentioned what can and should be done in the event of a boating accident, it is appropriate to mention some basic measures that should be taken by all boaters to reduce the chances of an accident[11,51]:

1. Before departing on any trip leave a "float plan" with someone on shore. It should include the description of your boat, the number of persons going with you, your route, destination, and expected time of arrival.
2. Know the "rules of the road" such as boat right-of-way, storm warning signals, meanings of buoys and markers, and distress signals. As an example:
   a. A boat being passed has the right-of-way.
   b. When meeting another boat head-on, keep to the right.
   c. A boat crossing your path from the right has the right-of-way.
3. Instruct at least one other person on board in the operation of your boat.

4. Show everyone on board where safety equipment is stowed and how it is properly used. This includes fire extinguishers, flares, horns, or whistles for signaling, and personal flotation devices.

5. Insist that all children and nonswimmers wear PFDs at all times. In cold-water boating everyone should wear a PFD.

6. On small boats (under 16 feet) carry a secondary means of propulsion such as a small second engine, oars, or paddles.

7. Have an anchor and sufficient line to hold in strong winds.

8. Make sure your boat is equipped with a bailer. It's a good idea to carry a hand bailer or scoop even when the boat is equipped with an electric bilge pump.

9. When underway:

    a. Watch your wake because you are responsible for any damage or injury caused by it.

    b. Be on the lookout for reckless boaters; not everyone plays by the rules.

10. With scuba diving gaining in popularity in recent years, boat operators should realize that a red flag with a white diagonal slash marks the approximate center of divers' activities. Give a wide berth in these areas.

11. If your group is water skiing, there should always be two people in the tow boat, one to watch skiers and one to operate the boat. Chances are your group will not be the only party skiing, so as you operate watch for other skiers who may be down in the water.

Boating and drinking. As with swimming, boating and drinking don't mix. Alcohol impairs coordination and greatly increases reaction time. Add to this a reduction in visual acuity and inhibition, and we now have a person who is less able to control the boat yet is willing to take more risks.

Coast Guard and state boating officials throughout the United States have recognized that the consumption of alcoholic beverages has become a widespread problem. Whether boaters are fishing, cruising, or sailing, there are lengthy periods of time when they are not fully occupied with operating their craft. The slower speeds of most boating activities, compared to those of automobiles, and the relatively unconfined nature of most waterways have also contributed to a lack of awareness of the risks involved with drinking and boating. Studies conducted by the Coast Guard suggest that alcohol may be involved in as many as 6 of 10 recreational boating fatalities.[53]

To reduce boating accidents caused by alcohol and drug misuse, the U.S. Coast Guard, in conjunction with the Department of Transportation, has proposed federal standards for determining intoxication in recreational boaters. Levels of intoxication will be based on blood alcohol concentrations similar to those applied to motor vehicle drivers (.10 BAC for operators of recreational boats) or on observations of the boat operator's demeanor or performance. In addition, there will be a provision for civil and criminal penalties for those found guilty of intoxication while operating a recreational vessel.

If there is going to be drinking on your boat, at least follow the one-drink-per-hour

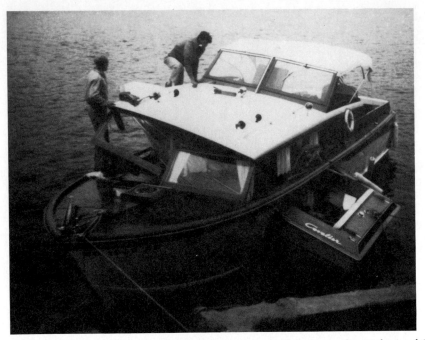

FIG. 10-13 This 16-foot runabout pierced the hull section of a 30-foot cabin cruiser in a collision on Lake of the Ozarks, Missouri.
Courtesy: Commander M. Thomas Woodward, U.S. Coast Guard.

rule. Better yet, assign a designated operator who will drink no alcoholic beverages during the outing (Fig. 10-13).

Waterskiing

Combining the elements of freedom of movement and high velocity, a water-related activity that has become a popular summertime sport is that of waterskiing. Part of the reason for its popularity is that beginners can succeed in a relatively short period of time. With minimal instruction new skiers can learn to get out of the water and keep their balance while being towed in a straight line. However, what many of them fail to realize is that this is only the beginning; proficiency in skiing, as with any activity, takes time to develop. Few participants prepare themselves by receiving formal instruction in skiing or basic water safety, nor do they condition themselves for the physical demands placed on them while skiing.

Although it is a relatively safe activity for the millions who participate, at least 50 deaths and as many as 25,000 injuries result each year from skiing accidents.[50] Most injuries to skiers occur in one of the following situations:[24]

1. A fall into unobstructed water.
2. Being hit by a boat propeller.

3. Collision with an obstacle.

4. Entanglement with the tow rope.

Waterskiing is by no means a simple activity. It takes at least three people to provide a maximum of safety: the skier, an observer, and the boat operator. Let's examine the responsibilities of each.

Since it is vigorous and physically demanding, waterskiing requires that both beginners and experienced skiers be in good physical condition. Preseason programs to develop strength and flexibility are essential. Even when this is done, skiers must exercise good judgment and stay within the limits of their abilities. Adequate preparation includes a clear recognition of the potential for injury in this sport. Skiers should:

1. Know how to swim.

2. Wear Coast Guard-approved personal flotation devices.*

3. Have the ability to communicate with those in the towboat via hand signals.

4. Avoid maneuvering near rocks, other boats, pilings, and buoy markers.

5. Keep the towline taut—a slack rope can get twisted around fingers, arms, or legs; if this occurs, a suddenly accelerating tow rope can cause massive trauma to these extremities.

6. Ski under control at all times. If you cannot control your movements easily, boat speed may be excessive, you may be fatigued, or you may be attempting skills beyond your current ability level

The observer's major responsibility is to stay in constant visual contact with the skier. This becomes especially important if a skier is disabled; the observer can direct the towboat operator for a rapid recovery of the skier. From his or her position, the observer can relay information to and from both the towboat operator and the skier concerning other skiers, boat traffic, or debris in the water.

When pulling skiers, boat operators' responsibilities significantly increase; they must take special care to avoid piers, beach areas, floating debris, and other boats. The operator must not only be aware of skiers he or she is towing, but must also watch for skiers from other craft in the area, particularly those who have fallen into the water. Finally, boat operators need to know and abide by the regulations governing waterskiing in their states.

Personal Watercraft

One of the newest and fastest growing recreational boating activities involves the use of personal watercraft. Personal watercraft are small, agile boats which are powered by an inboard engine and a jet pump mechanism. They are less than 13 feet in length and are designed to be operated by a person or persons sitting, standing, or

---

*Ski belts are not Coast Guard-approved, since they fail to provide adequate support for an injured skier. The waterskiing vest (Type III PFD) should be worn, because it has the capability to keep an injured person in a face-up position in the water.

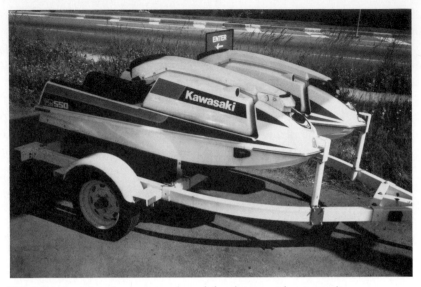

FIG. 10-14   One of a variety of models of personal watercraft.

kneeling, rather than within the confines of a hull.[29, 50] Sometimes called ''jet skis'' or ''waverunners,'' they are considered to be Class A inboard boats, and as such must meet the registration and safety requirements set forth by the U.S. Coast Guard (Fig. 10-14).

Since the mid-1980s sales of personal watercraft more than doubled; there are an estimated 250,000 of these boats in use. With their popularity have come problems; deaths and injuries involving personal watercraft (PWCs) have steadily climbed. In 1990 there were 29 deaths and more than 600 injuries resulting from the 1156 accidents involving PWCs. While the death rate per 100,000 registered boats in the United States is 5.0, the death rate for PWCs is 11.6.[50]

As with any other powerful, highly maneuverable recreational vehicle, the operation of a personal watercraft requires education and training. The Personal Watercraft Industry Association (PWIA) recommends that no privately owned personal watercraft be operated by anyone below the age of 14, and no PWC be rented to anyone under the age of 16. Because of a lack of responsible operation by numerous personal watercraft enthusiasts, a number of states have developed legislation which restricts the use of PWCs on lakes and waterways. Wake jumping, running too close to shore, running too near swimmers, and not yielding right of way to other boats are actions that have brought concerns from other boaters, fishermen, divers, swimmers, and concerned citizens.

To make sure that you and your personal watercraft will be welcome on the water, make sure that you and others who operate your boat follow manufacturers' recommendations, boating safety guidelines, and state boating regulations.

Skin and Scuba Diving

Skin diving and scuba diving are two distinct underwater activities that have gained immense popularity in the last 10 years. Skin divers use a face mask, snorkel, and fins as their basic equipment; their ability to hold their breath will determine how long they stay under. In scuba (self-contained underwater breathing apparatus) diving, tanks of compressed air carried with divers allow them to stay underwater for extended periods.

No one knows when humans first discovered that they could hold their breath and travel underwater, but the beginnings of the diving profession can be traced back more than 5000 years.[13] Early skin divers harvested a variety of materials including food, sponges, and coral. Records dating to the fifth century BC indicate the widespread use of divers in military and salvage operations.

Other than a few refinements in equipment, the skin diver of today has basically the same capabilities as his ancestors. There are three essential pieces of equipment: a face mask, fins, and a snorkel (Fig. 10-15).

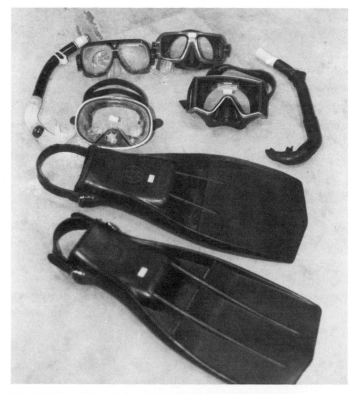

FIG. 10-15   Essential equipment for the skin diver.
Courtesy: Sea Ventures, Inc., Fairfax, Va.

The face mask primarily protects the diver's eyes and nose from the water. As a secondary function it provides maximum visibility by putting a layer of air between the lens of the eye and the water, thus permitting the eye to focus on the transmitted images. Regardless of the type of mask that is selected, its faceplate must be constructed of tempered or shatterproof safety glass. Although they are shatterproof, plastic faceplates are generally unsuitable because they are easily scratched and fog up often. One of the first skills a beginning diver should learn is how to clear a facemask of water that has seeped into it. To clear a flooded face mask, push gently on the upper portion of the mask and exhale through the nose into the mask. As water is forced out, tilt the head backward until the mask is clear.

Swimfins increase divers' efficiency by allowing them to move faster and farther with a lower expenditure of energy. There are a variety of styles and sizes. A longer, stiffer swimfin will transmit more power from the legs to the water, but it will take more leg strength to utilize these fins properly. It is a matter of what feels comfortable for the diver; as one becomes more proficient, equipment preferences will change.

A snorkel is a simple U-shaped breathing tube that allows a diver to swim along the surface scanning the area below without needing to lift the head from the water. Since a person's head weighs 15 to 20 pounds, repeatedly lifting the head out of the water can be quite fatiguing. As the diver descends into the water, the snorkel fills with water. On resurfacing, the diver blows water out of the snorkel and allows air to reenter by inhaling firmly. The more one practices and uses the mask, fins, and snorkel, the more one will enjoy the pleasures of diving.

Skin diving is a relatively safe sport, but it does have its hazards. Since part of the enjoyment of this activity depends on your ability to hold your breath, a certain amount of training is needed to improve this skill. With practice a person can stay under for 2 minutes or more; then as carbon dioxide levels increase in the bloodstream, the individual will find it necessary to surface for air. However, some divers can develop their capacity for breath holding so well that they can override this urge to surface. When that occurs the diver may black out and, on losing consciousness, inhale large amounts of water. The resulting blockage of air passages will quickly result in death from drowning, unless there is someone nearby to provide a prompt rescue.

Beginning divers may also find themselves in difficulty when they become exhausted from spending too long in the water. Suddenly they are some distance from shore and there is no place to rest before they swim back. A number of good swimmers who have overestimated their abilities have drowned under these circumstances.

There are a few specific rules of safety for the skin diver, but they must be followed[13]:

1. Never dive alone. Always have a buddy with you underwater. If a problem arises, time is of the essence.

2. Either have a boat or a floating apparatus anchored in the area where you are diving. It provides you with a base of operations from which to work. It can be used

as a resting station as well as a rescue device in an emergency. An inner tube with an affixed laundry basket for holding equipment makes an ideal floating platform.

3. Fly the diver's flag in the area where you are diving. This red flag with white diagonal stripe should be flown at least 3 feet above the water line, preferably attached to the floating platform or boat from which you are diving. It warns boaters in the area that divers are nearby.

4. Know the area in which you are diving. Be aware of particular hazards that may exist at the diving site.

5. Wear an inflatable vest when you dive. Known as "buoyancy compensators," these flotation vests can be inflated automatically by activating a small tank of compressed air or a CO_2 cartridge attached to the device, bringing a diver quickly to the surface in an emergency. Once on the surface, they will keep an exhausted or injured diver in a face-up, floating position. The vests also can be inflated by mouth.

Scuba. The most obvious and necessary step in broadening the diver's capabilities was to provide an air supply that would permit him to stay underwater. The earliest attempts involved hollow reeds or tubes extending to the surface of the water. However, at a depth of little more than 12 inches below the water line, it is essentially impossible to breathe through a tube using only the body's natural respiratory ability, since the weight of the water exerts a force of almost 200 pounds on a diver's chest. This force increases steadily with depth and is one of the most important factors in diving.

A technological breakthrough that occurred in the early 1800s was the development of a pump that was capable of delivering air under pressure. Shortly thereafter, the first practical diving helmets and suits came into existence. This was the forerunner of today's deep-sea diving suit. Man had gained a significant amount of freedom and flexibility underwater; however, the diver was tied to the surface by his air line.

As early as the late 1800s, practical self-contained breathing devices had been developed, but they were relatively dangerous because they used a 100%-oxygen concentration under pressure. A condition known as oxygen poisoning, which involves convulsions, was a common occurrence for divers who worked below a depth of 25 feet.[13]

It wasn't until World War II that the first truly efficient and safe **self-contained underwater breathing apparatus (scuba)** became a reality. Underwater explorer Jacques Yves Cousteau was a major contributor to the development of what was then known as the "Aqua-Lung." The high-pressure air tanks of the Aqua-Lung contained compressed air (that is, the air we normally breathe—79% nitrogen and 21% oxygen); consequently, there was no danger of oxygen poisoning for divers. This apparatus represents the most widely used and familiar piece of diving equipment (Fig. 10-16).

Today there are 3.5 million scuba enthusiasts in the United States; they dive in coastal waters, lakes, quarries, and rivers. As sport diving has become more popular, there has been an increasing incidence of serious diving accidents. Frequently the

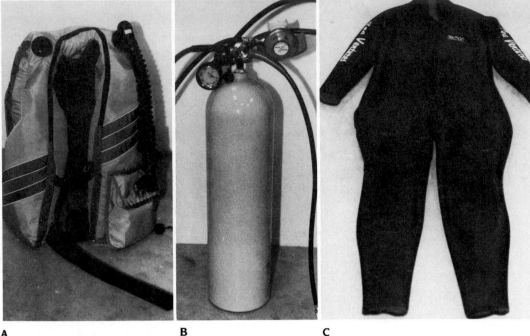

A   **B**   **C**

FIG. 10-16   Equipment used by scuba enthusiasts. **A,** Buoyancy compensator, **B,** Air tank and regulator **C,** Wet suit.
Courtesy: Sea Ventures, Inc., Fairfax, Fa.

victims are inexperienced people making their first or second dives. They also tend to dive in lakes and inland areas where scuba hasn't been a widespread activity, and they are unfamiliar with the dangers involved.[33]

Unlike the skin diver, who swims at relatively shallow depths for a short duration, the scuba diver can travel much deeper and stay down for long periods of time. With this extended capability, the scuba diver must be made aware of the effects of pressure on the body and its life-threatening potential.

Gas embolism. One of the first rules that a scuba diver must learn is: Never hold your breath during ascent from a dive in which breathing apparatus has been used. During an underwater dive, as the pressure on one's body increases, pressure on the lungs increases. It takes a greater number of molecules of air, the deeper one goes, to keep the lungs normally expanded. For example, at a depth of 33 feet, pressure on the lungs is twice that of the pressure at sea level. To keep the lungs properly inflated at this depth, it will take twice the number of air molecules that it would at sea level. If one went to 99 feet, the pressure would be four times that at sea level, and it would take about four times as many air molecules to fill the lungs.

When a diver holds his or her breath during an ascent, air trapped in the lungs expands as the water pressure decreases at shallower depths. Air in the lungs at a depth of 99 feet will expand fourfold by the time one reaches the surface. If exhalation does not occur, the increasing gas pressure in the lungs can rupture tissue and blood vessels. Ascent from even the shallow depths of a pool can cause these pressure problems. Air escaping from a lung can fill the chest cavity, which in turn causes the lung to collapse. This condition, known as pneumothorax, is a life-threatening situation, since it may affect both breathing and cardiac function.

A more dangerous situation can occur when air bubbles are forced into ruptured blood vessels in the lungs. These bubbles may be carried throughout the circulatory system and will continue to expand as the diver ascends. It becomes critical when one of these bubbles, known as an embolism, blocks blood flow to the brain, resulting in paralysis, blindness, coma, or death.

The dangers of pneumothorax and gas embolism can be avoided by breathing normally during the ascent, or if the ascent is made without an air supply, by continually exhaling the expanding gas that is already in the lungs.

Decompression sickness. With the increasing depth of an underwater dive, tissues in the body will gradually absorb larger quantities of nitrogen from the compressed air that enters the lungs and bloodstream. This process of nitrogen absorption under pressure is known as saturation; it occurs rather quickly as one descends in the water.

When a diver ascends to shallower depths, reducing pressure on the body, nitrogen will come out of solution in the tissues, enter the bloodstream, and then be released by the lungs. If the ascent is a slow and gradual one, there will be no problem with removal of nitrogen from the tissues. However, if the diver rapidly moves into shallow waters, the lungs will not be able to remove the nitrogen quickly enough, and it will form gas bubbles in the tissues. This condition is known as **decompression sickness** or "the bends."[13]

The joints and the spinal cord are most often affected in decompression sickness. Bubbles of nitrogen that have not been cleared from the bloodstream will accumulate in knee, shoulder, and elbow joints, causing swelling and acute pain. Nitrogen bubbles in blood vessels supplying the spinal cord can block the circulation, which may ultimately result in damage to the cord and paralysis of the diver.[29]

To reduce the likelihood of decompression sickness, all divers should follow the decompression tables that have been established by the United States Navy. The decompression tables specify the depths at which divers must stop and the length of time they will need to spend at each depth to allow the lungs to remove nitrogen from body tissues safely. For most scuba divers, the most important part of the decompression tables are the "no decompression" limits, which inform divers how long they can stay at a specific depth without the need for decompression.

National diving accident network. Whether it's a gas embolism or a case of "the bends," the definitive treatment for these pressure-related diving problems generally involves recompression. This is a process in which the diver is gradually returned to an atmosphere of increased pressure to reduce the size of gas bubbles to the point at which adequate circulation can return to blocked tissues. Recompression chambers are located throughout the United States at a number of military installations and university medical centers.

Since many physicians have had little experience in diagnosing and treating diving injuries, there was a need for centers that could provide treatment information as well as the location of the nearest facility with recompression capabilities. In January 1981 the National Diving Accident Network was established to provide this service.[33] Administered through the Duke University Medical Center, the Network has seven U.S. regional centers. A nationwide telephone number (919-684-8111) provides access to the system 24 hours a day. Because there has been a general lack of awareness about diving accidents, the Network has also become involved in the collection of data on the incidence and types of accidents.

Learning to scuba dive. The safest and smartest way to become involved with scuba diving is to receive training from a qualified instructor. Two organizations that provide educational programs for diving enthusiasts are the National Association of Underwater Instructors (NAUI) and the Professional Association of Diving Instructors (PADI). Because scuba diving is an activity that could be extremely hazardous for persons with no formal preparation, most dive shops and resort areas will neither sell nor rent equipment to individuals who have not received scuba instruction.

A Different Kind of Diving

Annually more than 700 swimmers are seriously injured in diving accidents; nearly half of them sustain some type of permanent disability, usually paralysis.[54, 60] Most injuries occur in the cervical vertebrae of the neck when the diver's head hits the bottom of a pool or lake. As the person's head suddenly stops on impact, the cervical vertebrae are compressed or crushed by the body's momentum. Depending on the force placed on the spinal cord, a diver may be lucky and suffer from numbness in the extremities for several days after a mild strain; however, if the impact causes the vertebrae to cut into the cord, tearing or severing it, the likely result is paralysis from the waist down or in more severe cases paralysis from the neck down.

The saddest part is that in almost every case the accident would have been totally preventable. Only about a quarter of all diving accidents occur in swimming pools; the majority involve natural bodies of water such as lakes, rivers, and quarries. Usually the person is diving into an area with which he or she is unfamiliar. If the water is murky or unclear, the bottom might be 15 feet away or it might be 3 feet away. Especially in stone quarries, there may be obstructions jutting from the sides just below the surface of the water.

Although pools provide a safety factor in greater clarity of the water, they do not provide an accident-free environment. Many of the in-ground pools found at apartment complexes, motels, or private residences provide a relatively small area for safe diving. The deepest part of these pools is generally about 9 feet. That is an adequate depth in which to dive from the sides of the pool, but it is not adequate for persons diving from a 1-meter board; in that case, pool depth should be a minimum of 11 or 12 feet. The addition of a diving board poses another problem at these small pools in that the deepest part lies at the end of the board or slightly in front of it. Most people will spring out and away from the board when they dive, and in smaller pools this means that they will actually be entering a shallower area. In a pool with a 1-meter board, there should be adequate depth for a distance of at least 25 feet from the end of the board. If a pool does not meet these depth and distance specifications, it should not have a diving board.

Another important element that must be considered for safe diving is the skill level of the diver. Often improper positioning of the arms and hands during the dive will cause the person's head to ram the floor of the lake or pool. Arms should be over the ears in a stretched position with the hands together. On contact with the bottom, the arms can dissipate the force and stop the head from hitting. For the noncompetitive diver, entry into the water should not necessarily be in a vertical position; although it may look pretty, it will bring a person into contact with the bottom of the pool very quickly. Using a flatter diving technique, a diver will not go as deep into the water, thus lessening the chances of injury.

Residential Pool Safety

Advances in construction technology have made the residential pool an affordable item for many American families; today there are more than 3.5 million home pools in the United States.[18] However, with this rapid increase in pool construction has come an equally rapid increase in residential pool drownings. Unlike public facilities, which provide lifeguards trained in rescue techniques, the home pool is generally left unsupervised. Additionally, most homeowners are not trained to handle a pool-related emergency.

Children under 5 years of age seem to be most at risk in these incidents; they account for nearly half of the drownings in the residential setting.[18] It takes only a few minutes out of a parent's sight and the results can be fatal; that 5- or 10-minute phone call can be just enough time for a little one to fall into the pool and drown. Young children must never be left unsupervised in or around a pool.

A relatively new safety apparatus that has been developed for residential pool owners is the in-the-water alarm. When a child falls in the pool, these devices detect changes in water surface motion or underwater pressure. They are battery powered and come with a remote receiver which sounds an alarm in the house. Though they can be adjusted for sensitivity to wave motion in the pool, windy environmental conditions are likely to cause false alarms.

Many communities have ordinances requiring fences around residential property that contains a pool, but few cities require that the entire pool area be enclosed by a fence. The National Spa and Pool Institute and the National Safety Council recommend that the entire pool be enclosed by a 5-foot fence and that the entry gate be self-closing and self-latching. Studies by these groups indicate that such ordinances could significantly reduce home pool drownings.[54]

COLD-WEATHER ACTIVITIES

Snowmobiling

Snowmobiles were introduced in the 1950s; however, it wasn't until the late 1960s, after a number of design changes, that they gained widespread popularity as recreational vehicles. Powered by an engine similar to that of a motorcycle, a snow-mobile is propelled by a wide, molded-plastic track and guided by a pair of front skis. Unlike a car or truck, its weight is distributed over a broader surface; thus, where a truck would bog down in the snow, a snowmobile is able to glide across the surface.

As the number of these vehicles increased, snowmobile-related accidents and injuries also increased. In the early 1970s more than 250 persons were killed per year while riding snowmobiles, and an additional 15,000 to 20,000 people were injured seriously enough to require emergency-room treatment.[20] Spectacular accidents in which snowmobiles collided with motor vehicles, trains, trees, and telephone poles, and incidents in which snowmobilers were decapitated by unseen fencing, guy wires, or chains across driveway entrances made for gruesome headlines.

Such reports began to worry and discourage prospective snowmobile enthusiasts, and sales declined; at the same time legislators and government officials called for strong measures to regulate the industry. Realizing that the snowmobile and the sport of snowmobiling were in jeopardy of being regulated out of existence, the International Snowmobile Industry Association (ISIA) developed a program to control its safety-related problems. It focused on three key areas: the machine itself, the operator, and areas where snowmobiles were used.

Machine safety. Sponsored by manufacturers, a nonprofit organization known as the Snowmobile Safety and Certification Committee (SSCC) was formed to address the issue of product safety. Through the efforts of this group, certification standards were developed for the manufacture of snowmobiles. Since 1975 all snowmobiles manufactured by member companies of the ISIA must meet these standards, which cover brakes, controls, seats, lights, shields, guards, hand grips, fuel systems, and sound levels. If you are thinking about buying a snowmobile, be sure that the model your purchase meets these safety standards. This is easily checked by locating the certification label of the SSCC on the right side of the vehicle (Fig. 10-17).

Rider safety. The second phase of the snowmobile industry's attempt to reduce accidents and injuries entailed the development of The Snowmobile Operator's Training Program, a 300-page manual that serves as a complete guide for safety training and instruction.[26]

Let's take a brief look at some of the important points that are stressed in most snowmobile safety classes[20,26,48]:

1. Always perform a prestart inspection of the vehicle before turning on the ignition. Check for such things as loose parts and adequate fuel supply. Be sure to test brake, steering, and throttle controls. Under certain conditions these systems are subject to freezing.
2. When starting the snowmobile, no one should be standing in front or in back of it. Serious injuries have occurred when bystanders have been run over by snowmobiles or they have been hit by debris thrown backward by the rotating track.
3. Before attempting to operate on more difficult terrain, the beginning driver should master the basic riding positions, turns, and weight-shifting techniques on a level area.
4. As with other winter sports, snowmobiling requires wearing apparel that provides adequate protection from the cold without preventing freedom of movement.

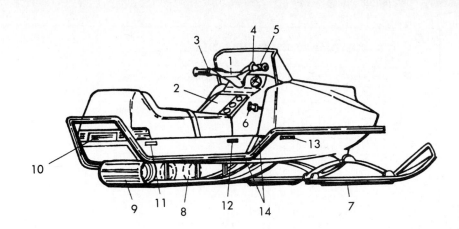

Nomenclature

1. Steering control (handlebar)
2. Console
3. Headlight hi-lo beam switch
4. Emergency stop switch (electrical cut-off for engine ignition)
5. Throttle control (lever type)
6. Manual starter handle
7. Ski wear rod, wear bar (reduces ski wear and greatly improves directional control)
8. Suspension (slide and/or bogie wheel types)
9. Track (cleated or moulded, propels vehicle)
10. Taillight/brake light
11. Reflectors/side marker lights
12. Vehicle identification number (right side of vehicle)
13. Reflectors/side marker lights
14. Running board and footrest

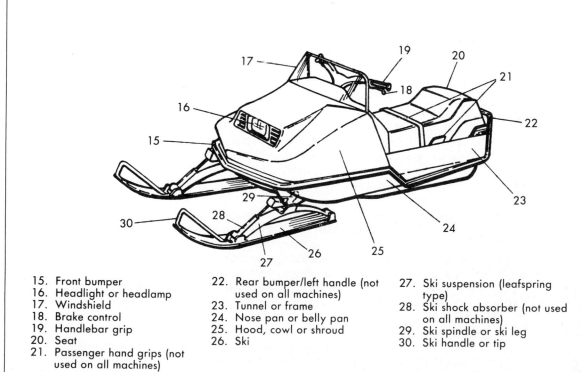

15. Front bumper
16. Headlight or headlamp
17. Windshield
18. Brake control
19. Handlebar grip
20. Seat
21. Passenger hand grips (not used on all machines)
22. Rear bumper/left handle (not used on all machines)
23. Tunnel or frame
24. Nose pan or belly pan
25. Hood, cowl or shroud
26. Ski
27. Ski suspension (leafspring type)
28. Ski shock absorber (not used on all machines)
29. Ski spindle or ski leg
30. Ski handle or tip

FIG. 10-17 Parts of a snowmobile.

Courtesy: Snowmobile Safety and Certification Committee, Inc., Annandale, Va.

U.S. CUSTOMARY WIND CHILL CHART

Combined speed of wind and snowmobile in MPH	Actual thermometer reading (°F)											
	50	40	30	20	10	0	−10	−20	−30	−40	−50	−60
	Equivalent temperature (°F)											
0	50	40	30	20	10	0	−10	−20	−30	−40	−50	−60
5	48	37	27	16	6	−5	−15	−26	−36	−47	−57	−68
10	40	28	16	4	−9	−21	−33	−46	−58	−70	−83	−95
15	36	22	9	−5	−18	−36	−45	−58	−72	−85	−99	−112
20	32	18	4	−10	−25	−39	−53	−67	−82	−96	−110	−124
25	30	16	0	−15	−29	−44	−59	−74	−88	−104	−118	−133
30	28	13	−2	−18	−33	−48	−63	−79	−94	−109	−125	−140
35	27	11	−4	−20	−35	−49	−67	−82	−98	−113	−129	−145
40	26	10	−6	−21	−37	−53	−69	−85	−100	−116	−132	−148
(wind speeds greater than 40 mph have little additional effect)	Little danger* (for properly clothed person)			Increasing danger*			Great danger*					
	*Danger from freezing of exposed flesh											

FIG. 10-18　U.S. customary wind chill chart.

Courtesy: Snowmobile Safety and Certification Committee, Inc., Annandale, Va.

Exposure to the cold is compounded by the speed of the snowmobile, which produces a wind-chill factor for its operator and passengers (Fig. 10-18). Insufficiently protected riders are likely to suffer frostbite. This condition occurs when the skin and underlying soft tissues freeze. Areas that are commonly affected are the fingers, nose, cheeks, ears, and toes. Symptoms include a numbing of the affected part and a white, waxy coloration of the skin surface. Often it is other members of the snowmobiling party who recognize the victim's problem. Treatment consists of the rapid thawing of tissues with a warm-water bath or warm, moist compresses. Never rub the frozen areas, because this may damage underlying tissues. One other word of caution is that damage to tissues becomes more severe if the frostbitten area that has been thawed is refrozen. Take special precautions to prevent the recurrence of frostbite.

In terms of protective clothing, helmets and faceshields are indispensable items; they provide both warmth from the cold and protection from objects such as low-lying branches or rocks kicked up by other snowmobiles. However, under no circumstances wear scarves or loose clothing which could become entangled in a snowmobile's moving parts.

5. Although they are capable of speeds in excess of 70 mph, snowmobiles handle more easily at speeds of 20 to 30 mph. Excessive speeds inhibit one's ability to identify potential hazards such as fences, posts, rocks, tree stumps, and sudden changes in terrain, especially at night.

6. As with any motor vehicle, operators of snowmobiles must realize the importance of moderation if they are going to drink and drive. In a 10-year study of snowmobile accidents in the state of Wisconsin, researchers found that over 60% of those fatally injured had elevated blood alcohol concentrations.[39]

7. When carrying a passenger, it is important to inform him or her about such things as leaning into turns, holding onto passenger grips, and keeping one's feet on the running board. Also,

reduced speed is essential, since a passenger cannot react as quickly to bumps in the trail, low-hanging branches, or sudden stops and starts of the vehicle.

8. Stay on established trails, never operate in unfamiliar territory, and know the state or provincial laws concerning the operation of snowmobiles. Be especially careful when operating vehicles on or near bodies of water such as lakes and rivers; studies indicate that nearly 20% of the fatally injured snowmobilers drown when their machines crash through the ice.

Trail development. Because of the lack of adequate riding and trail facilities in the early 1970s, many snowmobilers operated their vehicles on public roadways or over terrain that presented numerous hazards, such as fences, wires, tree stumps, and posts. During the past 10 years, an estimated 190,000 miles of public and private snowmobile trails have been developed in Canada and the United States. In the nonwinter months these same trails and paths may be used for bicycling, hiking, or horseback riding.

As we move into the 1990s snowmobiling remains a popular winter sport; yet deaths have decreased threefold and injuries have been reduced by half during the last decade. The primary factor in this steady reduction of accidents can be attributed easily to the combined efforts of snowmobilers and the industry in developing programs that have addressed the issues of machine safety, operator training, and trail development.

Snow Skiing

While downhill skiing is considered one of the most exhilarating and fast-paced recreational activities, the sport can present another side that is not so charming, especially for those who are not prepared for its challenges. In this section we will take a look at some of the injuries to which skiers are exposed and examine some of the ways to reduce these injuries.

With the advent of shorter skis, better release bindings, and improved grooming of slopes, the overall rate of injury for skiers appears to be on the decline.[10,27,31] The use of shorter skis has reduced the likelihood that a ski will act as a lever in bending or twisting the leg in a fall. At the same time, bindings—which hold the ski boot to the ski under normal operating conditions—have been designed to allow the boot to separate from the ski in a number of different directions when a fall occurs. Low-friction surfaces made of teflon, which are mounted on the sole rests of the bindings, allow for a quicker release during twisting falls. Modern snowmaking and grooming techniques also provide the skier a much smoother skiing surface, thus reducing the chances of hitting unseen rough spots and taking a hard spill.

However, even with these improvements injuries still occur; as in the past, the greatest proportion of them occur from the knee down. A number of studies have indicated that the knee is particularly vulnerable, especially when bindings fail to release and skis stay attached to boots. Another common skiing injury is fracture of the tibia (shin). These boot-top fractures occur when a ski tip dips into the snow or hits an obstruction. When the ski and attached boot suddenly stop, momentum carries the skier forward, thus creating a fracture point at the top of the boot. As manufactures have developed boots with higher tops over the years, these fractures have occurred higher up the leg. As with the knee injuries, failure of ski bindings to release plays a prominent role in this injury.

But shouldn't the improved design of bindings reduce these problems? Well, yes and no. Bindings will not provide adequate safety unless they are appropriately maintained. From the standpoint of safety, the ski binding is the most important piece of equipment for a skier. When purchasing new bindings, it is important to have a qualified ski-shop mechanic mount and adjust them. At least once a year bindings should be checked and serviced before the season; as with any device, corrosion and wear can lead to problems. Bindings should also be tested each day before heading for the slopes. Using slow leaning and twisting motions, the skier should be able to release the bindings in every direction in which they are designed to release. If a skier feels pain in the leg before the binding releases, the mechanism needs to be checked. If skiers paid more attention to proper binding functions, it is likely that lower-extremity skiing injuries would continue to decrease.

Another common injury is the thumb sprain or dislocation. While it may not be as traumatic as cartilage or ligament damage in a knee or a fracture of bones in the lower leg, severe dislocation of the thumb can be extremely painful and may require surgical intervention. When skiers fall forward, they extend their hands in front of them to cushion the impact. However, skiers have an added problem in that they have ski poles in their hands. What often happens is that the pole strap does not allow skiers to release their grip, and as they fall the pole itself forces the thumb back in a position of hyperextension. Even the newly designed saber-grip poles have a tendency to prevent the release of the pole during a fall, since they wrap around the hand. Although it may require an occasional climb back up a slope to retrieve a pole, the statistics indicate that a grip that does not employ ski pole straps is by far the safest to use.[10]

Although the rates for most skiing injures have declined in recent years, this does not seem to be the case for neurological injuries (head and spinal cord damage) suffered in skiing accidents. Likely candidates for these devastating injuries are those who challenge the tougher slopes or are attempting maneuvers such as aerial stunts and jumps without the necessary training and safety instruction. Often it's not the new skier who runs into trouble but the advanced beginner or intermediate skier who thinks that he or she is an expert, gets on an expert slope, loses control, and slams into a tree or another skier. Who is responsible for this skier's injuries and/or those of the victim? Is it the advanced beginner's fault for losing control on the expert run, or is the ski area responsible for allowing this person to attempt a run beyond his or her level of skill?

To reduce the chances of such an occurrence, an approach that has been taken by some ski resorts is to segregate skiers by ability level. Skiers who want to qualify for the expert slopes must get certified by an instructor. Needless to say, the instructor's decision is not always a popular one, but the initial results at ski areas using this screening method have shown promise in reducing the more severe injuries that occur on the slopes.

Sledding and Tubing

What happens on the evening of the first snow of the year at your school? Isn't it amazing how cafeteria trays suddenly disappear from the cafeteria? It's time to go sledding! Anything that can provide a slick surface can be used as a makeshift sled: cardboard, paneling, sheets of plastic, cafeteria trays, and inner tubes.

Sledding or tubing provides the thrill of high speeds with little or no skill required. So why mention such an innocuous activity in a safety text? While it may be simplicity itself, you can run into trouble unless you take precautions. If you like to tube or sled, go where there are no obstructions such as trees, fence posts, or stumps. By far the biggest danger is colliding with an obstruction; more than a few students have missed a semester as the result of fractures or internal injuries suffered when they hit an obstruction.

Take one other precaution—make sure there is an adequate area at the bottom of the hill to allow you to safely stop. Hills bordering busy streets can create severe hazards when sledding enthusiasts cannot stop and they continue into the street. Keeping these two things in mind, now go out and enjoy yourself!

BACKPACKING: HIKING AND CAMPING

Backpacking is an activity that tests the human body and spirit while offering a relaxing escape from the complexities of society. Defined as hiking while carrying essential equipment and camping overnight on the trail, backpacking is a good form of exercise.[24] It provides a means to explore areas of outstanding beauty and offers a variety of learning experiences for all members of the family. It can be a very fulfilling and gratifying experience, or it can be something that one would never again want to try.

To provide both a safe and positive experience, there are two basic considerations in backpacking—equipment and planning. Essential equipment includes such items as a backpack frame, sleeping bag and pad, tent, clothing, food, cooking equipment, and safety supplies. The safety supplies are materials that would be needed in an emergency situation: first aid kit, waterproof matches, flashlight with extra bulbs and batteries, compass, pocketknife, 20 feet of rope, extra food, extra clothes, and a water bottle.[24] To make sure of having the necessary equipment, the novice backpacker would do well to contact several experienced people for suggestions. Many communities have wilderness supply stores that cater to backpackers, hikers, and other outdoor enthusiasts; personnel at these stores are generally very helpful in advising people about their equipment needs.

The second important consideration for backpackers is that of planning: Where to go? When? Length of stay? Type and length of route to travel? These decisions must be made long before the journey begins. The best advice for the novice is don't overdo it your first time out. Just as there is a culture shock for many Americans who travel to foreign countries, there will be a form of culture shock when the city dweller enters the wilderness. Initial trips should last no more than several days, and the intended distances to be covered should be of reasonable length. Plan on covering about 1 mile per hour so that you can enjoy what you are doing. Having a planned, specific route and timetable provides an added measure of safety. Friends or relatives should have a copy of your travel plans so that if you do not return on schedule, assistance can be dispatched quickly. A well-planned trip usually results in a safe and enjoyable experience.

Hypothermia—a Special Problem for the Backpacker

Statistics indicate that nearly 80% of wilderness accidents involve lacerations or burns. Other common problems are fractures, infections, and eye injuries. Most of these occurrences are relatively minor or at least easily treated.

A problem that is often overlooked or disregarded by hikers and backpackers is that of overexposure to the elements. The condition resulting from this overexposure to wind, rain, and cool weather is known as **hypothermia.**[52] It is, in fact, the leading cause of wilderness deaths. Hypothermia occurs when there is a continued loss of heat from the body below 95°F. Factors that play a major role in this process are moisture, wind, fatigue, and improper clothing. Surprisingly, low temperatures are not necessary to induce hypothermia. Most cases occur when the temperature is between 30°F and 50°F.

The body loses heat in a number of ways:[22]

1. Respiration: During the process of breathing, the exhalation of warm air removes a small amount of body heat.
2. Radiation: Any uncovered body surface will give up heat to the surrounding air. As much as 40% to 50% of one's body heat can be lost from the head and neck regions.
3. Convection: Wind currents blowing across the body will accelerate temperature loss by quickly removing radiated heat.
4. Evaporation: As perspiration or moisture on the skin dries, there is a cooling effect. Wind currents enhance the process of evaporation and thus speed up heat loss.
5. Conduction: When sitting on the ground or leaning next to a cold or wet object, heat will be absorbed from the body.

To prevent hypothermia one must control these heat loss processes. Safety tips for the backpacker include the following:

1. Always keep your head covered.
2. If your clothes get wet, change into dry ones immediately.
3. Wear clothes in layers so that as you get warmer you can remove a layer at a time to control perspiration. Or if you begin to chill, you can add another layer.
4. When you take a break on the trail, do not sit directly on the ground.

5. If it starts to rain, set up a shelter so that you can remain dry.

6. Make camp before you become exhausted; do not wait until late in the evening.

7. While on the trail, continually nibble on high-energy foods (dried fruit, nuts, chocolates).

Always be on the lookout for the appearance of the signs and symptoms of hypothermia in your traveling companions. Its onset may be very gradual, and consequently people will not recognize that a person is in trouble. One of the initial signs of a drop in body temperature is shivering. This is the body's way of attempting to generate more heat. As the temperature continues to drop, the shivering will cease and the person may have problems walking and maneuvering. You may notice a slurring of speech and a certain amount of confusion in the victim. If the situation is not corrected, he or she will eventually lose consciousness as the cardiorespiratory system begins to slow down. A continuing drop in temperature will result in cardiac arrest and death.

Hypothermia is a very serious medical emergency that requires immediate action by the rescuers. The priority is to prevent further heat loss and attempt to rewarm the victim. The ideal treatment is to immerse the patient in a tub of warm water (100° to 104°F); however, this is not a realistic alternative when you're in the wilderness. Get the victim out of any wet clothes and set up a shelter to protect him against wind, rain, or cold air. If he is conscious and coherent, dress him in dry clothes, get him into a sleeping bag, and give him warm liquids to drink.

If the patient is semiconscious or stuporous, the problem is more severe. Remove all of his clothing and place him in a sleeping bag between two warm people; skin-to-skin contact offers the quickest method of rewarming in this case. If he is conscious and can take fluids, give him something warm to drink. Never give a hypothermia victim alcohol to drink; the alcohol will cause blood vessels to dilate, and the victim will lose further body heat.

Although hypothermia is a serious problem that may confront the backpacker, a victim's chances of recovery are excellent if the symptoms are recognized early and treatment is started immediately. However, the best way to handle hypothermia is to prevent its occurrence by planning your trip carefully and carrying the proper equipment.

ROLLER SKATING/IN-LINE SKATING

Although many consider roller skating a popular and trendy activity, its origins can be traced to the mid-1600s, when wooden spools were attached to strips of wood. The first roller skating boom occurred during the late 1800s, just before the turn of the century. It was during this era that a smooth-riding ball-bearing skate was developed. For the next 70 years the sport's popularity fluctuated with the times. With the Depression there was an increase in skate usage because many could not afford to drive; the introduction of the roller derby in the late 1940s was another period of renewed skating activity. During the 1950s and 1960s roller skating played a minor role in America's recreational picture. Skating was for children, not adults.

However, all that changed in the 1970s. The introduction of resilient polyurethane wheels provided a smoother, faster ride on rough surfaces. This allowed people to skate at locations other than a rink. It was also discovered that roller skating provided an excellent means of cardiovascular exercise while utilizing a significant number of calories. An older population began to roller skate; more than one fourth of the nation's skaters are over 25.[38] In most metropolitan areas, curbside stands do a brisk business renting skates to city dwellers during the lunch hour, evenings, and weekends.

In the 1990s a variation of the traditional roller skate is the "roller blade" or in-line skate. Instead of having two parallel pairs of wheels, in-line skates have four or five narrow polyurethane wheels in a single row. The technique for in-line skating is very similar to that of ice skating; however, stopping is a bit tricky since the rubber braking device is located at the rear of the skate instead of in the front like the traditional roller skate.

As roller and in-line skating have become more popular, injuries have increased significantly. In 1989 the U.S. Consumer Product Safety Commission estimated that 72,000 people were treated in hospital emergency rooms for skating injuries.[19]

Epidemiological studies have indicated several injury patterns that have implications for the safety educator. For instance, only 25% of the injuries occurred at rinks; the majority of them were in parks, on sidewalks, and in the streets. With in-line skates, 75% of injuries occurred on sloped surfaces.[19] In most cases excessive speed and uneven surfaces led to a loss of balance and the resultant injury.

An interesting finding was that the loss of balance usually resulted in a fall backward with the victims extending arms and hands to cushion the impact. Not surprisingly, 80% of skating injuries involve the upper extremities, with the majority being wrist fractures.

Although men are generally more injury prone than women in most recreational activities, that does not hold true for roller skating. Women are injured while skating twice as often as are men. As mentioned earlier, skating involves an older population than one might think; more than half of those injured are 15 or older.[38]

For people taking up roller or in-line skating one of the first priorities is to learn how to fall. Do not use the hand and arms to absorb the impact; the energy of the fall needs to be dissipated over a larger area. By tucking the arms in and rolling to the side, the impact can be absorbed by the buttocks, trunk, and shoulder. Safety gear such as knee pads, elbow pads, and gloves should be worn, but they do not afford a great deal of protection in a fall backward. Perhaps some type of padding could be designed to fit under one's clothing that would protect the hips and buttocks during a fall. Currently some manufacturers offer padded shorts for skaters.

Another important consideration for the safety of skaters is where they should skate. Whether it's inside or outside, the skating surface should be smooth. Sidewalks, with their uneven pavement, cracks, and curbs, do not fill the bill. City streets, cars, and skaters also do not mix (Fig. 10-19).

For the person who chooses to skate outdoors, there are several options. Asphalt-

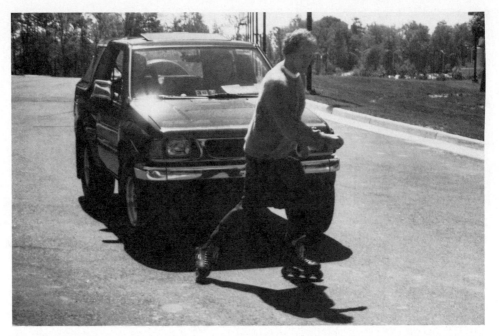

FIG. 10-19   This is not the place to skate. Also, the stereo headphones he is wearing will block out the sound of approaching vehicles.

covered bicycle and running paths provide a smooth and often scenic route for skaters. Parks and recreation centers may have outdoor rinks or special areas for skating. In some cities certain downtown areas are closed to vehicular traffic during weekends to provide a safe place to skate.

HANG GLIDING AND ULTRALIGHTS

One of the most unforgiving of recreational activities in the 1980s and 1990s has been the sport of hang gliding. Almost one fourth of the 1300 hang gliding injuries occurring each year require hospitalization. Additionally, at least 30 people per year have been killed since the sport's inception. The hang glider, consisting of a light tubular aluminum frame covered by nylon fabric, receives its power from wind and air currents and is steered by its pilot, who hangs underneath. Similar to a very large kite, the glider can be towed behind a car to gain altitude, or, more commonly, its pilot will leap from an elevated area to catch an air current. Once the glider is airborne, the pilot can control both altitude and direction by using body movements and a stabilizer bar.

The danger with these craft is that they allow little margin for error: Your first mistake may be your last. Wind gusts can also play havoc with one's ability to control the craft. A sudden strong wind can flip a hang glider over or send it into a stall. If the pilot cannot quickly recover, the glider will go out of control and plummet to the

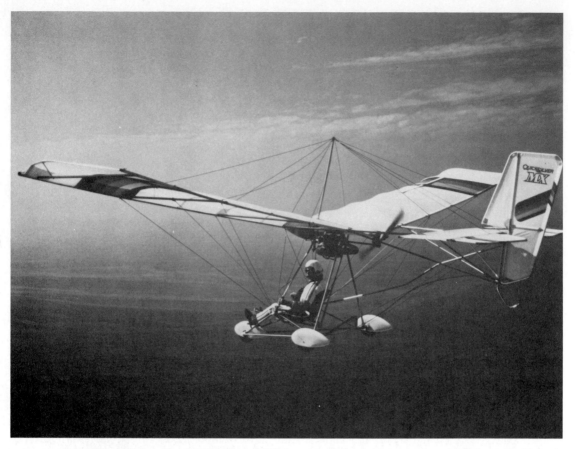

FIG. 10-20   The "Quicksilver MX" is one of the most popular ultralight craft. Note its tubular frame, fabric covering, and gasoline-powered engine.
Photograph by Eipper Aircraft, Courtesy of Sport Flight, Inc., Gaithersburg, Md.

ground. Poor judgments by pilots as they make their landing approaches have ended with fatal crashes into trees, power lines, and homes.

A relatively new variation of the hang glider, which has involved design changes and the addition of a motor, is the ultralight (Fig. 10-20). Using the same tubular frame and fabric covering, ultralights resemble planes that flew in the early 1900s. Unlike a hang glider, an ultralight does not depend on wind currents to keep it aloft. The small gasoline-powered engine can move an ultralight at speeds of 50 to 60 mph. Although little data have been collected about these motorized hang gliders, there are a number of potential problems that may threaten the safety of their operators as well as others. Although the Federal Aviation Agency (FAA) has strict regulations for the licensing of airplanes and their pilots, currently there are no regulations for ultralights or those who fly them. If you've got the money to buy it, you can fly it. Ultralight pilots are not required to receive any type of schooling or training before they fly.

A number of deaths have been caused by mechanical failures of ultralights in flight. Support lines used to guide the craft have broken, engines have failed, and wings have collapsed. However, on further investigation, most equipment failures have apparently occurred when pilots have exceeded the operating limits of the craft by taking them higher and faster than they were intended to go.[57]

Because of the exceptional risks involved in hang gliding and the flying of ultralights, purchasers of all such craft should be required to receive detailed instruction concerning their safe operation. During this instruction pilots should be made aware of the structural limitations of the craft as well as those procedures which should be used during an in-flight emergency.

ALL-TERRAIN VEHICLES

One of the most popular recreational machines of the 1990s has been the **all-terrain vehicle (ATV).** Produced in both three- and four-wheeled models, these motorized off-road vehicles travel on low-pressure tires and have a seat design that allows the operator to straddle the machine (Fig. 10-21). ATVs are not intended for use on paved surfaces, nor are they built to carry passengers.

Depending on their design, ATVs can vary significantly in terms of control and operation. Transmissions, throttle controls, suspensions, and braking systems differ

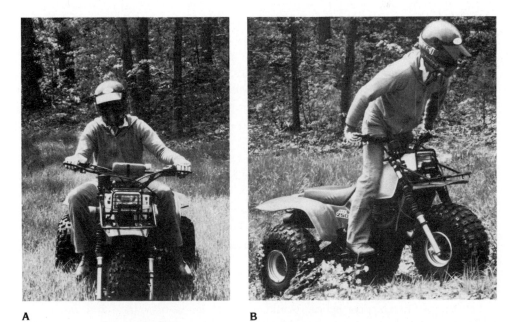

A   **B**

FIG. 10-21   A, Protective gear for the ATV rider includes: helmet, goggles, gloves, boots, jacket, and pants. **B,** With his weight shifted forward, this ATV rider demonstrates the proper technique for climbing a hill.

from model to model. Before riding any all-terrain vehicle it is important that one become familiar with the location of all controls and the handling characteristics of that particular model.

In recent years reports of excessive numbers of deaths and injuries of ATV riders have prompted the Consumer Product Safety Commission to evaluate this phenomenon. Since 1982 an estimated 500,000 injuries have been treated in hospital emergency rooms, and more than 1700 deaths have occurred as a result of ATV mishaps.[6]

Analysis of injury surveys has indicated that accidents involving three-wheeled ATVs appear to be similar to those involving four-wheeled ATVs. Hitting a terrain irregularity such as a bump, rock, or rut causes nearly a third of the incidents. Problems with turning, riding up or down a slope, and colliding with stationary or moving objects account for most of the other accidents. Although overturning or tipping is a common reaction of ATVs in such incidents, CPSC studies indicate that the dynamic stability of a four-wheeled vehicle is somewhat better than that of its three-wheeled counterpart. Because of the higher risk of injury associated with three-wheeled ATVs, in 1988 manufacturers agreed to no longer sell them in the United States.

Evaluations of driver-related factors have indicated that operators under 16 years of age riding adult-sized vehicles with engine displacements of 225 cc or more have shown an excessive risk of injury.[37] More than 45% of ATV deaths and injuries have been incurred by this age group. Driver inexperience was found to be a prominent issue; the risk of injury for those with less than 1 month of experience was 13 times the average.

Inappropriate riding behaviors such as not wearing a helmet, carrying passengers, riding on paved roads, and traveling at excessive speeds for the terrain contributed significantly to the number or severity of injuries. Nearly 80% of those injured had not worn helmets; consequently, it was not surprising to find that slightly more than 70% of ATV deaths resulted from head injuries. At accident speeds in excess of 25 mph, the percentage of occupants thrown from vehicles doubled, and their chances of severe injury quadrupled.

The evidence is clear: Because of the unique handling characteristics of ATVs, riding requires special skills that must be learned over a period of time. The Specialty Vehicle Institute of America (SVIA), a national nonprofit association representing manufacturers and distributors of all-terrain vehicles, has developed a comprehensive training course for ATV riders that is offered through local dealerships across the United States and Canada.

HOT TUBS

Although most people would not consider using a hot tub a water sport, it has certainly become a popular recreational and social activity. However, with this popularity some problems have arisen that have serious health and safety implications for their users. Introduced in the early 1970s, hot tubs were a West Coast phenomenon, with the majority of enthusiasts living in California. Basically a hot tub is an enlarged version of a whirlpool bath, with some models accommodating as many as eight people. A heating unit maintains a constant temperature as the water is continuously recirculated in the pool, which may have a depth of 2 to 4 feet.

Why the concern? In recent years the CPSC has estimated that 1700 people are injured each year while using hot tubs; more than 150 of these incidents are life threatening or fatal.[58]

The greatest danger for people using hot tubs is that of drowning. Heat, the suction created by water circulation pumps, and the use of alcohol while tubbing have been identified as contributing factors in many of these deaths. It is generally recommended that water temperature be set at approximately 100°F and should not exceed 104°F. Higher temperatures lead to excessive blood-vessel dilation, which reduces blood pressure and may cause a loss of consciousness. Add to the temperature factor a situation involving an excessive intake of alcohol, which can lead to further blood-vessel dilation, and there is an increased risk of drowning. The anesthetic effect of alcohol can inhibit one's ability to sense that there may be a problem.

A little-known danger of older hot tubs that makes women with long hair particularly susceptible to drowning is the suction created by recirculating pumps.[58] Water-intake ports are located at several places along the sides of hot tubs. At these locations, a fairly strong suction is created as water is drawn from the tub. In a significant number of instances, a woman's hair has been sucked into the water intake, forcefully pulling her head underwater. Without the assistance of others in the tub, this would mean sure death. Recognizing this problem, manufacturers have relocated intake ports near the bottom of newer tubs and have placed fine mesh grills over the coverings (Fig. 10-22). However, there is still a danger when small children are allowed to use the tub as a pool. If an intake covering is broken, a submerged child's

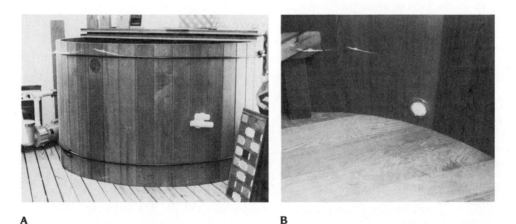

A   **B**

FIG. 10-22   A, Recirculating jets that force water back into the tub are placed approximately 2 or 3 feet below the water line. **B,** However, the drains, with their fine mesh grills, are placed at the bottom of the tub.

Courtesy: M.B.C. Aquatics, Fairfax, Va.

hair can be entrapped, or if the child is inquisitive and reaches into the intake, a hand or arm can be trapped.

A final note of caution about hot tubs. They can provide relaxation and pleasure, but like any water-related activity, tubbing should never be attempted alone.

TANNING SALONS

Let's face it; there is something attractive about that bronze look one gets from a good suntan, especially if it's mid-March and you haven't enjoyed sunny summer weather since September. But how can this happen if you haven't had the time or the money to spend 2 weeks in the Bahamas? The local tanning salon!

The use of tanning beds and tanning booths has become a popular way to get an out-of-season tan or to retain the one you got during the summer. However, with this quest for golden skin come the risks with which many students may not be familiar: premature aging of the skin, eye cataracts, and skin cancer.[21] Whether it's from the sun or from the fluorescent lamps in a tanning bed, long-term exposure to ultraviolet radiation can have serious effects on the skin and eyes. What may make an artificial tan even riskier is that ultraviolet radiation in a tanning booth is much more intense than that from natural sunlight; consequently, it has the potential to do more damage in a shorter period of time.

If you do decide to go to a tanning salon, it should not be for the purpose of long-term tanning. A common-sense approach is to use such facilities to prepare yourself for that spring trip to Florida, Mexico, or the Islands. Several weeks of short-term exposures at a tanning salon can help to reduce the likelihood of a severe sunburn once you're at the beach.

While the American Medical Association does not recommend the use of artificial tanning devices, it has developed guidelines for those who choose to use them[21]:

1. Do not use artificial tanning if you burn easily in normal sunlight or you are taking photosensitizing medications.

2. Do not overdo exposure time; start gradually and increase it slowly to about 20 minutes per session.

3. Always wear protective goggles that block out ultraviolet light; regular sunglasses, closing your eyes, or putting cotton balls over the eyelids will not protect you.

SUMMARY

Recreation in the 1990s has been geared toward the individual and his or her participation in lifetime activities. Major emphasis has been placed on the importance of becoming and staying physically fit.

On any given day nearly 20 million Americans run for their health; however, in some instances, that health can be jeopardized if they are not careful where, when, and how they run.

For many summertime sports enthusiasts, heat-related problems are quite common—especially for those who are not in shape. A general rule for all persons exercising vigorously during hot weather is to drink plenty of fluids before, during, and after exercising.

One of the fastest growing competitive recreational activities in the United States is racquetball. It offers the beginner an immediate opportunity for success while developing cardiovascular fitness. Although the racquetball is soft and the racquet used is short and easy to handle, these two pieces of equipment are responsible for most of the injuries. The greatest danger for the racquetball player is being hit in the eye with the ball. To prevent such a disaster, all players should wear eyeguards with impact-resistant lenses and frames.

While it is not a competitive activity, aerobic dance has developed into a highly popular form of cardiovascular exercise. People who have not exercised vigorously in some time should get a check-up by a physician before beginning an aerobic dance class.

Weight lifting for fitness has become a popular recreational activity. Like any fitness activity, there are certain hazards that must be controlled in weight lifting. The lower back and shoulder are particularly susceptible to training injuries, so it is important for both novices and experienced lifters to warm up properly and use correct technique when weight training.

An activity that provides both exercise and an economical means of transportation is bicycling. A top priority for a person purchasing a bicycle is to get one that fits the body. Saddle height, handlebar height, and stem length must be adjusted for each individual if the bicycle is to provide a safe and efficient means of transportation.

To provide maximum protection for the cyclist, certain accessories are suggested. Lights, reflectors, and riding vests can increase one's visibility, while a helmet provides both an increase in biker visibility and protection in an accident.

Water-related activities can offer numerous pleasurable experiences for their participants; however, they can also be quite dangerous. Each year nearly 5000 people drown in the United States, making this the second leading cause of accidental death for persons 5 to 44 years of age. Most of these drownings can be attributed to three factors: (1) inability to swim or poor swimming skills, (2) cold water immersion, and (3) consumption of alcohol.

Not all boating accidents can be prevented, but planning and preparation can eliminate many of them or at least lessen their consequences. Before leaving the dock, everyone on board should know where safety equipment is and how to use it. Also, a float plan should be left with someone on shore.

Skin and scuba diving have gained immense popularity in the last 10 years. With skin diving the essentials include a face mask, swimfins, and snorkel. The diver is limited only by his ability to hold his breath. Beginning skin divers must not overextend themselves; a diver who becomes exhausted and is a long way from shore may be in grave danger.

The increased capabilities offered a diver who uses scuba tanks with a compressed air supply may be offset by the dangers which they can present. The rapid expansion of gases during ascent can rupture lung tissue if the excess gas is not allowed to escape. If a diver rapidly moves into shallow waters, the lungs will not be able to remove nitrogen from the tissues adequately; the resulting nitrogen gas bubbles will accumulate in joints and blood vessels causing severe pain and possible blockage of normal blood flow.

A different type of diving accident, involving swimmers rather than skin or scuba divers, occurs when the swimmer strikes his or her head on a submerged object or hits the bottom of a lake or pool. Prevention of these injuries involves knowing about the water into which one is diving and using the proper diving technique.

A problem often overlooked by hikers and backpackers is exposure to the elements. Even on relatively warm days, exposure to wind and rain can lead to hypothermia. If heat loss is not controlled, the results can be fatal.

Although it has been around a long time, roller skating has had a great resurgence in the 1990s with the introduction of in-line skates. With this increased participation in skating has come an increase in injuries, especially among adults.

A variation of the hang glider is a motorized version known as an ultralight. Though few data are available concerning the safety of these devices, reports of most accidents indicate that pilots may have exceeded the operating limits of the craft. Because of the type of risk involved, pilots of both hang gliders and ultralights should receive extensive instruction before they attempt to fly these craft.

Another recreational pursuit that requires special skills that must be learned over a period of time is all-terrain vehicle riding. Driver inexperience and inappropriate rider behaviors play a prominent role in ATV injuries. The Specialty Vehicle Institute of America has developed a comprehensive rider-training course that is offered by ATV dealerships throughout the country.

A relatively new recreational pursuit involves the use of a hot tub. The greatest danger associated with them is drowning when the warm waters dilate the bather's blood vessels, causing a loss of consciousness. Many of these drowning deaths are alcohol related. The hot tub can provide many hours of relaxation, but like any other water-related activity, it should never be attempted alone.

The use of tanning booths and tanning beds has become a popular way to maintain a year-round tan; however, a person needs to know that long-term exposure to ultraviolet radiation can have serious effects on the skin and eyes. A safer and more practical way to use tanning salons entails several weeks of short-term exposure to reduce the likelihood of a severe sunburn once you're at the beach.

Key Terms

All-terrain vehicle (ATV)   A motorized off-road vehicle that travels on low-pressure tires.

Bicycle routes   Streets with reduced traffic flow that are marked with signs indicating that they are safe for bicycle travel.

Decompression sickness   Also known as "the bends," this condition occurs when bubbles of nitrogen gas accumulate in the joints and blood vessels of a diver who has surfaced too quickly.

Drownproofing   A technique of water survival that uses a person's buoyancy and the upward thrust of water against a body mass.

Handlebar palsy   Loss of sensation in the hands and an inability to coordinate finger movements as a result of ulnar nerve irritation. This condition results from excessive pressure being placed on the hands while riding a bicycle.

Heat cramps   Painful, involuntary muscle contractions resulting from the loss of body fluids and electrolytes during heavy exercise.

Heat-escape lessening position (HELP)   A floating position taken in the water to prevent heat loss from the body.

Heat exhaustion   A mild form of shock caused by a reduction in blood flow to major organs; this condition is caused by fluid loss during heavy exertion.

Heat stroke   Also known as sunstroke, this condition results from failure of the body's heat-regulating mechanism, resulting in temperatures reaching 105°F or higher.

Hypothermia   A condition in which a person's body temperature drops below 95°F; a continuing drop in temperature can affect breathing centers in the brain, resulting in respiratory arrest and death.

Mammalian diving reflex (MDR)   A complex series of body responses that reduce oxygen requirements of major organ systems when a person's face and head are submersed in cold water.

Self-contained underwater breathing apparatus (scuba)   A portable device with compressed-air tanks that allows a diver to stay submerged for extended periods.

Ultralight   A variation of the hang glider in which a gasoline engine is used to power this propeller-driven apparatus.

Valsalva maneuver   Blood pressure fluctuations resulting from air-pressure changes in the chest and abdominal cavities of a weight lifter who holds his breath during the performance of a lift.

References

1. Aerobics without the bounce, Taking Care 8(9), Sept. 1986, Reston, Va., The Center for Corporate Health Promotion.
2. Agne-Traub, C. E., and Traub, G. L.: Volksmarching: a popular leisure activity for the middle-aged, Journal of Physical Education, Recreation and Dance, Oct. 1987, p. 59.
3. Bettsworth, M.: Drownproofing: a technique for water survival, New York, 1977, Schocken Books.
4. Birenbaum, S., Lemberg, S., and Ewell, H.: Possible petition for mandatory standards for bicycle helmets, May 15, 1990, U.S. Consumer Product Safety Commission.
5. Bishop, P. J., Kozey, J., and Caldwell, G.: Performance of eye protectors for squash and racquetball, The Physician and Sportsmedicine 10(3):63, 1982.
6. Blechschmidt, C.: Update of all-terrain vehicle deaths and injuries, Sept. 1990, U.S. Consumer Product Safety Commission.
7. Burke, B.: The bicycle commuter, Family Safety, Spring 1982, p. 24.
8. Burke, B.: Two-wheel touring, Family Safety, Summer 1981, p. 16.
9. Burke, E. R.: Ulnar neuropathy in bicyclists, The Physician and Sportsmedicine 9(4):53, 1981.
10. Carr, D., Johnson, R. J., and Pope, M. H.: Upper extremity injuries skiing, The American Journal of Sports Medicine 9(6):378, 1981.
11. Commonsense approach to boats keeps your head above water, Recreational Newsletter, Chicago, May-June 1982, National Safety Council.
12. Dempsey, P.: The bicycler's bible, Blue Ridge Summit, Penna., 1977, Tab Books.
13. Department of the Navy: U.S. Navy diving manual, Washington, D.C., 1978, Naval Sea Systems Command.
14. Derven, J.: Power grips, Bicycle Guide, May 1991, pp. 109-111.
15. Dunn, K.: A tenuous partnership. novice runners and distance races, The Physician and Sportsmedicine 8(11):146, 1980.
16. Dunnett, W.: Running against the fall of night, Runner's World, November 1979, p. 85.

17. Easterbrook, M.: Eye injuries in racket sports: a continuing problem, The Physician and Sportsmedicine 9(1):91, 1981.

18. Elder, J., and Hoebel, J. F.: Estimates of residential swimming pool deaths and injuries, May 1990, U.S. Consumer Product Safety Commission.

19. Feineman, N.: Roll into shape: skating gets serious, Women's Sports and Fitness, Sept. 1990, pp. 50-53.

20. Glitz, W.: Decade of progress: highlights of the years 1972-1981 in the snowmobile industry and sport, Annandale, Va., 1982, International Snowmobile Industry Association.

21. Goldsmith, M. F.: The dark side of artificial tans, Family Safety and Health, Winter 1985-1986, p. 26.

22. Hafen, B. Q., and Karren, K. J.: First aid and emergency care workbook, ed. 3, Denver, 1984, Morton Publishing Co.

23. Hall, A., editor: Petersen's complete guide to the bicycle, Los Angeles, 1975, Petersen Publishing Co.

24. Hisk, P. H.: Outdoor safety and survival, New York, 1983, John Wiley & Sons, Inc.

25. Hummel, G., and Gainor, B. J.: Waterskiing-related injuries, The American Journal of Sports Medicine 10(4):215, 1982.

26. International Snowmobile Industry Association: Snowmobiling fact book, Annandale, Va., 1982.

27. Johnson, R. J., and Pope, M. H.: Ski binding biomechanics, The Physician and Sportsmedicine 10(2):49, 1982.

28. Kamela, W. C., and Demes, J. C.: Mandatory bike helmet legislation: a growing national trend, Childhood Injury Prevention Quarterly, Winter 1991, pp. 14-22.

29. Kawasaki Motors Corporation, U.S.A.: Personal watercraft: boating basics, Seattle, Washington, 1989, Outdoor Empire Publishing, Inc.

30. Lehrer, John: Bike helmets, Outside, April 1991, p. 125.

31. McKay, D. H.: Downhill skiing injuries, The Physician and Sportsmedicine 9(1):105, 1981.

32. Metcalf, J. A. and others: ECG effects of aerobic dance, Postgraduate Medicine 70(2):219, 1981.

33. Miller, J.: Management of diving accidents, Emergency Medicine, 1981, p. 314.

34. National Safety Council: Accident facts: 1990 edition, Chicago, 1990, The Council.

35. National Safety Council: Bicycles, Bulletin no 1, Chicago, 1985, The Council.

36. Naughton, T.: Are you fit for aerobic dancing? Family Safety and Health, Spring 1986, p. 8.

37. Newman, R.: Analysis of all-terrain vehicle-related injuries and deaths, Sept. 1986, U.S. Consumer Product Safety Commission.

38. Perlik, P. C., and others: Roller-skating injuries, The Physician and Sports Medicine 10(4):76, 1982.

39. Peters, R, and Wenzel, F.J.: A ten-year survey of snowmobile accidents, injuries, and fatalities in Wisconsin, The Physician and Sportsmedicine 14(1):140, 1986.

40. Present, P.: Diving study: report on injuries treated in hospital emergency rooms as a result of diving into swimming pools, Sept. 1989, U.S. Consumer Product Safety Commission.

41. Present, P.: Injuries involving pool and spa covers, Sept. 1989, U.S. Consumer Product Safety Commission.

42. Safety for the runner: Part I, Runner's World, February 1979, p. 83.

43. Safety for the runner: Part II, Runner's World, March 1979, p. 65.

44. Scheers, N. J., Fulcher, D., and Polen, C.: Four-wheel ATVs and lateral stability, Sept. 1990, U.S. Consumer Product Safety Commission.

45. Servine, R.: Mountaineering medicine, Emergency, July 1980, p. 70.

46. Smith, D. S.: Sudden drowning syndrome, The Physician and Sports Medicine 8(6):76, 1980.

47. Smith, D. S.: Drownproofing and the water safety spectrum, JOPERD, May 1982, p. 56.

48. Snowmobile Safety and Certification Committee, Inc.: Snowmobiler's safety handbook, Annandale, Va., 1978.
49. Specialty Vehicle Institute of America: ATV rider's course: student workbook, Seattle, 1985, Outdoor Empire Publishing, Inc.
50. U.S. Coast Guard: Boating statistics 1989, COMDTPUB P16754.3, Washington, D.C., June 1990.
51. U.S. Coast Guard. Federal requirements for recreational boats, Washington, D.C., 1979, United States Department of Transportation.
52. U.S. Coast Guard: Hypothermia and cold water survival, Washington, D.C., June 1980, United States Department of Transportation.
53. U.S. Coast Guard: Operation of a vessel while intoxicated; notice of proposed rulemaking, 52(26):4116-4124, Feb. 9, 1987, Federal Registry, U.S. Department of Transportation.
54. U.S. Consumer Product Safety Commission: Children and pool safety checklist, Publication No. 357, Washington, D.C., Spring 1988.
55. U.S. Consumer Product Safety Commission: Large buckets are drowning hazards for young children, Washington, D.C., July 1989.
56. U.S. Consumer Product Safety Commission: Minutes of commission meeting: Dec. 18, 1986, Washington, D.C., 1986.
57. U.S. Consumer Product Safety Commission: Reported incidents 1977 to present: hang gliding, Washington, D.C., July 1982, National Injury Information Clearinghouse.
58. U.S. Consumer Product Safety Commission: Reported incidents 1977 to present: hot tubs and whirlpools, Washington, D.C., July 1982, National Injury Information Clearinghouse.
59. U.S. Consumer Product Safety Commission: Injury estimates of weight lifting: 1981, Washington, D.C., July 1982, National Electronic Injury Surveillance System.
60. Yoxall, P.: Diving can be risky, Family Safety, Summer 1982, p. 8.

Resource Organizations

Amateur Athletic Union of the United States
3400 West 86th Street
Indianapolis, IN 46268

American Alliance for Health,
Physical Education, Recreation,
and Dance
1900 Association Drive
Reston, VA 22091

American Amateur Racquetball Association
815 North Weber Street
Colorado Springs, CO 80903

American Canoe Association
P.O. Box 1190
Newington, VA 22122

American College of Sports Medicine
P.O. Box 1440
One Virginia Avenue
Indianapolis, IN 46206

American Orthopaedic Society
for Sports Medicine
70 West Hubbard, Suite 202
Chicago, IL 60610

American Running and Fitness Association
2001 S Street N.W., Suite 540
Washington, DC 20009

Appalachian Mountain Club
Five Joy Street
Boston, MA 02108

Association of Physical Fitness Centers
600 Jefferson Street, Suite 202
Rockville, MD 20852

Bicycle Manufacturers Association of
America
1055 Thomas Jefferson Street N.W.,
Suite 300
Washington, DC 20007

Bikecentennial: The Bicycle Travel
Association
PO. Box 8308
Missoula, MT 59807

Council for National Cooperation in Aquatics
901 West New York Street
Indianapolis, IN 46223

Drowning Prevention and Beach Safety
Program
c/o Joe Pecoraro
Chicago Park District
425 E. McFetridge Drive
Chicago, IL 60605

Intercollegiate Outing Club Association
c/o Wesleyan Outing Club
WSA Office, Wesleyan Station
Middletown, CT 06457

League of American Wheelmen
6707 Whitestone Road, Suite 209
Baltimore, MD 21207

National Association of Underwater
Instructors
P.O. Box 14650
Montclair, CA 91763

National Athletic Injury/Illness Reporting
System
Pennsylvania State University
131 White building
University Park, PA 16802

National Athletic Trainers Association
2952 Stemmons Freeway, Suite 200
Dallas, TX 75247

National Campers and Hikers Association
7172 Transit Road
Buffalo, NY 14221

National Collegiate Athletic Association
P.O. Box 1906
Mall Avenue at 63rd Street
Mission, KS 66201

National Safe Boating Council
U.S. Coast Guard Headquarters
Commandant (G-NAB-3)
2100 Second Street, S.W.
Washington, DC 20593

National Spa and Pool Institute
2111 Eisenhower Avenue
Alexandria, VA 22314

Professional Association of Diving
Instructors
1251 E. Dyer Road, #100
Santa Ana, CA 92705

Roadrunners Club of America
c/o Henley Gibble
629 S. Washington Street
Alexandria, VA 22314

Underwater Society of America
P.O. Box 628
Daly City, CA 94017

United States Cycling Federation
c/o USOC
1750 East Boulder
Colorado Spring, CO 80909

United States Lifesaving Association
c/o Chicago Park District
425 East 14th Boulevard
Chicago, IL 60605

United States Power Squadrons
P.O. Box 30423
Raleigh, NC 27622

US Hang Gliding Association
P.O. Box 8300
Colorado Springs, CO 80933

CHAPTER 10

Applying What You Have Learned

1. Discuss the following temperature-related emergencies: heat exhaustion, heat stroke, and hypothermia. In your answer list causes, signs and symptoms, and specific emergency treatments for each condition.

a) Heat exhaustion:

b) Heat stroke:

c) Hypothermia:

2. In selecting a bike that fits your body, what elements would you need to consider?

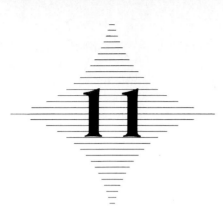

School Safety

Legal scholars estimate that 80% of all court cases involving alleged negligence for school-related injuries deal with some aspect of supervision.

Dr. Herb Appenzeller, Director of Athletics Guilford College, Greensboro, N.C.

Responsibility for the safety of students, faculty, and staff in our nation's schools involves a broad range of personnel. Typically, the majority of this responsibility lies with teachers and administrators; however, other personnel such as safety supervisors, physicians, athletic trainers, nurses, custodians, and bus drivers play an integral role in a school system's safety program.

RESPONSIBILITIES IN THE SAFETY PROGRAM

In this era of litigation consciousness, it is important for every school system to develop a detailed, written safety manual. Written policy statements provide procedural guidelines for both faculty and staff; they also serve as a checkpoint whenever a conflict arises. General areas of responsibility that may be covered in a school district's safety policies include safety instruction, first aid and emergency care, record keeping, disaster preparedness, plant inspections, in-service training, traffic control, bus transportation, and security.

The board of education and the superintendent have ultimate responsibility for carrying out the school system's safety policies; however, the actual development and control of the program is the responsibility of the director or supervisor of safety. A professional staff person appointed by the superintendent, the safety supervisor coordinates the efforts and programs of all divisions, schools, and departments in the system.

Using the school district's safety policies as a foundation, the director of safety can assist school principals, athletic directors, and academic and staff department heads in the development of specific safety guidelines for their particular situations. For example, a district policy concerning first aid may simply state that all teachers will be expected to render emergency care if the situation arises. In the case of junior and senior high school industrial arts departments, the safety supervisor, in conjunction with department chairpersons, may want to offer specific in-service training on how to handle severe lacerations, puncture wounds, and amputations, since industrial arts students are more likely to suffer these types of injuries.

To assist the safety supervisor, principals of the various schools have the responsibility for the development and implementation of their own safety programs. This works very well, because the principal may be aware of potential hazards that exist only at this particular school. Keys to the success of any school safety program are the principal-teacher and principal-staff working relationships. If the principal has a strong commitment to safety, teachers and staff are more likely to have a strong commitment, especially if the principal has established good rapport with personnel.

Teachers represent the front line of the school safety program. They have the responsibility for safety education and accident prevention. Teachers carry out policies that have been established for their school. Frequently, the teacher also acts as first responder. When a student is injured in a school-related activity, a teacher is usually the first person at the scene of the accident and must be prepared to render the appropriate aid. Not only are teachers expected to explain and demonstrate to students the safe performance of various skills and procedures in the classroom, they must also work with school custodial and maintenance personnel to ensure that all equipment and facilities are in good working order.

Custodial and maintenance personnel are responsible for controlling hazards and dangerous conditions inside and outside the school plant. There should be a close, positive working relationship between teachers and these staff members. With timely and accurate reporting of dangerous conditions by the faculty, custodial and maintenance personnel can promptly eliminate or correct the problems.

An often underutilized member of the school staff is the school nurse. Not only does the nurse act as the primary agent for treating students who become ill or injured at school, this individual can also play a major role as a safety consultant or resource person for the faculty. In-service first aid and CPR training for faculty and staff should come under the auspices of the school nurse. Since school accident reports can play an important part in litigation resulting from a student injury, the nurse can assist teachers who must complete these reports.

TRAFFIC AND TRANSPORTATION: A COMMUNITY-SCHOOL RESPONSIBILITY

Pupil transportation and traffic-control policies provide students with essential protection. With motor vehicle-related accidents leading the way as a major cause of death for school-aged individuals, it is important that the school system and the community work together to alleviate this problem. *Pupil transportation* in this case refers to more than cars, trucks, or motorcycles; it includes bus transportation and pedestrian movement as well.

Traffic Flow to and from School

The "great American dream" for most teenagers is to have a car to drive to and from school. With our highly mobile and vehicle-dependent society, that dream has come true for many students. The consolidation of smaller neighborhood schools into one or two large county facilities has made it necessary for students to arrange for alternative means of transportation in many areas.

With the influx of motor vehicles to school campuses, a certain amount of preparation is needed to handle vehicular flow. Traffic control for a school is usually a joint effort of school administrators, local police, and city or county engineers. Planning before the start of school should include the placement and posting of proper signs and devices and the assignment of officers to traffic duty before and after school.

Control of traffic flow on campus is the responsibility of school personnel—another area in which important decisions must be made. The use of speed bumps in parking areas and the restriction of student access to vehicles during the school day eliminates some of the control problem. The use of administrators to monitor on-campus traffic flow also reduces the accident probability.

Bus Transportation

School consolidations have not only increased the flow of automobile traffic to schools, they have also increased the use of buses for pupil transportation. The National Safety Council estimates that nearly one half of all students in public elementary and secondary schools are transported to school on buses owned or contracted for by boards of education.[16] In the 1990s this has meant that almost 22 million students have been transported daily.

Buses provide a much safer means of transportation for students than do automobiles; however, injuries and deaths can occur. Of the 50 students killed in bus accidents during 1989, 30 were pedestrians either approaching or leaving a loading zone. An additional 300 were injured in similar accidents.[15] Accidents during loading and unloading involved two problems: (1) other motor vehicle drivers who failed to see students and (2) bus drivers who did not see students. Over half of the pupils killed during loading or unloading were struck by the bus they were entering or leaving.

The safety of students transported by bus is a responsibility shared by students, bus drivers, school personnel, and motorists. An important first step in the development of a school busing program is to select and locate bus stops where students can be loaded and unloaded safely. A committee of parents, school officials, and state highway engineers should have input in establishing these points for boarding and departure.

Bus stop sites should require few students to cross the roadway during loading or unloading. The driver of a school bus should have 200 feet of clear visibility in front and to the rear of the bus at each stop.[16] Selection of these open areas as stopping sites also provides adequate warning for other motorists. In rural school districts, bus stops should not be located at sites where vehicle speeds are high and roadway hazards such as curves, hills, and trees restrict visibility. At the same time, reducing the number of stops through careful site selection will reduce hazards to pupils, speed up trip time, and save a school district considerable expense.

Another important consideration for bus safety is that students know the proper procedures for boarding and departing. The National Highway Traffic Safety Administration's Highway Safety Program Standard No. 17 (Pupil Transportation Safety) requires this instruction at least twice a year for all bus riders. Demonstrations provided by both teachers and bus drivers will enhance student learning. Since most bus-related facilities involve students crossing highways when boarding or leaving buses, special emphasis must be placed on making students more visible to bus drivers and motorists alike. Students crossing the road to get to or leave a bus should do so at least 10 feet in front of the bus so that the driver can see them. This will not only reduce the chances of a student's being hit by the bus, it will also allow the driver to assist students in safely crossing the road.

With the increasing number of states that have passed mandatory safety belt laws comes the question: "Should safety belts be required on school buses?" Although a number of school corporations (school districts) around the country have begun to retrofit older buses with safety belts and purchase newer buses with the devices already installed, researchers from the National Highway Traffic Safety Administration caution that such actions may be unwarranted.

The unique design of school buses provides a significant amount of protection to their riders. Unlike automobile occupants, bus passengers do not sit near doors that my fly open in a collision; windows in buses also provide protection against ejection from the vehicle. Federally mandated standards require that such structures as the bus roof and seat frames be able to withstand major impact forces so that the passenger compartment will stay intact. Multiple front and rear signal lights, buses' distinctive yellow color, and slower operating speeds provide additional protection for buses and their passengers.

Since it can cost as much as $2,000 to equip a bus with safety belts, a school corporation might be wiser to use that money to purchase special mirrors to help drivers see small children in front of buses and to improve bus driver education programs.

Buses provide an essential means of transportation for students participating in extracurricular activities as well as for those students attending regular classes. Many of the students involved in athletics or club activities may not ride a bus on a regular basis; therefore, teachers and coaches are responsible for giving them safety instruction concerning bus travel. A word to the teacher or coach who wants to transport students in his or her private vehicle to the site of a school-related activity: *Don't!* Too often school corporations fail to tell teachers that legal liability for student injuries becomes the teacher's responsibility when a personal vehicle is used. Whenever students are transported to an activity, a school-authorized vehicle (van or bus) should be used so that insurance responsibilities lie with the school, not the individual teacher.

Walking to School

Not everyone drives or takes the bus; there are still students who walk to school. Many state laws specify that transportation be provided only for students living outside a specified radius, such as 2 miles from the school. Since many elementary

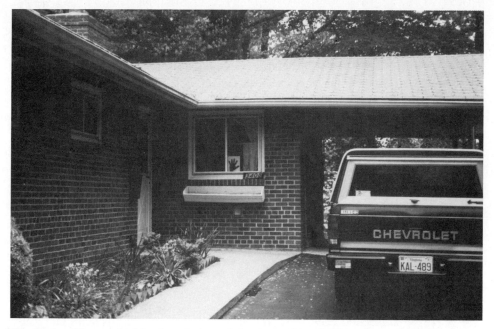

FIG. 11-1   The symbol in the window of this home lets children know that if they need help, they can stop here.

schools arc located in neighborhood settings, special attention must be given to the safety of the very young pedestrian.

Some school corporations establish route plans for many of their city schools. These plans consist of selected routes designated to minimize the potential risks for students when going to and from school. They try to use areas that have a reduced vehicle flow but have adequate sidewalks and traffic controls.

''Helping Hands'' is a program that has been introduced in may communities to help children if they run into difficulty while walking to or from school. Parents of school-aged children, PTA members, and local store owners working with local police departments provide a network of places where children can go if they get lost in a strange neighborhood or if they are threatened with violence. People participating in these programs register with the local police or a PTA group. They are given a brightly colored or designed card which informs children that if they need help they can stop at this house or store for assistance. The program is similar to the ''Neighborhood Watch'' that many cities have introduced to reduce crime in residential areas (Fig. 11-1).

LATCHKEY CHILDREN

The number of mothers of school-aged children who work outside the home has steadily increased. It is estimated that as many as 10 million children in the United States return to empty houses after school. Known as **latchkey children**, they take care of themselves and sometimes younger siblings for one to several hours each day until their parents return from work. Although most children adapt quite well to this unsupervised time, parents need to take certain steps to ensure their children's emotional and physical well-being:

1. Call home from work each day to let your children know that you are thinking about them. If you're going to be late, be sure to tell them.
2. Be sure children know your workplace address and phone number and how to use the 911 or local emergency system.
3. Teach them how to answer the phone safely, never saying that they are home alone. Delivery people and sales persons should be directed to a neighbor's or told to come back at another time.
4. Establish clear rules about homework, chores, playing outdoors, TV, and preparing snacks.
5. Have a trusted neighbor the children can call or visit if they become scared or upset.

SAFE SCHOOL ENVIRONMENT

A safe school environment consists not only of the physical plant (buildings and grounds), it also involves instructional areas that present specific hazards to students, such as chemistry and biology labs and industrial arts and physical education rooms. Extracurricular activities, especially interscholastic sports, further require administrators, teachers, and coaches to provide continued close supervision of students after the school day to maintain that safe environment. Also essential are emergency procedures for handling natural or human-made disasters and security procedures for controlling school violence and vandalism. As one quickly realizes, safety is a major theme throughout the entire school program.

Buildings, Grounds, and Equipment

Administrative actions should be designed to identify, eliminate, or minimize hazards through inspections of buildings, grounds, and equipment at regular intervals. A safety supervisor's responsibilities include planned inspections of schools and work sites to make sure that all codes and regulations are being observed. Requests from teachers and principals are also valuable in alerting safety personnel that immediate inspection of a site or equipment is needed to correct a potential hazard.

A number of state and federal Occupational Safety and Health Administration (OSHA) standards which protect workers in private industry are also applicable in the school setting. Use of equipment in industrial arts rooms and science labs must conform to OSHA guidelines. State and local building and fire codes provide guidelines for the construction of buildings and the selection and location of materials to be used. In some areas of the country another consideration for building safety involves disaster-resistant design information. In the tornado-prone Midwest, information provided by Federal Emergency Management Agency (FEMA) researchers has enabled architects and engineers to design new facilities that offer significant levels of protection against high winds from severe storms and tornadoes.[7] The FEMA research also makes it possible for engineers to determine which portion of older school buildings will offer the greatest protection to occupants if a tornado strikes. Taking this information into account, the safety supervisor would need to develop specific instructions for staff and students to ensure that the school building would offer maximum protection in such a disaster.

The safety of the school grounds is generally the responsibility of maintenance personnel. Staff duties include keeping well-traveled paths around the school clear from such obstacles as snow and mud. Maintenance of lighting on and around the school campus provides added security to people who use school facilities during the evening hours.

Playgrounds. An area of an elementary school's grounds that deserves special attention is the playground. Each year nearly 100,000 children 10 years of age or younger receive treatment at hospital emergency rooms for injuries suffered in playground accidents.[20] Many of the injuries require hospitalization; a few of the children die.

Falls from equipment to the surface below account for approximately 70% of playground injuries. Most of these injuries result from misuse of the equipment, such as pushing, shoving, and daredevil behavior. However, certain traditional playground equipment designs contribute to the problem. The height of apparatus on which children play is one of these factors. A slide that is 10 or 15 feet high not only presents a danger for children who have reached the top, but also presents dangers for children who are climbing. Another factor to be considered is the type of surface on which equipment is located. For ease of maintenance many playgrounds have asphalt or cement surfaces, even under swings, slides, and climbing apparatus.

Two steps that would likely reduce the number and severity of these injuries involve lowering equipment heights and providing surfaces that are more likely to dissipate some of the force as a child hits the ground. Wood chips or rubber mats placed under equipment are more likely to break falls and reduce the severity of injuries. Fig. 11-2, A-C demonstrates the use of cushioning material.

Close supervision by school staff can reduce the potential for injury. Discouraging horseplay and separating older and younger children on the playground can significantly reduce troublesome situations. In-class safety instruction about the correct use of playground equipment also provides a basis for the development of responsible student behavior.

Classroom safety. In the school setting, safety instruction comprises a number of phases. The primary phase involves safety in the classroom. Teachers must be familiar with the care and operation of equipment used in their specific areas of instruction, especially if the equipment is to be used by students in the educational process. Pupils should not be allowed to use equipment until they have received

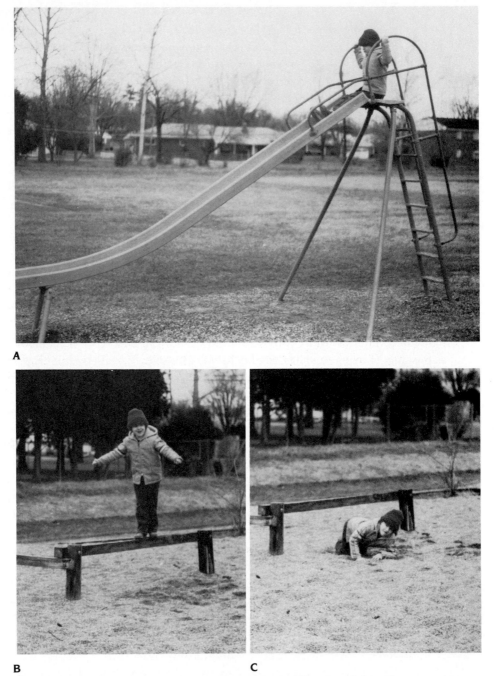

FIG. 11-2   A, A thick layer of wood chips placed under this slide will act as an energy-absorbing cushion. Also notice the protective handrails that have been attached to increase the safety of this apparatus. **B,** Surface of this play area consists of fine gravel. **C,** In a fall onto this surface a child is less likely to receive an injury.

Courtesy: Mark Bever Enterprises, Connersville, Ind.

instruction and training by the teacher on how to use it safely. Three instructional areas in which this is particularly applicable are science, industrial arts, and physical education classes.

Science. The science teacher must be concerned with two types of hazards—physical and chemical. Physical hazards include fires, explosions, electric shocks, and lacerations. Chemical hazards generally involve the toxic effects of substances that may lead to burns, tissue inflammation, and allergic responses.

From the beginning, students must realize that a number of chemicals stored in school laboratories may be flammable or explosive under certain conditions, especially in the presence of an open flame. While the introduction of electrical heating devices has eliminated some of this danger, there has been an increase in the number of electric shock injuries. When using any type of electric equipment in the lab, teachers should make sure that it is grounded properly.

Something as simple as handling glassware requires specific instruction for students. While not as dangerous as some of the other hazards, glassware that is improperly handled may result in painful cuts or burns. Most glass used in the laboratory is easily breakable and requires students to use a variety of techniques to handle it safely. Another problem may arise when the glass is heated; numerous students have painful memories of picking up a test tube that had just been heated by a lab partner.

Most chemicals have toxic effects if a person is exposed to a high enough dosage; consequently, a good strategy for controlling chemical hazards is to minimize exposure to them. Since most problems arise from the inhalation of substances or skin contact with them, procedures for the proper handling of chemical substances and the appropriate use of protective clothing are an important instructional responsibility of the teacher.

Students should be made aware of the importance of working in a ventilating hood while heating, handling, or mixing chemicals. It should also be stressed that equipment be placed as far back in the hood as possible to ensure that vapor concentration in the lab is kept to a minimum.[14]

Specialized protective gear can also minimize exposure to hazards. Safety glasses or goggles should be worn at all times. Depending on the types of chemicals used, protective clothing such as aprons, gloves, lab coats, or jump suits may become necessary to offer full protection.

Essential instruction for any laboratory safety program includes what to do in case there is an accident. Students need to know the location of safety showers, baths, and fire extinguishers and how they are operated.

Industrial arts. With its many pieces of sharp, high-speed equipment, the school shop presents a variety of potential hazards for industrial arts students. Power saws, drills, lathes, routers, and planing devices are just a few of the items that can be very destructive when used improperly. Detailed instruction and close supervision by teachers are essential to a safe shop program:

1. Before student operation, all machines and tools should be examined thoroughly to ensure that they are in safe working order and that guards are in place. Any

machine that does not meet local, state, or federal standards should be removed from the area until it is repaired.

2. Before students are allowed to use equipment, they should receive comprehensive instruction on safe and efficient operation. It should include demonstrations of both machine usage and protective gear. The instruction can be enhanced if the teacher sets the example for students to follow by personally obeying safety rules and practices.

3. Both written and practical tests in industrial arts classes should contain components for evaluating how well students have assimilated safety information and skills.

4. Use of color coding on and around machines to emphasize danger zones and the posting of signs warning of equipment hazards in conspicuous locations near each apparatus can further reinforce instruction.

5. The teacher must exercise continuous supervision to see that shop safety practices are observed, including the use of safety glasses or goggles at all times and the wearing of special clothing such as helmets, gloves, and aprons when necessary.

A positive use of peer group pressure can result when the teacher actively involves students in the shop safety program. Safety squads can assist the instructor in making sure that:

1. Equipment is maintained.

2. Tools and materials are properly stored.

3. Wastes and scraps are removed after each class.

The top students can be enlisted in helping other class members operate equipment in a safe and efficient manner.

A final consideration in any school shop safety program is that of students who do not follow the established practices and precautions. The industrial arts department needs a policy for handling people who are chronic abusers of safe practices. Because of the potential hazards involved in the operation of much of the equipment, students who do not cooperate should be removed from the class.

Physical education. According to statistics from the National Safety Council, physical education has the highest accident rate of any instructional area[15]; it is more than three times higher than the rate for shop and laboratory classes.

Obviously, it is impossible to eliminate all risks and hazards in physical education. The development of skills, whether they involve sports activities, machine operation, or foreign languages, depends on one's ability to reproduce patterns of motion consistently. As long as the human element is involved, mistakes will be made. Physical education students are going to trip, fall, and run into one another. Every type of human movement creates some potential for injury; the more rapid and vigorous the movement, the greater the potential for injury. Since physical education activities are characterized by movement that is frequently forceful and rapid, and since that movement may be opposed at the same time by similar movements of others, the potential for injury is proportionately high, even when rules are closely followed and protective equipment is used.

Are we saying that nothing can be done about these injuries? On the contrary! What has come to light in recent years is that many injuries to students have resulted not from the activity, but from a lack of supervision and instruction or from unsafe facilities and defective equipment.

The first dangerous area is supervision. Often the physical educator serves a number of roles in a school. Two duties often associated with this position are coaching and providing emergency medical care. Often the physical educator is the only person besides the school nurse who has a background in first aid, and it is likely that if an emergency arises he or she will be called to assist. During the various athletic seasons, game cancellations, scheduling problems, and transportation difficulties may require attention during a class period. Feeling reasonably certain that nothing will happen during their absences, many of these teacher-coaches leave their classes unsupervised from time to time. The tragic fact is that it takes only a split second for an injury to occur. As we will see in the next section, the courts have been exceptionally harsh in situations involving student injuries during a teacher's absence.

Given the fact that physical education is an activity-oriented class, the physical educator must take special care in the instruction of students. An incorrect list of dates given by a history teacher does not present the same dangers that occur if a physical educator has failed to adequately instruct students about the proper procedures for performing tumbling stunts. The physical education teacher is placed in a tenuous position; students' movement capabilities vary considerably, yet the teacher is required to provide a challenging experience for each person in the class (Fig. 11-3).

A realistic approach for the physical educator in this dilemma is to prepare students in a step-by-step progression going from the less complicated to the more advanced skills. Pupils should be assigned to activities commensurate with their size, skill, and fitness level. At the same time, as a part of adequate instruction, students

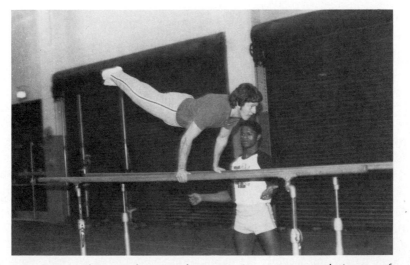

FIG. 11-3 This teacher is demonstrating proper techniques of spotting in his gymnastics class.

must be warned of the possible dangers of the activities they are about to perform. The incorporation of safety-related questions in class exams can be used to emphasize the importance of proper technique and performance.

Control and maintenance of physical education equipment and facilities is usually an overlapping responsibility of both the physical education faculty and athletic personnel. Playing fields (baseball diamonds, tennis courts, football and soccer fields) generally are used for interscholastic competition and activities classes. A specific person or department should be delegated the responsibility for inspecting these facilities regularly and seeing that necessary repairs are made. A detailed record of inspections can prove invaluable to a school district if an accident occurs.

Equipment and apparatus that are used on a regular basis should be checked on a regular basis. Protective items such as racquetball goggles, helmets, and padding around equipment should be examined before each use. If equipment is found to be defective or facilities are determined to be unsafe, the specific activities involving their use should be stopped until repairs can be made.

LEGAL LIABILITY IN THE SCHOOLS

In recent years many million-dollar settlements have been awarded to students injured in school-related activities. The basis for these court proceedings is that of **tort liability**—the responsibility placed by the law on one who commits a wrong against another person. In the school setting, the tort or wrongful act may have resulted in injuries to students, their property, or their reputations. It may have been an act of commission or omission, either intentional or unintentional.

Tortious acts fall into three categories:

1. **Malfeasance**: Performance of an illegal act (for example, physically abusing a student).

2. **Misfeasance**: Improper performance of a legal act (for example, making students do exercises that are not suitable to their age, sex, or physical capabilities).

3. **Nonfeasance**: Failure to perform a legal act that one ought to do (for example, failing to instruct students about the safe use of machinery and chemicals).

In school liability cases, the major consideration in court proceedings usually involves misfeasance or nonfeasance. An all-encompassing term that is popularly used is **negligence**. *Negligence* has been defined as the failure to conduct oneself in conformity with standards established by law for the protection of others against unreasonable risk of injury.[5,13] Simply stated, it means that a teacher or school official has failed to act as a reasonably prudent person would in the same situation.

Who determines how a "reasonably prudent person" should act? This involves an ideal or model of community conduct that is determined by a jury. If a court decides that a reasonable man or women would have foreseen the danger of a situation and the teacher in this instance did not, then he or she is usually held responsible for damages. Injury is generally foreseeable: (1) in situations where large crowds of students are gathered without supervision, (2) in specialized activities in physical education, vocational education, and science classes, or (3) in cases where a teacher is absent from the room for an unreasonable amount of time.[5]

There are certain conditions under which a teacher is likely to be considered negligent should an injury occur to a pupil. The most significant is teacher absence from the classroom while school is in session. Investigations have indicated that as many as half of all school liability cases involve lack of supervision as grounds for litigation. Generally it is claimed that if a teacher were in his or her appointed place, student injury would not have occurred.

Other conditions that have resulted in litigation against school personnel include use of faulty or unsafe equipment, lack of proper instruction, lack of care with regard to the age and maturity of pupils, and failure to provide adequate medical assistance.

In the cases in pp. 438-439 we examine some situations that ultimately led to serious legal difficulties for school personnel as a result of their negligence.

Liability Protection

In the past, school districts were protected by the doctrine of governmental immunity from lawsuits involving the negligence of their personnel. Immunity from suits was based on English law, in which "the King could do no wrong." State governments applied this same concept to school corporations since they were an arm of the state and performed a service essential to the welfare of the people.

One point that frequently came as a shock to teachers and other school personnel was that immunity from liability enjoyed by school corporations did not extend to many of their employees. The only members of a school corporation who were protected by immunity clauses were the superintendent and members of the school board, since they were considered to be officers of the state and thus immune to suit when acting in their official capacities.

Principals, assistant principals, and corporation administrative personnel were technically classified as school employees and did not have immunity from suit; however, records indicate that seldom were these employees sued. The same held true for custodians, secretaries, school nurses, and other nonteaching personnel, since they were seldom placed in situations that could lead to legal difficulties. By far the most vulnerable employees were teachers, because they have been considered "substitute parents" in the eyes of the law.

Until 1959 the doctrine of governmental immunity protected school corporations in most states; during that year the Illinois Supreme Court abolished this rule in school liability cases. In the past 33 years numerous states have followed in the direction of Illinois, thus allowing school districts to be held liable for the negligent acts of their employees. Known as "save harmless" legislation, these statutes allow school districts to defend and/or pay damages awarded against any school employee who has been sued in the performance of school-related duties. Laws vary from state to state; in some the teacher is protected, whereas in others it is not mandatory for a

Case Examples of Legal Liability

Case No. 1—*Lack of Supervision*

At the beginning of a class period, a high school science teacher/wrestling coach received a message that he was to call the school's athletic director as soon as possible concerning his team's first meet of the season, which was to occur that night. Since his students were taking a quiz and working quietly, he went to the principal's office and phoned the athletic director. The important message was that the team bus would leave a half hour later for the meet that evening. On his return to the classroom approximately 10 minutes later, he found the students quite shaken and a pool of blood at the back of the room. A student in the last row had been leaning back in her chair and had tipped over and hit her head on the radiator. Another student in the class escorted her to the school nurse's office. Her injuries included a mild concussion and a scalp laceration that required 15 stitches to close.

The girl's parents sued the teacher for negligence, since he had left the room unattended. The teacher claimed that he had repeatedly warned this particular student about the dangers of leaning back in her chair, and that it would have been impossible to prevent her fall. Although this may have been true to a degree, the court awarded the girl's parents damages, stating that the teacher's presence more than likely would have deterred the girl from leaning back in her chair in the first place.

Case No. 2—*Unsafe Equipment*

A group of students was allowed access to a university's recreation center after hours by a student janitor. During a game of "ultimate frisbee" in which the ends of a basketball court were used as goal lines, one of the students fell through the glass paneling of a door at one end of the court. As he fell through the glass, he received a number of severe lacerations.

Subsequently the student sued the university, claiming that unsafe facilities provided by the university had been the direct cause of his injuries. For a person or organization to be held liable for an injury suffered by a student, the plaintiff must prove that a substantial connection existed between the wrongful act and the student's injury. In legal parlance this is known as the "proximate cause."

The court finding in the student's favor decided that the university should have foreseen that glass-paneled doors placed in close proximity to the end of the basketball court posed a danger to students using the recreation facility and therefore should have made the necessary changes to eliminate this hazard.

Case No. 3—*Lack of Proper Instruction*

Two recent cases in Minnesota and Michigan have indicated that proper instruction is not just the responsibility of a teacher or coach. School administrators such as athletic directors and principals may need to take a closer look at the development, planning, and administration of educational and athletic programs in the school.

In Minnesota a first-year physical education teacher was found 90% negligent and his principal was found 10% negligent after an eighth-grade student broke his neck doing a headspring over a rolled mat during a tumbling class. The sum awarded to the student and his family was in excess of $1 million.

The court supported claims by the student and his family that class members were permitted to perform the headspring well before they had the opportunity to progress through a series of preliminary exercises. The court further concluded that the teacher was not spotting the exercise properly at the time the student was injured. Judgment against the principal was based on the conclusion that his failure to closely supervise an inexperienced instructor and administer the curriculum created the opportunity for the accident to occur.

In the Michigan case a 15-year-old football player who was seriously injured in a weight-lifting accident during an organized summer training program sued not only the coach, but also the school's athletic director and principal. The coach was charged with failure to instruct players about proper lifting techniques and with pressuring them to attempt lifts beyond their abilities. The principal was charged with negligence for allegedly ignoring a Michigan High School Athletic Association rule prohibiting football players from participating in organized summer training programs involving school coaches. The athletic director was also named a defendant in the lawsuit, because he was responsible for all athletic programs at the school. It was claimed that he had special training for the job and had both the knowledge and authority to eliminate any unsafe practices in the athletic program.

Although the principal was not held liable, the final disposition of the case found both the coach and athletic director guilty of negligence. The court stated that the coach had failed to provide adequate instruction, while the athletic director had failed to control unsafe practices that existed in a sports program for which he was ultimately responsible.

These findings have demonstrated a need for strong lines of communication between teachers, coaches, and administrators. At the same time they indicate a growing need for school personnel to have a strong background in safety if they are to provide adequate instruction for students.

Case No. 4—*Failure to Provide Proper Emergency Care*

Only in rare cases do states require individuals to administer emergency care at the scene of an accident. In most states doctors, nurses, and rescue personnel have a legal obligation to stop at the scene of an emergency; however, laymen are not under this obligation.

In the school setting many teachers are under the mistaken impression that they are laymen in terms of emergency care and thus have no obligation to provide medical care for an injured student. First aid knowledge and skills are expected and required of teachers in student emergencies. In fact, teachers can be held liable for injuries suffered by students resulting from incorrect treatment or delays in seeking medical assistance.

A North Dakota court held a teacher liable for increasing the severity of neck injuries of a student involved in a trampoline accident. Instead of using proper techniques for immobilizing a suspected spinal injury or waiting for rescue personnel, the teacher, with the assistance of several students, pulled the victim off the trampoline after his fall.

Two Louisiana football coaches were found negligent in the death of a high school player who died from heat stroke. During the court proceeding it was found that the coaches delayed seeking medical assistance for 2 hours after the player exhibited symptoms of heat stroke. To make matters worse, their initial treatment of the victim included covering him with a blanket.

Being a teacher makes one responsible for students' instruction, supervision, and safety. If teachers do not fulfill the responsibility, they may be held liable. The duty of school personnel to exercise reasonable supervisory care for the safety of students entrusted to them and their accountability for injuries resulting from failure to discharge that duty are well recognized.

school district to provide this type of employee protection. It is extremely important for new teachers to understand the policies of their school district and the state in which they are teaching.

In today's complex legal system, the normal course of litigation is for the plaintiffs (usually the student and parents) to sue not only the teacher but the principal, superintendent, members of the school board, and the school district itself to ensure that someone has the funds with which to pay if damages are awarded. This is known as the "deep pocket" doctrine. The courts then go through the list of defendants and assess whether this or that individual is to be held liable for the injuries suffered by the student. As we have seen previously, school administrators, such as principals and athletic directors, have become more vulnerable to litigation since a close working relationship is expected between teachers and these personnel.[3,4] And it would not be surprising to see this trend continue in future years.

What is the answer? How can school personnel adequately protect themselves? The days of "governmental immunity" for school systems and their personnel are gone. Probably the most realistic approach in handling lawsuits involving negligence of school personnel involves setting limits on the amount that can be awarded. This legislation would be similar to that pending in a number of states concerning malpractice suits against physicians.

After reviewing court cases involving teacher and administrator liability, one finds that many of them are poorly prepared for the responsibilities they must fulfill. Following is a list of recommendations for the legal protection of school personnel:

1. All personnel should be familiar with the liability laws of their state and be aware of the type of insurance policy provided by the school district. If the school system has no policy, then teachers and administrators must invest in personal liability policies for their own financial protection. Policies may be purchased from such groups as the American Federation of Teachers, the National Education Association, or most insurance companies.

2. Teachers should have some training in first aid, since they are likely to be the first ones to respond to an injured student and since most states expect them to have specific skills to handle an emergency involving student injury.

3. The teacher should exercise reasonable care in:
   a. Supervising student activities.
   b. Informing students of the dangers involved and keeping the activity within their abilities.
   c. Making sure that equipment is in good working order.
   d. Giving detailed instruction before permitting performance by students.

4. A school administrator should:
   a. Assign only qualified personnel to perform any service under his or her supervision.
   b. Closely supervise new personnel to ensure their familiarity with the school district's policies and programs.

c. Have an awareness of the various curricular and extracurricular programs that use school district facilities.

d. Provide adequate in-service training for school personnel regarding the handling of emergency situations.

MEDICAL RECORDS AND ACCIDENT REPORTS

As a matter of concern for student protection as well as the legal protection of school personnel, it is important that teachers and coaches know the health status of those under their supervision. Students with prior histories of illness, such as allergic reactions to bee stings, diabetes, and epilepsy could be in danger if a teacher is unaware of their conditions. Delay in seeking emergency medical assistance for a child exhibiting symptoms of anaphylactic shock after being stung by a bee or wasp could have fatal consequences. At the beginning of each semester instructors should check the medical records of their students to identify those with potential problems. This awareness of a particular condition enables a teacher to react appropriately in an emergency.

Medical records of students also can be helpful in developing and modifying activities that they might not normally be able to perform safely. A child with a handicap such as cerebral palsy, which affects balance, coordination, and body movement, may need some assistance in performing certain skills or using dangerous equipment. For too long individuals with disabling conditions were not allowed to participate fully in the school curriculum. However, Public Law 94-142 (the Education for All Handicapped Children Act), guarantees that every child, regardless of the handicapping condition, will have access to all school programs and activities.[19] Through students' medical records teachers can better understand the students' handicaps and thus ensure a safe yet rewarding experience for them.

Accident reports serve two functions in the school safety program: (1) They are used to protect the school corporation and its employees in liability suits involving student injury, and (2) they can be used to identify and correct hazardous conditions in the school environment.

Prompt, accurate, and permanent records of all accidents should be kept for future reference. This is particularly important because of students' powers of delayed suit. What may have seemed trivial or of little importance some months before could become a key issue of contention in a liability case. Detailed reports are essential if intelligent conclusions are to be drawn and applied. As an example, a high school chemistry teacher was sued at the end of the school year by the father of a student who had been injured during the second week of school. The student had received second degree burns across the palm of his hand when his lab partner handed him a test tube that had been held for an extended period over a glass flame. Scar tissue that formed over the wound ultimately reduced the range of motion in his hand.

A problem that arose during litigation was that the teacher's only comment on the

Report of Accident to the Superintendent

Name _____ Home address _____
School _____ Sex M F Age _____ Grade _____
Time accident occurred Hour _____ AM _____ PM _____ Date _____
Location of accident School building _____, Room _____, School grounds _____
Home _____ Elsewhere _____ To or from school _____
_____

Nature of injury

Abrasion	____	Concussion	____	Puncture	____
Amputation	____	Cut	____	Scalds	____
Asphyxiation	____	Dislocation	____	Scratches	____
Bite	____	Fracture	____	Shock (el)	____
Bruise	____	Laceration	____	Sprain	____
Burn	____	Poisoning	____	Other	____

Description of the accident. How did accident happen? What was student doing?
Where was student? List specifically unsafe acts and unsafe conditions existing.
Specify any tool, machine or equipment involved. _____
_____
_____
_____

Part of
body
injured

Abdomen	____	Ear	____	Foot	____	Knee	____	Scalp	____
Ankle	____	Elbow	____	Hand	____	Leg	____	Tooth	____
Arm	____	Eye	____	Head	____	Mouth	____	Wrist	____
Back	____	Face	____	Knee	____	Nose	____	Other	____
Chest	____	Finger	____	Leg	____				

_____

Teacher in charge when accident occurred (Enter name) _____
Present at scene of accident? No _____ Yes _____
Immediate   First aid treatment ____ By (Name) _____
action   Sent to school nurse ____ By (Name) _____
taken   Sent home ____ By (Name) _____
             Sent to physician ____ By (Name) _____
             Physician's name _____
             Sent to hospital ____ By (Name) _____
             Name of hospital _____
_____

Was parent or other individual notified? No _____ Yes _____ When _____
How _____
Name of individual notified _____
By whom? (enter name) _____
Witnesses Name _____ Address _____
           Name _____ Address _____
_____

Signature Principal _____ Teacher _____

FIG. 11-4 School accident report.

accident report concerning how the incident occurred was "Student burned hand." Although the actual description of an accident is the most vital information in an accident report, this is the one most frequently given minimal attention.[9] Luckily for the teacher, the case was dismissed after further testimony indicated that the injured student had failed to follow detailed oral and written instructions that had been provided to the class. Had more information been given in the original report, it is unlikely that a suit would have been filed. Fig. 11-4 is a copy of a standard accident reporting form. Some of the essential components include:

1. Time and place of the incident.
2. Activity involved.
3. Identification of participants.
4. Description of the injury:
   a. Mechanism of injury.
   b. Body part damaged.
   c. Initial care given.
5. Detailed description of what happened.
6. Final disposition:
   a. Medical diagnosis.
   b. Date of student's return to activity.

Probably the most important use of accident reports involves the correction of hazards. The periodic summarization of accident data by the safety supervisor can be used to determine injury trends and identify dangerous equipment, procedures, and locations in the school district. Monthly or semester accident summaries might indicate that a particular type of slide has caused the majority of elementary school playground injuries. An analysis of football injuries may indicate that a new blocking technique has significantly increased neck and shoulder injuries of players during the season. A yearly report of motor vehicle accidents involving students may identify a relatively hazardous intersection near a high school.

For accident reports to be effective in eliminating and modifying hazardous conditions, the data collected on these forms must be disseminated to school employees and presented in an understandable form. If this is done, administrators, teachers, and staff are more likely to become actively involved in school safety.

SCHOOL SAFETY AND THE ATHLETIC PROGRAM

During the past 15 years the number of students participating in high school athletics has increased significantly. Even during times of financial difficulty, communities have produced the revenue to support their favorite teams. Much of this increase has been a result of the expansion of women's programs.

As participation has increased, so have injuries. With more than 5 million students competing in interscholastic sports annually, a conservative estimate of injuries runs into the hundreds of thousands.[8] In spite of improvement in equipment, training methods, and medical care, injury rates have remained the same or in some cases have increased. Why, in the high-technology decade of the 1990s, have we not been able to control this injury problem? And is there anything that can be done to solve this dilemma?

The answer to the first question involves several factors. Although improvements have been made in technology, such as new equipment and medical care, many school systems simply cannot afford to use it. When bond issues fail and money is tight, coaches either use their old equipment or a particular program is dropped. Likewise, the position of the school athletic trainer (a specialist in the prevention and treatment of sports injuries) is one of the first to go when school funds are limited.

A second factor involves safety education. Many coaches may not have had academic or in-service training in sports safety, coaching theory, emergency medical care, or sports medicine. Participation in a sport does not prepare one to coach it. As funds have become scarce, many school districts have used part-time coaches from the community who have absolutely no educational background or coaching credentials.

When unqualified personnel are hired, serious liability problems can arise for school administrators. A frequently used rationale for litigation in athletic injury cases involves the absence of proper instruction as the cause of injury. The fact that coaches have volunteered their services does not reduce liability if athletes are injured as a result of their negligence.[4]

With the increased vulnerability of school districts to liability suits, it is essential that athletes receive adequate supervision and injury protection during practices and games. At the same time it must be realized that many school districts have been forced to operate under considerable economic adversity. Let's look at some realistic options that must be considered.

Care and Protection of Athletes: Whose Responsibility?

Physicians can provide a number of important services for school athletic programs, but they are just one part of an integrated system of protection for athletes. Athletic trainers, coaches, and emergency personnel play key roles as well. The team doctor is often a volunteer or is paid a minimal fee, so schools should use his or her services wisely. Since most states require that students receive medical clearance before participating in athletic programs, one of the first priorities for a school is to see that all athletes have a preseason physical examination. With a minimal amount of planning, school officials can schedule examinations by the team physician over 1 or 2 days. By using allied health professionals such as nurses and emergency medical technicians to do basic screening, the physician will be able to spend more time in the physical evaluation of each athlete.

Because of the constant threat of injury in most sports, continuous medical observation should be a primary consideration; however, a team physician or physicians cannot be expected to attend all athletic events. Traditionally, varsity basketball and football games have had more coverage by community physicians than any other sports. What about junior varsity, freshman, and girls' athletic events? A physician is seldom in attendance at these contests. And although it has been indicated by Garrick and Requa[8] that more athletes are injured at practice than in games, one is not likely to see a physician at practice.

For these reasons a valuable member of any athletic department is the athletic trainer. The trainer is qualified to establish conditioning programs, provide emergency care to injured athletes, and follow through with rehabilitative therapy. With their thorough background in sports medicine, trainers can provide an important link between athletes, their families, the coach, and the attending physician. Because they are sensitized to the potential problems that may arise from athletic injuries, trainers are usually responsible for referring an injured athlete to a physician for additional evaluation or treatment. They also are given the authority to determine when and if an athlete is ready to return to competition after an injury. By having trainers make such decisions, coaches are not forced into a conflict-of-interest situation involving whether to let an injured player stay in the game (Fig. 11-5).

Even if every high school had an athletic trainer, there are still too many sports and athletes to be served by one person. It is not unusual for a high school to have more than 20 athletic teams, including varsity, junior varsity, and freshman squads.

This brings us to the cornerstone of any school athletic program—the coaches.

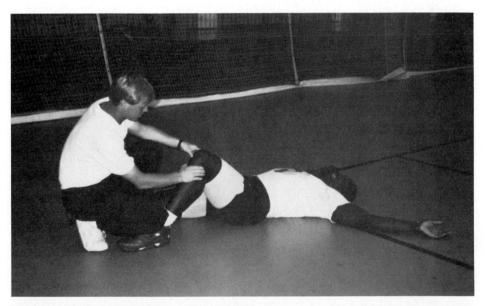

FIG. 11-5 After the trainer examines this athlete, he will make the decision as to whether or not this young man will continue to practice.

Coaches and only coaches are responsible for players before, during, and after both games and practices. In a recent investigation of medical care provided for Chicago high school athletes, researchers found that in 80% of the schools the coach was responsible for on-field care of injuries during games and practices. Only 42% of the schools had a physician attending games, generally varsity contests, and only 25% of the schools had a full-time athletic trainer.[10] While most authorities agree that athletes in practices and games should receive treatment from a certified (National Athletic Trainers Association—NATA) trainer who is supervised by a physician, it is an unrealistic expectation given the current financial situation of many school districts in the United States.

Recognizing the importance of their roles in providing for the safety of athletes, prospective coaches should complete coursework in such areas as emergency medical care, athletic training, coaching theory, and sports safety. With such training, coaches are more likely to use proper techniques of instruction for all athletes, which could prevent injuries. At the same time they would be able to ensure a better standard of care for those who do become injured, and in so doing, reduce the likelihood of liability problems.

In conducting any sports-related activity, coaches should consider the following points:

A. Adequate instruction—
   1. Understanding the participants:
      a. Age and size.
      b. Skill and maturity.
   2. Communication at participant level:
      a. Progression of instruction.
      b. Adherence to safety practices:
         i. Warning of dangers.
         ii. Required use of protective devices.
B. Facilities and equipment management—
   1. Equipment in good repair.
   2. Playing and practice areas:
      a. Natural hazards.
      b. Man-made hazards.
C. Provision for emergency care—
   1. Team physician or athletic trainers.
   2. First aid-certified coaches and supervisors.
   3. Quick access to emergency medical transport.

As with teachers, an additional protection for coaches is the purchase of liability insurance. In the past, coaches were usually thanked for helping an injured athlete; today they are just as likely to be sued for negligence. Whether working as a full-time teacher/coach or a part-time coach from the community, this individual must be well qualified and prepared for the responsibilities he or she has accepted.

SCHOOL SECURITY

Not only have property crimes such as vandalism been on the upswing, but violent crimes including assault, rape, and robbery have also increased in the schools. In one recent academic year more than 5000 teachers received injuries from student attacks; 280,000 students were assaulted, and over 100,000 of them were robbed.[1]

Many people have the mistaken impression that school security problems exist only in the larger cities. Although more violence occurs in city schools, property damage from vandalism is greater in suburban areas. Another misconception is that parents of vandals are responsible for the damages caused by their children. Only in rare cases is this true; most states limit to several thousand dollars the amount for which a parent is liable. The remaining amount of damages must be covered by a school's insurance company—that is, if the school has a policy that will cover the particular damages. Because of the high premiums many schools limit their insurance coverage. In reality every taxpayer will end up paying a share of those expenses (Fig. 11-6).

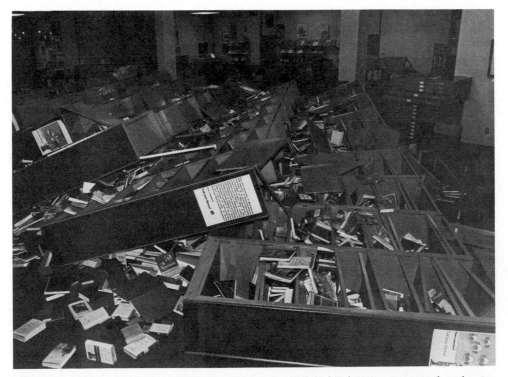

FIG. 11-6   Damages from vandalism of this new high school were estimated to be in excess of $500,000 dollars.

Courtesy: Jack Brockley, Connersville News-Examiner, Connersville, Indiana.

What is the answer to this security problem which over 80% of school administrators list as their top priority? There is no single, simple answer to the problem of school crime, but there are several major areas of emphasis which must be considered.

The first of these is school design. Architects and school officials must devote attention to the targets selected by vandals. To reduce the damages from glass breakage, newer schools are designed with fewer windows and glass doors. To provide some natural lighting, skylights made of unbreakable plastic are placed above school corridors and hallways.

Another design modification involves the development of specially coated inside and outside wall surfaces that resist penetration by paints and dyes. These surfaces, which can be wiped clean with a damp cloth, could significantly reduce the costs for repairing walls marred by graffiti.

Just as Neighborhood Watches have reduced crime in residential areas, a similar format can be used in the school setting. Professional security services are used by many metropolitan school districts to protect school facilities as well as students; however, they generally do not provide sufficient personnel to maintain a safe school environment. The key to adequate protection involves the use of community volunteers, preferably the parents of students attending these schools.

Parents living nearby can patrol school grounds on a regular basis, especially when the facility is closed (for example, after school and during vacations). An even more important role for these parent/volunteers is to assist educators and administrators in providing security at schools. Each year a significant number of students and teachers are assaulted, raped, and robbed, and much of the vandalism is committed during the school day. Teachers who are expected to supervise 35 to 40 students for six periods in the classroom cannot cover the hallways and outside grounds as well. The parent or volunteer who patrols hallways and outside areas while classes are in session provides a high-visibility deterrent effect that cannot be overemphasized.

One other group that must become actively involved in a school's security is its student body. This can be accomplished by giving students some of the authority for protecting their school. Students and parents can work together to patrol locker rooms, empty classrooms, and parking lots. Some schools use police department personnel to teach students about law enforcement and police work in such classes as history, government, and sociology. Such programs help students to overcome their prejudices against authority and, in particular, police officers.

Since it is easier to establish positive attitudes than to attempt to change negative ones, school and crime-prevention authorities in many cities have concentrated their efforts at the elementary school level. Some programs have been quite successful in reducing vandalism and improving student behavior. A poem written by a fifth-grade boy says it all very clearly:

Ralphie, Ralphie hit the teacher
Broke her nose and marred her features
He hurt the teacher seriously
Now he's doing 1 to 3.

SCHOOL DISASTER PLAN

Whether it is a natural disaster such as a tornado or a disaster of human origin such as a fire, the school setting may be the location in which students experience such an occurrence. To enable them to react properly in these emergency situations, each school must develop and regularly test its particular disaster plans.

Depending on the area of the country in which a person lives, the types of disaster plans will vary. While every school system must have detailed fire plans, schools in the South and Midwest are apt to have an additional tornado disaster plan, whereas schools on the West Coast are likely to implement an additional plan for protecting students during an earthquake.

Using the four phases of disaster planning discussed in Chapter 9, let us attempt to develop a school fire-safety plan. The first phase to consider is hazard reduction. This would entail determining which areas of the school pose the greatest fire risk. Industrial arts rooms, science labs, bookstores, and storage facilities may contain a variety of flammable materials and consequently deserve special consideration in the installation of smoke detectors, sprinkling devices, and fire extinguishers.

Preparedness activities involve identifying what would need to be done if a fire did occur. The top priority here is the development and planning of escape routes from the facility.

In each room, escape routes should be posted. Teachers should review them with students regularly. Meeting places for students should be established away from the building so that individuals would not be in the way of incoming fire-rescue equipment. Certain faculty or administrative personnel should be designated as the persons who will be responsible for notifying the fire department and ensuring that the building has been evacuated by all students and staff. In the event of a fire, this detailed planning could reduce casualties and damage significantly.

To limit the possibility of chaos and confusion in an actual fire, escape procedures should be practiced on a regular basis. When and if the need arises, students, faculty, and staff will be able to respond more efficiently since they will be thoroughly versed in the escape procedure.

The fourth phase of the school fire-disaster plan is recovery. If a fire does occur and damage is extensive, school officials will need to develop contingency plans for continuing the educational process. If the school corporation is a large one, certain facilities should be designated as host schools to handle the displaced students. If the system is smaller, local churches or public buildings may be used as temporary school settings.

SUMMARY

Although the majority of the responsibility for school safety lies with teachers and administrators, other personnel such as nurses, custodians, and bus drivers play an integral role. To provide procedural guidelines for both faculty and staff, it is important for every school district to develop a written safety manual. Specific areas that may be covered include emergency care, disaster preparedness, record keeping, in-service training, transportation, and security.

While the board of education is ultimately responsible for a school system's safety policies, the supervisor of safety is the professional staff member directly in control. Using the district's safety policies as a foundation, the safety supervisor assists the staff of various schools in developing programs to fit their specific needs.

Teachers represent the front line of the school safety program; they are responsible for the safe instruction of students, maintenance of safe equipment, and provision of emergency care to injured students. In maintaining a safe environment, teachers rely heavily on the assistance of custodial and maintenance personnel.

The advent of school consolidations has greatly increased the number and traveling distances of students, thus creating an influx of motor vehicles to campuses. Traffic control must be a joint effort between school officials and city or county personnel. Not only must plans be established for student vehicles, but also numerous considerations are necessary for developing a safe and effective bus transportation system.

The safety of school buildings and grounds is generally the responsibility of maintenance and custodial staff. In conjunction with the school safety supervisor, they make periodic inspections of buildings to ensure that all codes and regulations are being observed and that damaged equipment is repaired or replaced. In some areas of the country safety of buildings may entail special design modifications to ensure the integrity of the structure against weather phenomena such as hurricanes and tornadoes.

To provide adequate classroom safety, teachers must be familiar with the care and operation of equipment in their specific areas of instruction. Three areas in which this is particularly applicable are science, industrial arts, and physical education.

As litigation has become more common in the school setting, with settlements sometimes exceeding $1 million, school administrators and teachers have been forced to closely evaluate their duties and responsibilities. A term popularly associated with these school-related lawsuits is *negligence* (one's failure to act as a reasonably prudent person).

Investigations have indicated that as many as half of all school negligence cases involve lack of supervision as grounds for litigation. Other situations that have led to serious legal difficulties for school personnel include the use of unsafe facilities and equipment, lack of proper instruction, and failure to provide adequate medical assistance.

School administrators should assign only qualified personnel to work with students and closely supervise new teachers and coaches. At the same time they must have an awareness of both curricular and extracurricular programs that use school district facilities.

Although most authorities agree that athletes in games and practices should receive treatment from a certified trainer who is supervised by the team physician, it is an unrealistic expectation given the current financial situation of many school districts. As recent investigations indicate, medical care for athletes is most frequently provided by coaches. Recognizing the importance of their roles, prospective coaches should receive instruction in emergency medical care, athletic training, and coaching theory.

In an age in which there has been a continued increase of crime in the United States, school systems have been affected in much the same way as their communities. Most school administrators now list security problems as their top priority.

While there is no single solution to the problem of school crime, several approaches have been taken by educators to lessen its negative effects. The use of community volunteers to patrol both inside and outside school facilities shows great promise for decreasing violence in and around campuses.

The student body must also become actively involved before school crime can be controlled. This can be accomplished by giving students some of the authority for protecting their own schools. When school authorities, students, and parents share the responsibilities of the educational process, the problem of school crime will diminish quickly.

Key Terms

Latchkey children Children who spend one to several hours each day at home alone, until their parents return from work.

Malfeasance Performance of an illegal act.

Misfeasance Improper performance of a legal act.

Negligence The failure to conduct oneself in conformity with standards established by law for the protection of others against unreasonable risk of injury.

Nonfeasance Failure to perform a legal act for which one is responsible.

Tort liability The responsibility placed by the law on one who commits a wrong against another person.

References

1. Alliance of American Insurers: Civil Justice enactments: 1986, Schaumburg, Ill., July 11, 1986.
2. American Tort Reform Association: Fault-based liability standards and defenses, Washington, D.C., 1986.
3. Appenzeller, H., and Ross, C. T., eds.: Sports and the courts, Physical Education and Sports Law Quarterly 2(1), Winter 1981.
4. Appenzeller, H, and Ross, C. T., eds.: Sports and the courts, Physical Education and Sport Law Quarterly 2(4), Fall 1981.
5. Bailey, J. A., and Matthews, D. L.: Law and liability in athletics, physical education, and recreation, Boston, 1984, Allyn & Bacon, Inc.
6. Dougherty, N.: An analysis of negligence claims in educational programs, School Safety World Newsletter, Summer 1985, p. 5.
7. Federal Emergency Management Agency: Tornado protection: selecting and designing safe areas in buildings, 0-620-672/760, Washington, D.C., 1980, U.S. Government Printing Office.
8. Garrick, J. G., and Requa, R.: Medical care and injury surveillance in the high school setting, The Physician and Sportsmedicine 9(2):115, 1981.

9. Haering, F. C.: School safety handbook, Chicago, 1977, Association of School Business Officials.

10. Hage, P., and Moore, M.: Medical care for athletes: what is the coach's role? The Physician and Sportsmedicine 9(5):140, 1981.

11. Insurance Information Institute: The lawsuit crisis, 110 William Street, New York, N.Y., April 1986, The Institute.

12. Jungle gyms and school sidewalks, Fairfax County Public Schools Bulletin 18(4):14, 1982.

13. Kaiser, R. A.: Liability and law in recreation, parks, and sports, Englewood Cliffs, N.J., 1986, Prentice-Hall, Inc.

14. McKusick, B. C.: Prudent practices for handling hazardous chemicals in laboratories, Science 211 (4484):777, 1981.

15. National Safety Council: Accident facts, 1990 ed., 444 N. Michigan Ave., Chicago, Ill., 1990, The Council.

16. National Safety Council: School transportation: safety bulletin no. 11, Chicago, 1985, The Council.

17. Redfearn, R. W.: The physician's role in school sports programs, The Physician and Sportsmedicine 8(9):67, 1980.

18. Rossol, M.: Here's help getting toxic art supplies out of school, School Safety World Newsletter, Winter 1983, p. 2.

19. Schaller, W. E.: The school health program, ed. 5, Philadelphia, 1981, W. B. Saunders Co.

20. Too many playgrounds are unsafe: Changing Times, May 1981, p. 70.

21. U.S. Chamber of Congress: The liability crisis: an overview, Washington, D.C., 1986, National Clearinghouse on the Liability Crisis.

22. U.S. Department of Justice: Report of the tort policy working group on the causes, extent, and policy implications of the current crisis in insurance availability and affordability, Washington, D.C. Feb. 1986, Office of Policy and Legislation, Civil Division.

Resource Organizations

American Alliance for Health, Physical
Education, Recreation,
and Dance
1900 Association Drive
Reston, VA 22091

American Association of School
Administration
1801 North Moore Street
Arlington, VA 22209

American Industrial Arts Association
1914 Association Drive
Reston, VA 22091

American School Health Association
P.O. Box 708
7263 State Route 43
Kent, OH 44240

Campus Safety Association
c/o National Safety Council
444 North Michigan Avenue
Chicago, IL 60611

National Association of School Security
Directors,
c/o Edgar B. Dews, Jr.
P.O. Box 31338
Temple Hills, MD 20748

National Association of Secondary School
Principles
1904 Association Drive
Reston, VA 22091

National Council of Secondary
School Athletic Directors
1900 Association Drive
Reston, VA 22091

National School Transportation Association
P.O. Box 2639
Springfield, VA 22152

National Science Teachers Association
1742 Connecticut Avenue N.W.
Washington, DC 20009

CHAPTER 11

Applying What You Have Learned

1. Define the following terms and cite one example for each:

a) Negligence _____

_____

_____

b) Misfeasance _____

_____

_____

c) Malfeasance _____

_____

_____

d) Nonfeasance _____

_____

_____

2. If you were put in charge of your university's weight-training facility, how would you address the following safety-related issues?

a) Student instruction and training:

_____

_____

_____

b) Facilities and equipment management:

_____

_____

_____

c) Provision for emergency care:

_____

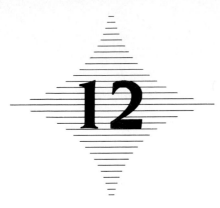

12 Where Do We Go From Here?

CAREERS IN SAFETY

As injury has received increased emphasis as a major public health problem in this country, federal and state agencies, local municipalities, and corporate entities have begun to develop career opportunities for qualified individuals who can address a vast array of safety-related issues.

At the federal level, agencies such as the National Highway Traffic Safety Administration (NHTSA), National Institute for Occupational Safety and Health (NIOSH), Occupational Safety and Health Administration (OSHA), Federal Emergency Management Agency (FEMA), Consumer Product Safety Commission, Environmental Protection Agency (EPA), the United States Department of Justice, and the National Institute of Mental Health (NIMH) have positions which address injury and violence prevention.

On the state level, departments of public health are hiring injury specialists to investigate funded projects which deal with issues such as farm related-injuries, gang violence, unintentional and intentional injuries in minority populations, and the effectiveness of safety-belt, child-restraint, and helmet laws. State OSHA programs utilize personnel to investigate safety in industries and businesses, and divisions of employment have a need for safety specialists who address workers' compensation and insurance issues. The fire marshal's office, state police, and departments of transportation and construction at the state level have career opportunities in the area of safety as well.

At the local level, there is an increasing trend for communities both large and small to hire safety personnel. The chief safety administrator in most municipalities is the risk manager. Injury investigations, workers' compensation, hazard analysis surveys, and property damage/vehicle accident involving municipal workers are the responsibility of the risk manager. He or she will also have a number of safety supervisors who assist with these various duties.

As fire and police departments across the country have expanded their emphasis on public education and citizen safety, there has been an increasing need for these public safety agencies to hire health and safety educators.

With the continuing escalation of insurance costs for industries and businesses, companies have had to take a serious look at controlling worker injuries and illnesses. Risk management for corporations is a necessity, if they want to maintain an adequate margin of profit. As in the case of municipalities, risk managers in the private sector must address worker health and safety issues. National trade associations and unions also have benefited from the hiring of injury-prevention and safety specialists.

Into the year 2000 we are going to see an increasing need for injury-prevention and safety specialists. Our nation's colleges and universities need to develop curricula and programs for the training and education of these professionals.

INTO THE TWENTY-FIRST CENTURY

As we have seen, the field of safety involves a broad range of topics. With this text we have only scratched the surface. Our purpose has been to stimulate readers and to make them aware of the way in which safety issues affect everyone's life.

Safety is not a matter of luck; it involves careful planning. In minimizing the risks of injury, illness, and property damage from a wide variety of hazards, we must continually address the four factors of safety: (1) understanding the difficulty of the activity, (2) ability level of the performer, (3) immediate state of the performer, and (4) condition of the environment. Whether it concerns nondeliberate acts such as accidents or deliberate acts such as violent crimes, these four closely interrelated factors must be controlled.

The concept of safety does not eliminate risk taking; it involves a dynamic equilibrium in which we attempt to perform an action or skill consistently—even in the face of possible unplanned interruptions. The safe individual is one who can enjoy the greatest benefits at the lowest possible risk and cost. To achieve this, we must personally focus on our own safety. Regardless of how much the environment is changed to protect us, human interaction and involvement will play the key roles in minimizing risks and maximizing the quality of life.

It should be further noted that significant overlap exists between the fields of health education and safety education. Do we call chronic lung disorders such as pneumoconiosis (black lung disease) and asbestosis health problems because they are illnesses, or do we consider them safety problems, because they are occupationally induced? What about the drunk driver with three previous DWI convictions who has a fatal traffic accident—isn't his alcohol abuse (a health problem) directly related to the fatal accident (a safety issue)? Even with recreational activities the health-safety interrelationship can be illustrated. A runner suffering from heat stroke after a 20-kilometer race has a life-threatening health problem; however, from the standpoint of safety, this situation would not have occurred had the proper preventive measures been taken.

Isn't it amazing how pervasive safety-related issues are in our lives? Yet they have not generated the concern from the public that would lead to a focused, coordinated research effort which could save lives, improve productivity, and reduce costs and long-term losses to the injured, their families, and society. There is a misperception in this country that most people should be able to cope with the safety-related aspects of their lives without education or training. Everyone knows how to use a fire extinguisher, make an emergency phone call, handle a rape attack, or use appropriate protective gear in the workplace—don't they?

The sad answer is "no." Nearly 100,000 die each year in a variety of accidents. Annually more than 1 million Americans are victims of violent crime. The relative importance of injury has increased to the point that it is now the most prominent cause of death for more than half the human lifespan (ages 1 to 44). More years of future worklife are lost to injury than to heart disease and cancer combined! These are only a few of the reasons why the Surgeon General of the United States has stated that injury, in all of its aspects (both accidental and deliberate), has become one of the major health problems in American society today.

In the early 1980s, as motor vehicle death rates began to escalate, the violent crime rate continued its upward trend, and the all-terrain vehicle controversy gained national attention, Congress authorized the Department of Transportation to request a study on injury by the National Research Council and its Institute of Medicine. A Committee on Trauma Research was established to determine what is known about injury, what research should be done to learn more, and what arrangements the federal government could make to increase and improve the knowledge of injury. Their final report, entitled *Injury in America*, was published in 1985.

The committee found two recurrent themes during its examination of the injury problem:

1. The lack of a single, coordinated focus of activity that would distinguish injury as an important public health issue.
2. The lack of financial support for research on injury.

In its final report to Congress, the committee recommended the establishment of a center for injury control within the Department of Health and Human Services' Centers for Disease Control in Atlanta. It was further recommended that funding for research on injury be significantly increased.

In response to the *Injury in America* report, the Centers for Disease Control (CDC) established the Division of Injury Control within the Center for Environmental Health. This new injury-control unit serves as a national clearinghouse for agencies or organizations interested in injury prevention and research. It has also been responsible for collecting and analyzing national injury data and developing education and training programs.

The CDC addressed the National Research Council's recommendation for increased funding by announcing a new grant program to fund injury-control research and demonstration projects beginning in 1987. Currently, injury-control research centers are funded across the country.

Injury control gained further prominence as a public health priority when Congress passed The Injury Prevention Act (Public Law 99-649) in 1986. This law mandated the development of injury-control activities in state and local public health agencies that are coordinated with CDC's Center for Injury Control. Special emphasis has been placed on the analysis of childhood injuries and subsequent recommendations for legislative action.

During the 1990s the Division of Injury Control and the National Institute for Occupational Safety and Health (NIOSH) of the Centers for Disease Control will be developing a national agenda for injury control. Areas to be addressed include unintentional, motor vehicle, and occupational injury prevention, violence prevention, acute-care treatment, trauma care systems, and rehabilitation. This national agenda will help to shape the future of injury-control research into the twenty-first century.

Although Congress has taken a step in the right direction with the Injury Prevention Act, it must increase funding and support for such regulatory agencies as the Consumer Product Safety Commission, the U.S. Fire Administration, the National Highway Traffic Safety Administration, and the Occupational Safety and Health Administration if they are to continue playing a major role in identifying and correcting hazards that threaten large segments of our society. Directly and indirectly, millions of Americans have benefited from the research and regulatory activities of these and other federal agencies; however, without adequate funding, these organizations will be unable to provide for the safety of the nation.

In recent years these federally funded agencies have had to reduce or curtail many of their functions as a result of major budget cuts. A period of fiscal uncertainty in our economy and an administration that favors the interests of big business rather than the needs of the public have compromised the effectiveness of these agencies.

Time and again, history has indicated that private industry cannot regulate itself adequately, especially when it involves a conflict between profit and safety. Repeatedly, the tendency has been to minimize safety to maximize profit; for example, although passive-restraint technology has been available since the early 1970s, auto manufacturers failed to install passive restraints in vehicles until the National Highway Traffic Safety Administration mandated their installation in all new cars manufactured after September 1989.

The Comprehensive Environmental Response, Compensation, and Liability Act and the Resource Conservation and Recovery Act represented the first major governmental response to the hazardous waste crisis, which became a concern in the late 1970s. This legislation was enacted to protect people against the dangers posed by hazardous wastes that had been abandoned at sites across the nation, most of which had been created by the chemical and petroleum industries. Today companies that produce hazardous waste are responsible for the proper packaging, transportation, and safe disposal of these materials. No longer can a manufacturer give its wastes to a ''midnight dumper'' who flushes them illegally into the nearest stream.

Money is not the only factor that has generated conflicts of interest in safety. Americans have a tradition of freedom of choice; this freedom and the free enterprise system have made North America a land of opportunity and growth. Nevertheless, without some controls and rules to follow, freedom becomes chaos; common sense must play a role in developing the choices we make.

In 1966, the Highway Safety Act included a federal mandate that all states establish legislation requiring motorcycle riders and their passengers to wear helmets. During the next 10 years, the fatality rate declined 50% while the number of riders nearly doubled. The significant reduction in motorcycle fatalities was attributed to the mandatory helmet laws. However, the good news was not to continue; groups opposed to mandatory helmet laws on the grounds of personal freedom campaigned successfully to have this law overturned by Congress in 1976. Although not all states have repealed their helmet laws, there has been a significant increase in the fatality rate for motorcycle riders in states that have done so. It is estimated that an additional 1500 people die each year as a result of the repeal of mandatory helmet laws.

Who will be responsible for these 1500 needless deaths? Is it true that we must ''let those who ride decide?'' What about the relatives and friends of these 1500 people who will die this year, how do you measure their grief and suffering?

The same misguided thinking that was used to repeal motorcycle helmet laws is being used today by persons who want to repeal the new mandatory safety-belt use laws. Opponents of these statutes do not question the efficacy of safety belts; their only argument is that the law infringes on individual freedom.

Accountability and cost-benefit analyses are being used in the decision-making process; these same methods ought to be considered in the development of cost-effective legislation to save lives and reduce injuries. Obviously, it is not possible to place a dollar value on grief and suffering; however, it is possible to place a dollar value on the medical expenses, lost wages, and increased insurance costs that result from a person's failure to use safety belts or helmets.

Until a common-sense approach is used in developing safety legislation, laws and mandates will be based on the political pressure of special interest groups rather than on the needs of citizens. What many of us fail to realize is that the responsibility for legislating protection is not limited to a small group of elected officials; each of us has a duty to become actively involved.

If you believe strongly that a particular safety issue is important, write to your congressman, senator, or state representative and let him or her know how you feel. Become actively involved with voluntary agencies and citizens' groups that support the issue. The more pressure that can be exerted on elected officials, the more likely they are to listen to our position. For example, more and more communities are developing local ordinances concerning the installation of smoke alarms and sprinkler systems in newly constructed dwellings. Such codes have developed as the result of pressure from a variety of groups, concerned citizens, fire-fighting organizations, and insurance companies. Each of these groups has an interest in reducing the death toll, injuries, and property damage from fires. Through a concerted effort, individual citizens can do much to change the safety picture in this country. However, legislative efforts alone will not solve the injury crisis in this country. If we are to have an impact on the injury problem, especially with the young, safety and health education must become a significant part of the school curriculum at all levels—elementary, secondary, and postsecondary.

Most injuries are the result of a combination of factors: (1) a lack of knowledge and (2) a failure to apply what is known. Learning is an active process and requires a hands-on approach. Whether it is a fire extinguisher, protective gear (such as a respirator), a chain saw, or an all-terrain vehicle, people will utilize this equipment in a safer, more productive manner if they have had previous hands-on training experiences in a controlled educational setting.

We have discussed a variety of options that have been developed to increase the safety of the nation. In some cases, the use of automatic protection such as air bags, ground fault circuit interrupters, and sprinkler systems may provide the best protection. In other circumstances, legislative or administrative rules such as mandatory helmet laws and federal motor vehicle safety standards may be the answer. The third option, education, may be the most important component, since it can affect the knowledge, attitudes, and skills of an individual, thus allowing him or her to perform safely and enjoy a maximum of success with a minimum of risk.

Regardless of the means used to protect us—automatic devices, legal mandates, or education—*safety involves a personal focus!*

Appendix

Throughout Chapters 1 through 12, this text has emphasized a variety of prevention and mitigation strategies to reduce injuries and property damage. Regardless of the protective methodologies used, there eventually will be situations which will require you to provide basic emergency care as a first responder. It may occur on a roadway, in the home, in the occupational setting, or at a recreational facility. Once you have utilized the cursory exam (illustrated in Chapter 3) and activated emergency medical services, you may need to provide first aid to the victim or victims until rescue personnel arrive.

In this appendix, first aid procedures have been illustrated for four of the more commonly occurring emergencies:

1. Airway obstruction
2. Respiratory arrest
3. Cardiac arrest
4. Soft-tissue injuries

The first aid and CPR procedures in this book are based on the most current recommendations of the American Red Cross, the American Heart Association, and the National Safety Council. However, the author and the publisher make no guarantee as to, and assume no responsibility for, the correctness and/or completeness of such information. Additional emergency care procedures and treatments may be necessary in certain situations.

1. Airway Obstruction

Although some authorities may disagree as to the procedures to be used in treating a complete airway obstruction, the American Heart Association and the American Red Cross recommend the following sequence in such emergencies (see Fig. 1, A-H):

Once the obstruction has been cleared, the rescuer will need to monitor the victim's respiratory and cardiac function. If need be, he or she may have to perform rescue breathing and/or cardiopulmonary resuscitation.

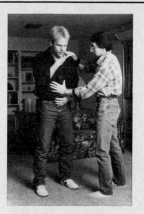

FIG. 1-A, Identify complete airway obstruction by asking the victim: "Are you choking?"

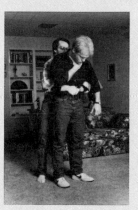

FIG. 1-B, Move behind the victim, wrapping your arms around his waist. Make a fist and place the thumb-side just above the navel in the soft, fleshy part of the abdomen. Grasp the fist with your other hand and thrust inward and upward in rapid succession. Each thrust should be distinct and delivered with the intent of relieving the obstruction. This procedure forces the abdominal contents and the diaphragm upward against the lungs, thus compressing them. The residual air in the lungs flows through the trachea and into the throat with sufficient force to expel most obstructions.

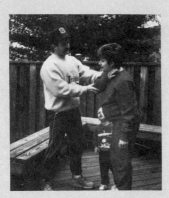

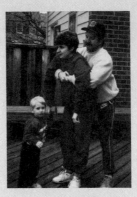

FIG. 1-C & D, For the obese individual or a person who is pregnant, a modification known as the chest thrust may be used. The rescuer's fist, thumb-side in, is placed on the victim's sternum at nipple level. As each chest thrust is applied to the sternum, the lungs will be compressed and residual air will be forced through the trachea to expel the blockage. Repeat thrusts until either the foreign body is expelled or the victim becomes unconscious.

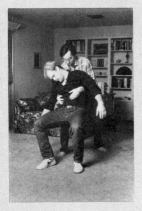

FIG. 1-E, If the choking victim loses consciousness, carefully place him or her on the floor in a face-up position. Be sure to protect the person's head and neck.

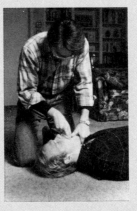

FIG. 1-F, Using a jaw lift maneuver, open the victim's mouth. With the index and middle fingers, sweep deeply into the oral cavity to remove the foreign body, if possible.

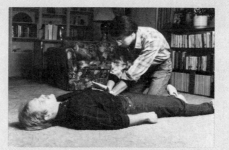

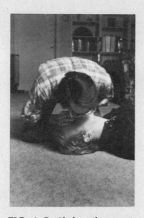

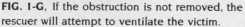

FIG. I-G, If the obstruction is not removed, the rescuer will attempt to ventilate the victim.

FIG. I-H, If the obstruction is not removed or attempts at ventilation indicate a continued obstruction, the rescuer must then straddle one or both of the victim's thighs and perform 6 to 10 abdominal thrusts. (Place the heel of one hand on the abdomen just above the navel; then place your other hand on top of it. Give 6 to 10 quick, upward thrusts into the abdomen.) The sequence of foreign-body check, breathing attempt, and abdominal thrusts should be continued until the obstruction is cleared.

In the case of a pregnant choking victim who becomes unconscious, the rescuer would perform 6-10 chest thrusts by utilizing a technique similar to that illustrated in Fig. 3-G of the Appendix.

2. *Respiratory Arrest*

Respiratory arrest is a condition in which breathing stops but the heart continues to function. Common causes of respiratory arrest include drowning, airway obstruction, suffocation, inhalation of poisonous gases, drug overdose, electric shock, head injuries, and allergic reactions. With a cessation of breathing, body systems are no longer being supplied with the oxygen that is crucial for their survival. Without oxygenation the heart will begin to slow and eventually stop. Other organ systems, including the brain, will fail to receive adequate amounts of blood. Cells in the brain will begin to die within approximately 4 to 6 minutes of being deprived of oxygenated blood. If this occurs, irreversible brain damage will result and the victim will die.

The key for the first responder is to be able to correctly identify that the victim is in respiratory arrest. After assuring him or herself that there is no further risk to the victim or potential rescuers, the first responder should perform the following sequence of steps (see Fig. 2, A-D):

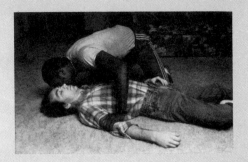

FIG. 2-A,   To determine the level of consciousness, gently grasp the victim's arms just above the elbows; lean over closely to his or her ear and ask in a loud voice, "Are you okay? Can you hear me?" Attempts to open the eyes and movement of the limbs and/or head are signs of responsiveness. In some cases the person who is regaining consciousness may become combative; that's why you gently hold the arms down. If there is no response, shout "Help" to get someone to assist you.

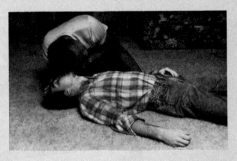

FIG. 2-B, When the victim is unresponsive, you need to open the airway and check for breathing. Place your hand nearest the top of the victim's head on his or her forehead. With the other hand, place two or three fingers on the bony tissue at the tip of the lower jaw. Push down on the forehead and lift at the chin to open the airway. While maintaining the open airway, place your ear close to the victim's mouth and nose. **Look** for respiratory movement of the chest and abdomen. **Listen** for breathing. **Feel** for an air exchange with your ear and cheek.

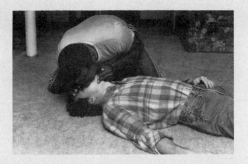

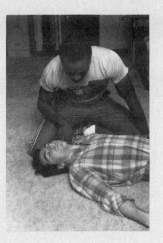

FIG. 2-C, If the victim is breathing, continue the cursory exam that you learned in Chapter 3. If he or she is not breathing, maintain the head-tilt, chin-lift position, pinch the nostrils closed, seal your mouth tightly over the victim's mouth, and deliver two rescue breaths. Each breath should be approximately 1 to 1.5 seconds in duration; you should be able to see the patient's chest cavity rise as you ventilate. Between each breath, break your seal with the victim's mouth to allow for exhalation.

   If you feel resistance to the airflow from your mouth as you attempt to ventilate, reposition the head and neck and try to ventilate again. Continued inability to ventilate the victim indicates the likelihood of an airway obstruction; utilize the emergency procedures that have been illustrated for clearing the obstruction (Fig. 1, A-H).

FIG. 2-D, After completing two successful ventilations, locate the victim's carotid artery and check for a pulse. When you are on the patient's right side, find the right carotid artery; when you are on the left side, use the left carotid. The pulse check should take approximately 10 seconds. If the victim has a pulse, tell someone to phone EMS personnel and tell them that a victim is in respiratory arrest and that rescuers are performing rescue breathing. After activating EMS, continue rescue breathing on an adult victim at a rate of 12 breaths per minute (once every 5 seconds). For children under 8 years of age, use a breathing rate of 20 breaths per minute (once every 3 seconds). Recheck the victim's pulse every minute. Rescue breathing should be maintained until the victim begins to breathe on his or her own, or until emergency personnel take over.

3. Cardiac Arrest

Many of the conditions that cause respiratory arrest may also lead to cardiac arrest. In a cardiac arrest, not only has the victim stopped breathing, but the heart is beating too weakly to circulate blood effectively or has stopped altogether. Initially victims of drowning or carbon monoxide poisoning will go into respiratory arrest. As time passes and they are not rescued, their hearts will also cease to function and they will be in cardiac arrest.

However, the most common cause of cardiac arrest is the heart attack. A blockage (usually a blood clot) in one of the coronary arteries shuts off oxygenated blood flow to the heart. This, in turn, leads to damage of heart muscle tissue, which causes the heart to beat erratically and ineffectively; or it may cause the heart to stop completely. In both of these cases, blood will not be circulated to the brain; the victim will lose consciousness, stop breathing, and have no pulse. **The absence of resperations and pulse are the key factors in determining that a person is in cardiac arrest.**

When a victim is not breathing and has no pulse, he or she is said to be clinically dead; however, the brain and other vital organs can survive a short period of time (approximately 4 to 6 minutes) before oxygen in the tissues is depleted. During this short period it is critical that the circulation of oxygenated blood be restored. If this cannot be done, cells (especially those in the brain) will die rapidly; this irreversible damage is termed biological death or brain death.

With cardiopulmonary resuscitation (CPR) the first responder has the opportunity to supply the brain and other organs with oxygenated blood until advanced life-support personnel arrive and attempt to restore the victim's cardiac and respiratory functions. Cardiopulmonary resuscitation is an emergency care procedure which utilizes rescue breathing and chest compressions to take over the function of the heart and lungs. Rarely will CPR, by itself, restore a functional heartbeat and breathing in a victim suffering from cardiac arrest. Generally, advanced life-support procedures, which are provided by paramedics, are needed. When paramedics arrive at the scene, you may see them perform a number of the following procedures: defibrillation, endotracheal intubation, and the administration of cardiac drugs.

In defibrillation an electrical device known as a defibrillator sends an electric current through two conducting paddles attached to the victim's chest. The current is used to stimulate the heart into a functional rhythm.

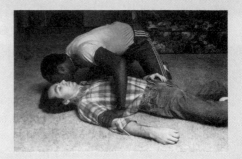

FIG. 3-A, Determine the victim's level of consciousness. If there is no response, shout "Help" to get someone to assist you.

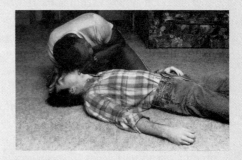

FIG. 3-B, Open the airway using the chin-lift, head-tilt method. While maintaining an open airway, **look, listen,** and **feel** for an air exchange or respiratory movement.

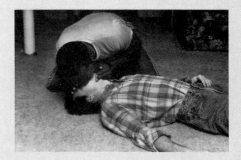

FIG. 3-C, If the victim is breathing, continue the cursory exam that you learned in Chapter 3. If he or she is not breathing, maintain the head-tilt, chin-lift position, pinch the nostrils closed, seal your mouth over the victim's mouth and deliver two full rescue breaths, each lasting 1 to 1.5 seconds.

Endotracheal intubation involves the insertion of a tube through the mouth and into the trachea or airway. This procedure provides high concentrations of oxygen directly to the victim's lungs, thus enabling the blood to be oxygenated more quickly.

Additionally, you may see paramedics place an intravenous line or IV into the patient's arm or hand. This will allow them to inject a variety of drugs to stimulate the heart.

However, none of this advanced life-support technology will work if the victim is already biologically or brain dead. You, the first responder, are the key to a cardiac arrest victim's survival. In a cardiac arrest emergency, the first responder performs three critical functions: (1) determining that the victim is in cardiac arrest, (2) calling for help and activating the emergency medical response system, and (3) through the use of CPR, keeping the victim's brain and vital organs supplied with oxygenated blood until emergency personnel can respond.

Figs. 3-A to 3-G illustrate the basic steps for performing one-rescuer adult CPR. Notice that Fig. 3, A-D illustrates the same assessment techniques that are used with victims of respiratory arrest (Fig. 2, A-D).

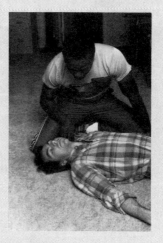

FIG. 3-D, Locate the victim's carotid artery and check for a pulse. Take at least 10 seconds to feel for the pulse; it's not always easy to find, especially in older individuals. If he or she has a pulse, activate EMS and continue rescue breathing. However, if there is no pulse, tell someone to phone EMS personnel and inform them that you have a victim in cardiac arrest and that rescuers are performing CPR.

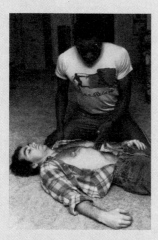

FIG. 3-E, Once the assessment has been made that the victim is in cardiac arrest, CPR should be started promptly. Make sure the victim is face-up on a hard, flat surface; chest compressions are ineffective if the person is on a soft surface such as a mattress. Position yourself on the side of the victim near his or her shoulder; this allows you to move easily from chest compressions to ventilations. Open the victim's shirt or blouse so that you can achieve proper hand placement for chest compressions. Slide your fingertips upward along the edge of the ribcage until you locate the lower tip of the sternum called the xiphoid process. In some cases you will be able to feel the pointed tip of the xiphoid; in other cases you will feel a notch or indentation at the bottom of the sternum.

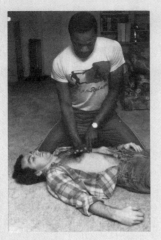

FIG. 3-F

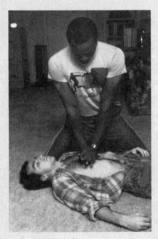

FIG. 3-G

FIG. 3-F, Once you have located the xiphoid, slide your index and middle fingers up onto the bony surface of the lower sternum. Place the heel of your hand closest to the victim's head next to the index finger of the other hand. The heel of the hand is now approximately two finger-widths above the tip of the sternum. This hand positioning reduces the risk of breaking off the xiphoid and lacerating underlying organs once compressions are begun. Before every set of chest compressions, use this landmarking procedure.

FIG. 3-G, Place your second hand on top of the one that is in contact with the sternum. To reduce the risk of rib fractures during CPR, interlace your fingers so that only the heel of the hand is in contact with the sternum. With your hands in position on the sternum, straighten your arms, lock your elbows, and move your shoulders so that they are directly over your hands. Now you are ready to begin chest compressions.

With a smooth downward pressure, depress the sternum 1.5 to 2.0 inches, then release the pressure and return to the starting position. A series of 15 compressions should be performed in approximately 10 seconds, with the relaxation phase (upstroke) being equal to the compression phase (downstroke). Count aloud, "1 and 2 and 3 ... " to 15; this will help to keep your compressions at a rate of 80 per minute. The heel of your hand remains in contact with the sternum throughout the compressions.

At the end of each cycle of 15 compressions, deliver two breaths. When you have completed four cycles of 15 compressions and two breaths, check the victim's carotid artery for a pulse. If there is no pulse, ventilate the victim two more times and continue CPR. Thereafter, do a pulse check every 4 to 5 minutes. If at some time during cardio-pulmonary resuscitation you find that the victim does have a pulse, stop the chest compressions, continue with rescue breathing, and intermittently monitor the pulse. Otherwise, continue CPR until rescue personnel arrive and take over, until another CPR-certified rescuer relieves you, or until you are too exhausted to continue.

Infants (under 1 year) and children (ages 1 to 8) require slightly different CPR procedures when they are in cardiac arrest. For further information and training, contact your local chapter of the American Heart Association or the American Red Cross.

4. Soft-Tissue Injuries

Soft-tissue injuries involve damage to the skin, underlying blood vessels, muscles, and in some cases, ligaments and tendons. There are generally two types of soft-tissue injuries: closed wounds and open wounds.

Closed wounds involve damage to underlying tissues but the skin remains unbroken. Classic closed wounds include bruises, muscle strains, and sprains. All three of these involve localized pain and swelling. If blood vessels under the skin have been broken, you will notice a black and blue discoloration at the injury site. Initial treatment for any of these injuries involves **RICE: rest, ice, compression,** and **elevation.** If swelling can be controlled quickly, pain will be reduced and healing time will be shortened. The compression of damaged tissues with a loosely applied elastic wrap prevents the seepage of fluid into the area, while the application of cold over the elastic wrap constricts damaged blood vessels and provides an anesthetic effect for the injured tissues. Never apply ice directly to the skin over the area of damage; place it in a towel or washcloth before application. Ice should be applied for approximately 20 minutes at a time, with a break of 15 to 20 minutes between each application. Use the application of cold three or four times a day for the first 48 to 96 hours after the injury. In the case of soft-tissue damage in an extremity, elevation will slow down blood flow and assist in reducing swelling. Resting of the damaged tissues will reduce pain as well the risk of aggravating the injury.

If a soft-tissue injury, especially in an extremity, involves deformity, inability to bear weight, or intense pain upon movement, there may be a more serious underlying problem. Consult medical personnel immediately.

In the case of open wounds, there is a tearing or breaking of the skin surface as well as underlying tissue and blood vessel damage. Open wounds are identified easily by the loss of blood externally. For the first responder, there are three procedures which should be used to control external bleeding: (1) direct pressure, (2) elevation, and (3) pressure points. Fig. 4, A-G illustrates these techniques:

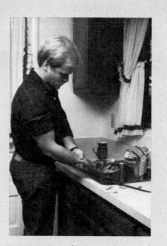

FIG. 4-A, This open wound involves damage to the skin, underlying tissues, and blood vessels.

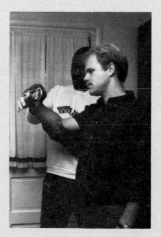

FIG. 4-B, The best method for controlling bleeding is to use direct pressure and elevation. The rescuer has applied a sterile gauze pad to the wound, and he has elevated the injured hand. If you don't have sterile material, any clean cloth such as a handkerchief, washcloth, or towel can be used. By the way, any material applied directly to a wound is called a **dressing,** while the material that holds a dressing in place is called a **bandage.**

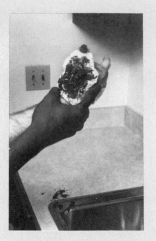
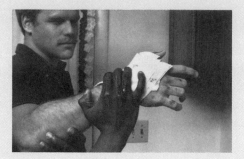

FIG. 4-C & D, If blood soaks through the dressing, do not remove it; the dressing helps with the clotting process. Place another clean dressing over the top of the bloody one and continue direct pressure and elevation.

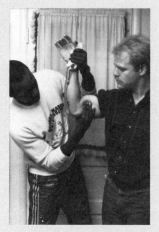

FIG. 4-E, If bleeding continues, an additional method of wound control involves the use of pressure points. Pressure points are areas of the body where large arteries run along bony tissue and lie close to the surface of the skin. When pressure is applied, the artery is squeezed against the underlying bone and blood flow to the wound is reduced. The two most commonly used pressure points are the brachial artery in the upper arm and the femoral artery in the groin area. In Fig. 4-E the rescuer continues to use direct pressure and elevation as he applies pressure to the brachial artery in the upper arm.

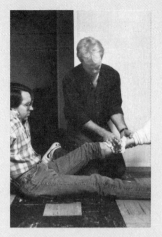

FIG. 4-F, For an open wound of a lower extremity, direct pressure and elevation should be used initially.

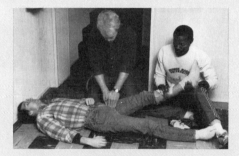

FIG. 4-G, If bleeding cannot be controlled with direct pressure and elevation, utilize the femoral pressure point to slow blood flow to the damaged area. The femoral artery crosses the bony pelvic girdle at the crease in the groin area. This rescuer is applying fingertip pressure on the artery to reduce blood flow, while a second rescuer maintains direct pressure and elevation.

Courtesy Manuel, Morton, and Spelman, Inc.

Index

t indicates table.
f indicates figure.